Radiation Oncology Review for Boards and MOC

Radiation Oncology Review for Boards and MOC

Editors

Tithi Biswas, MD
Clinical Associate Professor
Associate Residency Program Director
Department of Radiation Oncology
Case Western Reserve University
Cleveland, Ohio

George Rodrigues, MD, PhD, FRCPC
Professor
Departments of Oncology/Epidemiology and Biostatistics
Western University
Clinician Scientist, Radiation Oncology, LRCP/LHSC
London, Ontario, Canada

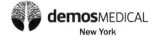

demosMEDICAL
New York

Visit our website at www.demosmedical.com

ISBN: 978-1-6207-0063-1
e-book ISBN: 978-1-6170-5228-6

Acquisitions Editor: David D'Addona
Compositor: diacriTech

Medicine is an ever-changing science. Research and clinical experience are continually expanding our knowledge, in particular our understanding of proper treatment and drug therapy. The authors, editors, and publisher have made every effort to ensure that all information in this book is in accordance with the state of knowledge at the time of production of the book. Nevertheless, the authors, editors, and publisher are not responsible for errors or omissions or for any consequences from application of the information in this book and make no warranty, expressed or implied, with respect to the contents of the publication. Every reader should examine carefully the package inserts accompanying each drug and should carefully check whether the dosage schedules mentioned therein or the contraindications stated by the manufacturer differ from the statements made in this book. Such examination is particularly important with drugs that are either rarely used or have been newly released on the market.

Library of Congress Cataloging-in-Publication Data
Names: Biswas, Tithi, editor. | Rodrigues, George, editor.
Title: Radiation oncology review for boards and MOC / editors, Tithi Biswas
  and George Rodrigues.
Other titles: Radiation oncology review for boards and maintenance of
  certification
Description: New York : Demos Medical, [2017] | Includes bibliographical
  references and index.
Identifiers: LCCN 2016024474| ISBN 9781620700631 | ISBN 9781617052286 (e-book)
Subjects: | MESH: Neoplasms—radiotherapy | Radiation Oncology—methods |
  Certification | United States | Examination Questions
Classification: LCC RC271.R3 | NLM QZ 18.2 | DDC 616.99/40642—dc23 LC record available
at https://lccn.loc.gov/2016024474

Special discounts on bulk quantities of Demos Medical Publishing books are available to corporations, professional associations, pharmaceutical companies, health care organizations, and other qualifying groups. For details, please contact:

Special Sales Department
Demos Medical Publishing
11 West 42nd Street, 15th Floor, New York, NY 10036
Phone: 800-532-8663 or 212-683-0072; Fax: 212-941-7842
E-mail: specialsales@demosmedical.com

Printed in the United States of America by McNaughton & Gunn.

16 17 18 19 20 / 5 4 3 2 1

To my parents without whom I would not have become the person that I am today
—Tithi Biswas

I would like to dedicate this book to my wife Melanie, my daughter Amelia, and my son Owen. Their continuing support has been instrumental in achieving my academic goals in radiation oncology and personal goals in life.
—George Rodrigues

Contents

PART II

Contributors

Christie Binder, MD, PhD Resident Physician, Department of Radiation Medicine, Oregon Health and Science University, Portland, Oregon

Tithi Biswas, MD Clinical Associate Professor, Associate Residency Program Director, Department of Radiation Oncology, Case Western Reserve University School of Medicine, Cleveland, Ohio

Alec M. Block, MD Radiation Oncology Resident (PGY-4), Department of Radiation Oncology, Stritch School of Medicine Loyola University Chicago, Cardinal Bernardin Cancer Center, Maywood, Illinois

Simon Brown, MD Resident Physician, Department of Radiation Medicine, Oregon Health and Science University, Portland, Oregon

Jeffrey Q. Cao, MD, MBA, FRCPC Assistant Professor, Department of Oncology, Schulich School of Medicine & Dentistry, Western University; Radiation Oncologist, London Regional Cancer Program, London, Ontario, Canada

Mehee Choi, MD Assistant Professor of Radiation Oncology, Department of Radiation Oncology, Stritch School of Medicine Loyola University Chicago, Cardinal Bernardin Cancer Center, Maywood, Illinois

Aidnag Z. Diaz, MD, MPH Associate Professor of Radiation Oncology, Department of Radiation Oncology, Rush University Medical Center, Chicago, Illinois

Clifton D. Fuller, MD, PhD Assistant Professor of Radiation Oncology, Department of Radiation Oncology, The University of Texas, MD Anderson Cancer Center, Houston, Texas

Emma B. Holliday, MD Radiation Oncology Resident (PGY-5), Department of Radiation Oncology, The University of Texas, MD Anderson Cancer Center, Houston, Texas

Arthur Y. Hung, MD Assistant Professor, Associate Residency Program Director, Department of Radiation Medicine, Oregon Health and Science University, Portland, Oregon

Randall Kimple, MD, PhD Assistant Professor, Department of Human Oncology, University of Wisconsin School of Medicine, University of Wisconsin Carbone Cancer Center, Madison, Wisconsin

David B. Mansur, MD Associate Professor of Radiation Oncology and Pediatrics, Vice Chairman for Proton Therapy, Director of Pediatric and Hematologic Radiation Oncology, Department of Radiation Oncology, Case Western Reserve University School of Medicine, University Hospitals Seidman Cancer Center, Rainbow Babies and Children's Hospital, Cleveland, Ohio

Allison M. Quick, MD   Assistant Professor of Radiation Oncology, Department of Radiation Oncology, The Ohio State University Comprehensive Cancer Center, Arthur G. James Cancer Hospital and Richard J. Solove Research Institute, Columbus, Ohio

George Rodrigues, MD, PhD, FRCPC   Professor, Departments of Oncology/Epidemiology and Biostatistics, Western University; Clinician Scientist, Radiation Oncology, LRCP/LHSC, London, Ontario, Canada

Suzanne Russo, MD   Associate Professor, Department of Radiation Oncology, Case Western Reserve University School of Medicine, University Hospitals Seidman Cancer Center, Cleveland, Ohio

Neelesh Sharma, MD, PhD   Assistant Professor, Division of Medical Oncology, Department of Medicine, Case Western Reserve University School of Medicine, University Hospitals Seidman Cancer Center, Cleveland, Ohio

Tracy Sherertz, MD   Assistant Professor, Department of Radiation Oncology, University of California San Francisco School of Medicine, San Francisco, California

Timothy N. Showalter, MD, MPH   Associate Professor of Radiation Oncology and Residency Program Director, Department of Radiation Oncology, University of Virginia Health System, Charlottesville, Virginia

Daniel M. Trifiletti, MD   Resident Physician, Department of Radiation Oncology, University of Virginia Health System, Charlottesville, Virginia

Stephanie E. Weiss, MD   Associate Professor and Chair of CNS Tumors and Radiosurgery, Department of Radiation Oncology, Fox Chase Cancer Center, Philadelphia, Pennsylvania

Julia White, MD, FACR, FASTRO   Professor and Vice Chair, Department of Radiation Oncology, The Ohio State University Comprehensive Cancer Center, Arthur G. James Cancer Hospital and Richard J. Solove Research Institute, Columbus, Ohio

Preface

The continued practice of radiation oncology requires clinicians to integrate a variety of disciplines including basic science knowledge, clinical skills/practice, and treatment planning. As radiation oncology is an ever evolving field of medicine due to technological improvements and the generation of evidence, clinicians need various educational materials to keep up with practice changes.

Radiation Oncology Review for Boards and MOC was specifically written to efficiently review high-yield clinical concepts and knowledge for trainees studying for radiation oncology specific board examinations as well as established clinicians who need a quick review for maintenance of certification examinations. Ideally, this book should be used in concert with *Radiation Oncology Primer and Review: Essential Concepts and Protocols* (Rodrigues/Velker/Best, Demos Medical Publishing) in order to ensure a complete coverage of basic science concepts and treatment planning approaches.

Both the editorial team and individual authors were assembled for this book in order to provide a consistent presentation of clinical information to the reader. The book also contains end of chapter multiple choice questions with annotated answers to maximize learning for the reader. Two full practice tests (including annotated answers) on basic science, clinical science, and treatment-planning concepts covering both *Radiation Oncology Review for Boards and MOC* and *Radiation Oncology Primer and Review: Essential Concepts and Protocols* are included in this book to maximize the utility of covering this material prior to any board examination. Although pre-examination preparation is the main focus of the book, residents may also find the content of this review useful for teaching interactions and internal program examinations.

Ultimately, the primary goal of *Radiation Oncology Review for Boards and MOC* is to successfully prepare trainees or practicing clinicians for either primary board examinations or maintenance of certification examinations that are required for licensure in radiation oncology.

Finally, the authors would like to thank Rich Winters, David D'Addona, and Norman Graubart from Demos Publishing for their assistance and encouragement during the book writing and editing process.

Tithi Biswas, MD
George Rodrigues, MD, PhD, FRCPC

1

Pediatric Malignancies

David B. Mansur

1.1 Tumors of the Central Nervous System

Epidemiology and Risk Factors

- Tumors of the central nervous system (CNS) are the most common solid tumors in children.
- There are several syndromes that predispose children to develop tumors of the CNS including neurofibromatosis types I and II, tuberous sclerosis, von Hippel-Lindau syndrome, and Gorlin syndrome.

Anatomy and Patterns of Spread

- The infratentorial compartment (inferior to the tentorium crebelli) includes the cerebellum and brain stem and rests within the posterior cranial fossa. The remaining parts of the intracranial brain are referred to as supratentorial.
- The majority of tumors occur intracranially, with only 5% of tumors originating in the spinal cord or cauda equina. Extra-CNS spread is quite rare, but is described especially in embryonal tumors.
- In contrast to adult tumors, several histologies that are common to pediatrics have a high propensity to seed distantly through the cerebrospinal fluid (CSF). These include the embryonal tumors, germ cell tumors, ependymal tumors, and less commonly astrocytomas.

Presentation, Diagnosis, and Workup and Staging

- The presenting signs and symptoms result from mass effect, associated vasogenic edema, hydrocephalus, and resulting increased intracranial pressure or a combination of these factors.
- Supratentorial tumors commonly present with either seizures or focal neurologic symptoms.
- Infratentorial tumors often present with gait disturbance, cranial nerve palsy, and nausea and vomiting.
- World Health Organization classification of brain tumors:
    Astrocytomas
    Grade I
        Pilocytic astrocytoma
        Subependymal giant cell astrocytoma
    Grade II
        Diffuse astrocytoma
        Pilomyxoid astrocytoma
        Pleomorphic xanthoastrocytoma
    Grade III
        Anaplastic astrocytoma
    Grade IV
        Glioblastoma (and variants)

Oligodendrogliomas
Grade II
   Oligodendroglioma
Grade III
   Anaplastic oligodendroglioma
Ependymomas
Grade I
   Subependymoma
   Myxopapillary ependymoma
Grade II
   Ependymoma
Grade III
   Anaplastic ependymoma
Embryonal tumors (All Grade IV)
   Medulloblastoma
   Primitive neuroectodermal tumor (PNET)
   Atypical teratoid rhabdoid tumor (ATRT)
Pineal tumors
Grade I
   Pineocytoma
Grade II to III
   Pineal parenchymal tumor of intermediate differentiation
   Papillary tumor of the pineal region
Grade IV
   Pineoblastoma
Neuronal and mixed neuronal-glial tumors
Grade I
   Ganglioglioma
   Dysembryonic neuroepithelial tumor (DNET)
Grade II
   Central neurocytoma
Grade III
   Anaplastic ganglioglioma
Suprasellar tumors (All grade I)
   Craniopharyngioma
   Pituicytoma
Germ cell tumors
   Pure germinoma
   Other germ cell tumors
      Teratoma
      Yolk sac tumor
      Embryonal carcinoma
      Choriocarcinoma
Meningeal tumors
Grade I
   Meningioma
   Hemangioblastoma
Grade II
   Atypical meningioma
   Hemangiopericytoma

Grade III
>   Anaplastic meningioma
>   Anaplastic hemangiopericytoma

Other tumors

(Choroid plexus tumors, oligoastrocytomas, schwannoma, neurofibroma, primary CNS lymphoma)

- The wide range of diagnoses means that tissue is almost always indicated for diagnosis. There are a few well-described exceptions in which radiologic appearance of tumor is nearly pathognomonic, and biopsy is associated with significant risk such that in these instances biopsy is often *not* indicated:
    - o Diffuse intrinsic pontine glioma (DIPG)—associated with a short symptom duration and an expansile, minimally enhancing MRI signal changes in the pons. Clinically a high-grade tumor with very poor overall survival.
    - o Optic pathway glioma (OPG)—often (not always) in the setting of neurofibromatosis, expansile tumors of the optic nerves, chiasm, and or tracts. Clinically a low-grade tumor usually with indolent natural history.
- Majority of tumors should undergo maximal safe surgical resection.
- Tumors where biopsy alone is sufficient and thus not requiring maximal resection include germinomas and primary CNS lymphoma.
- The workup is designed to accurately delineate the extent of the primary tumor and tumor resection and, if indicated, determine if any CSF seeding is present.
- Evaluation of the primary site requires MRI with images in multiple planes and sequences (T1, T2, FLAIR, etc.). Postoperative imaging of the primary should be done within 48 hours of surgery. After this interval, the postoperative bed can begin to enhance, which can be hard to distinguish from residual tumor.
- Some tumor histologies have significant risk of CSF dissemination; therefore, MRI of the spine and lumbar puncture for CSF cytology are indicated for these tumors which include embryonal tumors, ependymal tumors, and germ cell tumors. Serum and CSF levels of alpha feto-protein and beta human chorionic gonadotropin (HCG) must be drawn in patients with germ cell tumors. Any elevation in alpha feto-protein indicates the presence of nongerminomatous elements and therefore changes management.
- The use of systemic chemotherapy is common in pediatric brain tumors:
    - o Up front chemotherapy in babies and very young children in order to delay the use of curative radiation therapy (RT). This approach has been used in a wide range of histologies and must be individualized.
    - o Concomitant chemotherapy with RT.
    - o Adjuvant chemotherapy.

Low-Grade Astrocytoma

- OPG is commonly diagnosed without tissue based on imaging characteristics alone. Management of this often indolent tumor begins with close observation with serial MRIs and formal vision testing. Treatment is indicated if the tumor is progressive (either on imaging or with worsening vision). Chemotherapy is often used initially. RT is considered if chemotherapy does not halt tumor progression.
- Note that children with neurofibromatosis often have tumors that are more indolent. They are also at increased risk of RT complications including vascular complications (i.e., Moyamoya syndrome) and second malignancies (threefold increased risk).
- Other low-grade astrocytomas should be treated with maximal safe surgical resection.
- Following resection most children are observed with serial MRIs.
- Gross total resection of grade I tumors is usually curative.
- Additional treatment is indicated in the setting of progressive residual/recurrent tumor.
    - o In children younger than 10 years, chemotherapy (carboplatin and vincristine) has been commonly used as initial treatment, with RT held in reserve for tumors that progress despite chemotherapy. Progression free survival (PFS) with chemotherapy in this setting is 40% to 50%.
    - o In children 10 years or older, RT is often used as initial management with PFS rates of 70% to 80%.

Radiation Therapy Techniques—Low-Grade Astrocytoma

- Simulation includes immobilization mask and head rest. For supratentorial tumors, tucking the chin helps facilitate use of Antero-posterior beams (AP) by keeping the eyes inferior to the beam axis.
- No dose response has been observed in randomized trials. The usual dose is 50.4 to 54 Gy in 1.8-Gy fractions.
- Target volume should include the residual tumor and cavity with a 1- to 2-cm margin.

High-Grade Astrocytoma

- High-grade astrocytomas are more rare in children.
- Initial management should include maximal safe surgical resection.
- Postoperative therapy always includes RT plus concomitant temozolomide followed by additional temozolomide. Overall outcome is poor with few long-term survivors.

Radiation Therapy Techniques—High-Grade Astrocytoma

- Simulation is similar to low-grade astrocytoma.
- Total dose is 59.4 Gy in 1.8-Gy fractions.
- Volume includes initially the T2 abnormality with 2- to 3-cm margin to be followed by a cone-down to the T1 enhancing portion and/or tumor cavity with a 1- to 2-cm margin. Tolerances of the optic chiasm and nerves are 50 to 54 Gy and should be respected.

Ependymoma

- A small subset of children with ependymoma will present with disseminated disease. If present, this radically changes treatment to include craniospinal RT, whereas conformal fields are used if disease is localized. This means that proper workup to detect dissemination must be done. This includes spinal MRI and CSF cytology.
- Grade I tumors are usually treated with surgical resection followed by observation. Unresectable tumors can be closely followed in very young patients. RT is reserved for residual tumor, especially if there is demonstrated progression after surgery.
- Grades II and III ependymomas are approached similarly. Treatment should include maximal safe resection, with gross total resection being an important prognostic factor.
- The standard of care is postoperative RT even in the setting of gross total resection (GTR) for children older than 3 years. PFS is as high as 70%.

Radiation Therapy Techniques—Ependymoma

- Simulation should include immobilization mask and head pad. Head position can be neutral or with chin tucked for supratentorial tumors. If craniospinal RT is indicated, the chin should be extended so exit dose from the spinal beam will avoid the mouth.
- There is little consensus regarding dose in the literature. Standard dose is 54 to 59.4 Gy in 1.8-Gy fractions. If craniospinal axis should receive 36 Gy if indicated.
- Ependymomas of all grades have pushing rather than infiltrative borders; therefore, treatment volume is tumor and/or cavity with 1-cm expansion to clinical target volume (CTV). Even smaller CTV expansion of 5 mm is being investigated in clinical trials.
- Craniospinal RT is used only if disseminated disease is present. See embryonal tumor techniques in the following.

Craniopharyngioma

- Surgical resection of these often large suprasellar tumors can be associated with significant morbidity. Since these are highly radiosensitive tumors, the morbidity of RT should be carefully weighed against the morbidity of achieving GTR. Repeated debulking surgeries should be avoided since this likely will result in higher morbidity than modern conformal RT.

- Gross total resection is usually considered curative, though recurrences can occur. Following GTR, patients should be serially imaged.
- Following subtotal resection, close observation or RT can be considered. RT should be used if there is demonstrated tumor progression. Control rates are excellent with RT with greater than 90% progression-free survival.

Radiation Therapy Techniques—Craniopharyngioma

- Simulation should include immobilization mask and head pad. Multiple beams (at least three) should be used. Use of opposed lateral beams alone is discouraged since it results in poor conformality and can result in significant heterogeneity with "hot spots" in the temporal lobes. Tucking the chin and/or use of a "pituitary board" can help facilitate vertex beams.
- Dose is 50.4 to 54 Gy in 1.8-Gy fractions.
- Volume should include gross disease with a 0.5- to 1.0-cm expansion to CTV.

Germ Cell Tumors

- Germ cell tumors arise in the midline structures of the brain specifically the pineal and suprasellar regions.
- Pure germinomas must be distinguished from germ cell tumors with nongerminomatous elements since the treatment is different. This is usually done based on histopathology. However, due to sampling error, a biopsy specimen that is histopathologically pure germinoma does not rule out the possibility of nongerminomatous elements being present. Therefore, in addition to tissue diagnosis, both serum and CSF should be tested for both alpha fetoprotein and beta HCG. Any elevation of alpha feto protein or marked elevation of beta HCG indicates the presence of nongermanomatous elements and should be treated as such.
- Disseminated disease is common in germ cell tumors so workup also includes spinal imaging and CSF for cytology.
- Pure germinomas are extremely radiosensitive. Surgery can be limited to biopsy only and patients are treated with RT alone with excellent outcomes of over 90% relapse-free survival.
- Other germ cell tumors have poorer outcome with RT alone so they are treated with maximal safe surgical resection and systemic chemotherapy in addition to RT resulting in progression-free survival of 75%.

Radiation Therapy Technique—Pure Germinoma

- Simulation should include immobilization mask and head pad. Head position can be neutral, unless craniospinal RT is indicated. In this case, the chin should be extended.
- In patients with localized pure germinoma, the standard volume remains prophylactic whole ventricle RT followed by a conformal boost to the primary site. Patients with disseminated disease require craniospinal RT followed by a boost to the primary.
- Subclinical sites at risk (whole ventricle or craniospinal axis) can be treated with 24 Gy with the primary tumor or other gross disease boosted to 45 to 50 Gy in 1.8-Gy fractions.

Radiation Therapy Technique—Other Germ Cell Tumors

- Simulation includes immobilization mask and head pad and all patients should have chin extension to facilitate craniospinal RT.
- Volume includes the entire craniospinal axis prophylactically with a boost to the primary site and any other areas of gross disease.
- Initial dose is 36 Gy to the craniospinal axis, followed by a boost of the primary tumor to 54 Gy in 1.8-Gy fractions. Areas of spinal seeding should be boosted to spinal cord tolerance (45–50.4 Gy).

Embryonal Tumors

- This group of tumors includes medulloblastoma, ATRT, PNET, and pineoblastoma.
- This group of tumors shares the propensity to seed throughout the CSF so spinal MRI and CSF cytology are important in staging.
- Surgical approach should be maximal safe resection.
- All patients require postoperative RT and chemotherapy.
- With the exception of average risk medulloblastoma, the prognosis is poor for these tumors.
- Average risk medulloblastoma includes patients with each of the following features:
  - Patient age ≥3 years old
  - ≤1.5-cm^2 residual tumor after resection
  - No evidence of dissemination
  - Not anaplastic histology
- Outcome with craniospinal RT and systemic chemotherapy is in the range of 80% in this subset of patients.
- Unfortunately, high-risk medulloblastoma and the other embryonal tumors have a worse prognosis with PFS ranging from 30% to 60%.

Radiation Therapy Technique—Embryonal Tumors

- Simulation should immobilize the patient with the chin extended and the shoulders pulled inferior to facilitate craniospinal RT. Prone or supine positions have been used at different institutions. This will require a mask and head pad.
- The spine is typically treated with a posterior beam (PA) that includes 2-cm lateral margins on the spinal canal. Note should be made of the positions of the kidneys to be out of the beam as much as possible. The inferior port edge should include the entire thecal sac with margin. The inferior edge of S3 will usually include the entire thecal sac, but verification of this on sagittal MRI is encouraged. In older children, the spine will need to be treated with two matched PA beams. The junction of these two beams should be inferior to the level of L2 so the match is not in the spinal cord. These beams will diverge and meet at the anterior spinal canal. The brain will be treated with lateral beams with a collimator rotation to match the divergence of the superior edge of the spinal beam. To match the divergence of the lateral beams to the spine beam the couch is "kicked" approximately 7° to 8° toward the treatment machine. The anatomic position of the junction of the cranial and spine beams is determined by default—the lateral beams should not enter the shoulder, and the spine port should not exit the mouth. This junction should be moved or "feathered" in 1-cm increments approximately three times over the course of the craniospinal treatment.
- Standard therapy is craniospinal RT to a dose of 23.4 Gy (average-risk medulloblastoma) or 36 Gy (all other) with a boost to the primary to a total dose of 54 to 55.8 Gy in 1.8-Gy fractions. Boosting the entire posterior fossa in medulloblastoma has largely been replaced with conformal boosts (tumor and tumor cavity plus 2 cm).
- The treatment of babies and very young children with embryonal tumors is particularly difficult since they are at very high risk for neurocognitive decline following treatment. Current protocols are investigating local field only RT with omission of the craniospinal portion. The decision to treat local field only off of protocol must be made carefully and take into account the age of the child and balance the concern for late neurocognitive effects with the possibility for reduced PFS with such an approach.

Follow-Up and Late Effects—CNS Tumors

- Follow-up should involve a multidisciplinary approach including neurologists, neuropsychologists and endocrinologists, social workers, and school liaisons. Serial physical examination and neurological imaging are central.
- Many children with brain tumors have a good prognosis and are therefore at risk for multiple late effects:
  - Neurocognitive decline can occur and its cause is multifactorial. The presence of the space-occupying tumor, hydrocephalus, and craniotomy can result in decline.

- o RT factors associated with neurocognitive decline include younger age at RT, larger target volume (especially craniospinal volume), and higher radiation dose.
- o Endocrinopathies are common when dose to the pituitary/hypothalamus exceeds 30 to 35 Gy. Most common are growth hormone deficits and secondary hypothyroidism.
- o Second malignancies begin to appear after a latency of approximately 8 to 10 years. These can range from highly curable such as skin cancers or low-grade meningiomas, to very aggressive tumors such as sarcomas or high-grade astrocytomas. Patients with neurofibromatosis have a threefold higher risk of second malignancy.

1.2 Wilms' Tumor

Epidemiology and Risk Factors

- An embryonal tumor of the kidney named for Dr. Max Wilms following his 1899 description.
- Most common kidney cancer of childhood, but makes up only 6% of childhood cancer.
- Associated congenital anomalies are present in 10% of cases secondary to several syndromes that predispose to the development of Wilms' tumor:
  - o Denys–Drash (mesangial sclerosis and renal failure, intersex disorders). Most will develop Wilms' tumor.
  - o **W**ilms', **A**niridia, **G**enitourinary abnormalities, mental **R**etardation (WAGR). Approximately 50% will develop Wilms' tumor.
  - o Beckwith–Weidemann (macrosomia, hemihypertrophy, macroglossia, ear pits, abdominal wall defects). Ten percent risk of childhood cancers including Wilms'.
  - o Simpson–Golabi–Behmel (macrosomia, macrostomia, ocular hypertelorism, multiple others). Ten percent risk of Wilms' or neuroblastoma.

Anatomy and Patterns of Spread

- Tumors can spread by direct extension beyond the renal capsule into surrounding organs, to regional lymph nodes, or to distant sites (primarily to the lungs or liver).

Presentation

- A palpable abdominal mass in an otherwise well-appearing child is a common presentation.
- Less common presentation is hematuria, flank or abdominal pain, or symptoms from metastatic disease (lungs).

Diagnosis and Workup

- o History and physical examination
- o Routine laboratory studies
- o CT of chest, abdomen, and pelvis
- o Ultrasound of abdomen/kidney
- o Bone scan
- Histologic classification of renal tumors treated on Wilms' tumor protocols
  - o Favorable histology Wilms' tumor
  - o Anaplastic Wilms' tumor (focal or diffuse)
  - o Rhabdoid tumor of the kidney
  - o Clear cell sarcoma of the kidney

Staging

- Most often these tumors are staged postoperatively based on pathologic features and operative note. One exception is a tumor deemed to be unresectable that is treated with chemotherapy prior to resection. In this case, the tumor is considered stage III.

Stage I	Complete resection, tumor limited to kidney, capsule intact
Stage II	Complete resection, but tumor beyond kidney (capsule penetration, other extension beyond kidney including through renal vessels)
Stage III	• Positive lymph nodes or surgical margins • Gross residual • Tumor deemed unresectable • Tumor in separate nodules • Extension to peritoneum • Any operative spill ("flank" or diffuse) • Biopsy prior to resection
Stage IV	Distant metastases or involved nonregional nodes
Stage V	Bilateral disease

Treatment Overview

- Treatment requires a coordinated multidisciplinary approach.
- Initial management is surgical resection of the primary tumor with sampling of regional lymph nodes. Risk stratification is then determined based on tumor size, stage, and loss of heterozygosity at 1p and 19q.
- With the exception of small (<550 g) stage I tumors in children younger than 2 years, all patients are treated with adjuvant chemotherapy with vincristine and actinomysin D with or without doxorubicin.
- RT is given to all patients except stages I and II with favorable histology.
- When indicated, RT should start by postoperative day 14.
- Though not Wilms' tumor, rhabdoid tumor of the kidney and clear cell sarcoma of the kidney are treated on Wilms' tumor protocols.

Radiation Therapy Techniques

- Indications and dose (in Gy) of RT are determined independent of risk stratification based on abdominal stage and histology.

Stage	Histology				
	Favorable	Focal Anaplasia	Diffuse Anaplasia	Rhabdoid Tumor	Clear Cell Sarcoma
I	0	10.8	10.8	10.8/19.8[a]	10.8[b]
II	0	10.8	10.8	10.8/19.8[a]	10.8
III	10.8	10.8	19.8	10.8/19.8[a]	10.8
IV	Based on Abdominal stage and histology				

[a] If >1-year old.
[b] If node sampling not done.

- Flank RT should encompass the entire preoperative tumor and kidney bed with a 1- to 2-cm margin. The field typically extends medially to include the vertebral bodies in their entirety, but excludes as much of the contralateral kidney as possible. Laterally, the field should flash.
- Indications for whole abdomen RT are diffuse intraperitoneal spill or other extensive peritoneal involvement. Whole abdomen really refers to whole abdomen and pelvis. The field should include the entire peritoneum. Superiorly, this will include the domes of the diaphragms with margins to account for respiratory excursion. Inferiorly, the beam should extend to include the obturator foramen, but exclude the femoral heads.
- Current protocols utilize whole lung irradiation reserved for patients with lung metastases who have less than a complete response by week 6 of chemotherapy. These fields include the entirety of the lungs including the posterior/inferior extent of the diaphragm (costophrenic recess).
- Generally APPA beams are sufficient for treating these fields.

1.3 Neuroblastoma

Epidemiology and Risk Factors

- Neuroblastoma is a malignant tumor arising from the sympathetic nervous system.
- It is the third most common malignancy in childhood, behind leukemia and brain tumors.
- It is the most common malignancy in children younger than 12 months of age.
- It typically occurs in very young children with a median age of diagnosis of approximately 2 years.

Anatomy and Patterns of Spread

- Most common sites of origin are adrenal medulla, posterior mediastinum, and other paraspinal ganglia.
- Metastatic disease is very common, occurring in approximately 70% at diagnosis.
- Common metastatic sites are lymph nodes, bone and bone marrow, liver, orbits, and skin.

Presentation

- Most patients present with signs and symptoms of metastatic disease. Pain is common and in contrast to Wilms' tumor presentation, children with neuroblastoma appear ill at presentation.
- Neurologic compromise can occur secondary to the paraspinal location of primary tumors that can invade into the spinal canal.
- Abdominal masses from adrenal primaries or liver metastases are common.
- Respiratory compromise from large posterior mediastinal masses can occur.
- Skin lesions can appear raised and purple (blueberry muffin sign).
- Orbital metastases can result in proptosis or periorbital ecchymoses.
- Occasionally neuroblastoma is associated with the paraneoplastic syndrome of opsoclonus myoclonus.
- Calcification of masses as seen on CT or radiographs is very common.

Diagnosis and Workup

- Diagnosis is usually made with biopsy of primary mass or metastatic sites.
- Workup should include:
  - Physical examination and routine labs
  - Urine catecholamine levels
  - CT scan of neck, chest, abdomen, and pelvis
  - Bone scan
  - Meta-iodobenzyl guanidine (MIBG) scan
  - Bone marrow biopsy and aspirate

Staging

- Staging is based on the International Neuroblastoma Staging System (INSS):

Stage 1	Localized tumor and complete gross excision
	With or without positive surgical margins
	Ipsilateral nodes negative (unless positive nodes are attached to and removed with the primary tumor)
Stage 2A	Localized tumor, gross residual
	Ipsilateral nodes negative
Stage 2B	Localized tumor with or without gross excision
	Positive ipsilateral nodes
Stage 3	Unresectable tumor
	Unilateral tumor with extension over midline
	Midline tumor with bilateral extension
	Positive contralateral nodes
Stage 4	Metastatic disease
Stage 4S	Localized primary (1, 2A, 2B) in patients <1 y, AND mets limited to skin, liver, and limited bone marrow (<10% of nucleated cells)

Treatment Overview

- Management of neuroblastoma is based on risk stratification into low-, intermediate-, and high-risk groups.
- Risk is stratified based on INSS stage, N-myc amplification, age, tumor histology, tumor ploidy, and extent of resection.
- Unlike rhabdomyosarcoma (RMS) and Wilms' tumor, the risk stratification determines which patients will be irradiated in neuroblastoma.

Neuroblastoma Risk Group	5-y survival	Chemotherapy	RT
Low • All stage 1 • Stage 2, N-myc non-amp, and <50% resection • Stage 4s, <1-y old, non-amp, favorable histology (FH)	 90%	Taylor intensity of chemotherapy to specific risk categories: 0–8 cycles	No routine role for RT.
Intermediate • Any not low or high risk			
High • N-myc amplified (stage 2–4s) • N-myc non-amp, >1-y old, stage 4	30%	All have high-dose chemotherapy and autologous stem cell transplant (SCT). (Randomized to single vs. tandem SCT) Cis-retinoic acid after SCT	All patients irradiated to primary site and select metastatic sites.

- Patients with low- and intermediate-risk neuroblastoma have an excellent prognosis and are treated with either observation or limited chemotherapy.
- Patients with high-risk disease, however, have a poor prognosis and are treated with intensive chemotherapy with autologous stem cell rescue. In addition, all patients with high-risk disease are treated with irradiation to the primary site and to select metastatic sites.

Radiation Therapy Techniques

- Simulation is dependent on the area of the body to be treated taking into account primary site and metastatic sites to be treated. Usual immobilization and sedation are used as required.
- The primary site volume treated includes the postchemotherapy (prestem cell transplant) residual disease. This gross tumor volume (GTV) is expanded by 1.5 to 2 cm to form the CTV.
- Metastatic sites are also treated if they do not completely respond to chemotherapy prior to stem cell transplant. For patients with multiple metastatic sites that do not respond, approximately five of the sites are treated. It may not be feasible to treat every metastatic site.
- Dose to the primary is 21.6 Gy in 1.8-Gy fractions to subclinical disease with a boost of 14.4 Gy to gross residual disease.
- Metastatic sites are treated to 21.6 Gy (if indicated).
- Both primary and metastatic sites are typically treated following autologous stem cell transplant.

1.4   Rhabdomyosarcoma

Epidemiology and Risk Factors

- RMS is the most common soft-tissue sarcoma in children.
- It arises anywhere in the body from embryonal mesenchyme.
- Some syndromes are associated with increased risk of RMS including Beckwith–Wiedemann syndrome, Costello syndrome, neurofibromatosis type I, and Gorlin syndrome (basal cell nevus syndrome).

Anatomy and Patterns of Spread

- RMS occurs anywhere in the body. Common locations include:
  - Genitourinary 30%
  - Parameningeal 25%
  - Extremity 13%
  - Orbit 9%
  - Head and neck (nonparameningeal) 7%
  - Trunk 5%
- Lymph node involvement at diagnosis is overall 15%, but depends on the location of the primary. Lymph node involvement is rare in orbital primaries, but occurs in approximately 25% of extremity, trunk, and paratesticular primaries.
- Overall, there is a15% risk of metastatic disease at presentation.

Presentation

- Because RMS can arise anywhere in the body, signs and symptoms are highly varied depending on anatomic location. Pain and mass effect are common.

Diagnosis and Workup

- Initial workup includes biopsy, with assessment of resectability.
- Classification of RMS:

- o Embryonal (including botryoides and spindle cell variants)
- o Alveolar
- o Pleomorphic variants
- Botryoides and spindle cell variants have the best prognosis while alveolar and pleomorphic variants have the worst. Prognosis of embryonal tumors is intermediate.
- Staging workup:
  - o History and physical examination (examination under anesthesia for gynecologic or genitourinary primaries)
  - o Routine laboratory studies
  - o MRI of primary tumor
  - o PET/CT for metastatic workup
  - o Bilateral bone marrow biopsy and aspirate
  - o Lumbar puncture for CSF cytology (parameningeal primaries)

Staging

- Staging system:

Stage	Site	Size	Node	Metastasis
1	Orbit H&N (nonparameningeal) GU (nonprostate or bladder) Liver/biliary tract	Any	Any	M0
2	Everyone else		≤5 cm and N−	
3			>5 cm or N+	
4		ANY METASTATIC		M1

- Postoperative grouping:

Group I	Localized Tumor, Complete Resection
A	Confined to organ of origin
b	Outside of organ of origin
Group II	**Gross Total Resection, but Residual Disease**
a	Positive surgical margins
b	Positive lymph nodes
c	Both positive margins and nodes
Group III	**Gross Residual Disease**
a	Biopsy only
b	Subtotal resection (>50%)
Group IV	**Metastatic Disease**

Treatment Overview

- Treatment requires close multidisciplinary coordination. If the primary tumor is amenable to complete surgical resection without excessive morbidity, this is the initial treatment of choice. However, depending on location, many tumors are unresectable in which biopsy alone is performed and RT is used for definitive local control.
- All patients receive systemic chemotherapy with vincristine, actinomycin D, and cyclophosphamide (VAC). Additional agents are being investigated for poorer prognosis patients on current protocols.
- Current risk stratification:
  - High risk
    - Any metastatic
  - Intermediate risk
    - Any nonmetastatic alveolar
    - Group III embryonal in an unfavorable site
  - Low risk
    - All other patients
- Use and dose of RT is independent of this risk stratification and is determined by histology, group, lymph node status, and location.

Radiation Therapy Techniques

- All patients receive RT except group I embryonal tumors.
- Summary of RT use in RMS:

Group	Histology	
	Embryonal	Alveolar
I	0	36
II Node −	36	36
II Node +	41.4	41.4
III (orbit)	45	45
III	50.4	50.4

- Simulation is dependent on the primary site and should include adequate immobilization (mask, head pad, vacuum bag, or alpha cradle, etc.) to facilitate reproducibility of setup. Sedation or anesthesia should be used as needed.
- RT volume includes a GTV consisting of primary tumor and or residual tumor and a CTV expansion of 1 to 1.5 cm is used and is limited by anatomic constraints.
- Metastatic sites are treated to similar volumes if amenable to RT. Doses range from 36 to 50.4 Gy depending on response to chemotherapy and anatomic location.

1.5 Ewing's Sarcoma

Epidemiology and Risk Factors

- The Ewing's sarcoma and soft-tissue PNET family of tumors arise from neuroectodermal precursor cells.
- Ewing's sarcoma is the second most common bone tumor of childhood. Most, but not all, cases are associated with translocation between chromosome 11 and 22, t(11;22).
- These tumors are more common in Whites and quite rare in children of Asian or African descent.

Anatomy and Patterns of Spread

- Ewing's sarcoma can originate in any bone or soft-tissue site. More common primary sites are:
  o Pelvis 25%
  o Femur 20%
  o Chest wall (Askin tumor) 15%
  o Spine 6%
- Metastatic disease occurs in approximately 25% of children at diagnosis. Most common metastatic sites are lung, bone, and bone marrow. Lymph node and liver metastases are rare (Bernstein et al., 2006; doi:10.1634/theoncologist.11-5-503).

Presentation

- Bone pain and mass are the most common presenting symptoms.
- Occasionally patients present with neurological compromise from spinal primary tumors.

Diagnosis and Workup

- Diagnosis is made by incisional biopsy or core biopsy.
- Diagnostic workup to determine the local extent of disease and to detect metastatic disease should include:
  o MRI of the primary site
  o CT scan of the lungs
  o Bone scan
  o Fluorodeoxyglucose (FDG)-PET
  o Bone marrow biopsy and aspirate

Staging

- There is no specific staging system for Ewing's sarcoma. The main distinction for prognosis and protocol treatment is metastatic versus nonmetastatic disease.

Treatment Overview

- All patients receive systemic chemotherapy with vincristine, actinomysin D, cyclophosphamide, and doxorubicin or a variation. Chemotherapy is usually the initial modality, with local control modalities used after several weeks.
- Use of high-dose chemotherapy and stem cell rescue in high-risk patients (metastatic disease) continues to be investigated in clinical trials.
- Local therapy of the primary site can consist of surgery, RT, or a combination of both. The decision of which local control modality to use requires cooperation between surgical and radiation oncology specialists in a multidisciplinary setting. Surgical resection of tumor with negative margins results in good local control so postoperative RT is indicated only for positive surgical margins. However, Ewing's sarcoma is a radiosensitive tumor and RT is often used for definitive local control in situations where resection would be excessively morbid (pelvic or base of skull primary sites for instance).
- Whole lung RT is standard for patients with lung metastases. In addition, other metastatic sites are often irradiated as well.

Radiation Therapy Techniques

- Simulation should include adequate immobilization with sedation used as necessary for younger children.
- Timing of RT is usually several weeks after initiation of systemic chemotherapy. Primary site irradiation volume should include the prechemotherapy gross tumor volume (GTV) with an expansion of 1 to 2 cm for CTV.
- Postoperative RT is indicated for positive surgical margins. GTV should include the preoperative tumor site and operative bed with a 1 to 2 cm expansion for CTV.

- Dose for definitive RT is 55.8 Gy in 1.8 Gy fractions.
- Postoperative doses are usually 45 to 50.4 Gy in 1.8-Gy fractions.
- Whole lung irradiation is indicated in children with lung metastases at diagnosis.
- A dose of 15 Gy in 1.5 Gy per fraction is usually used.
- Treatment of metastatic sites is routine.
- Dose of 55.8 for gross residual disease is recommended with a reduction of dose to 45 to 50.4 if complete response to initial chemotherapy.
- Newer protocols utilize stereotactic body radiation therapy (SBRT) for smaller metastatic sites.

Follow-Up and Late Effects—Non-CNS Tumors

- The prognosis is good for many pediatric malignancies. Therefore, surviving children are at high risk of developing late effects from treatment.
- Late effects of treatment have multiple etiologies including:
  - Intensity of chemotherapy (especially alkylating agents and anthracyclines)
  - RT
  - Morbidity caused by the tumor itself
  - Surgery
  - Underlying genetic predisposition syndromes
- Use of RT is associated with multiple late effects in the tissues treated. The nature and intensity of these effects are determined by the age at the time of treatment, volume of treated tissue, and dose. Common late effects include:
  - Impaired growth and development of mesenchymal tissues that can result in kyphosis or scoliosis (Wilms' tumor), hypoplastic flat bones resulting in facial asymmetry, and shortened extremities.
  - Cataracts
  - The 20-year rate of congestive heart failure is 4% to 5% in Wilms' tumor survivors treated with anthracyclines and/or RT.
  - Impaired fertility in girls treated to the pelvis can include primary ovarian failure, increased rates of spontaneous abortion, and restricted fetal growth.
  - Renal insufficiency is common in Wilms' tumor survivors though end-stage renal failure is much less common. Note that patients with Denys–Drash syndrome have very high rates of renal failure secondary to their underlying syndrome.
  - Second malignancy rates are between 1% and 2% at 10 to 15 years of follow-up for Wilms' tumor and RMS survivors. Higher risks are expected in patients with predisposition syndromes such as neurofibromatosis (NF), WAGR, Li–Fraumeni, and so on.

Chapter 1: Practice Questions

1. Orbital rhabdomyosarcoma (RMS) is considered what stage?

   A. 1
   B. 2
   C. 3
   D. 4

2. A neuroblastoma with positive surgical margin is classified as what stage?

   A. Stage I
   B. Stage IA
   C. Stage 2
   D. Stage 2A

3. The following are all embryonal tumors EXCEPT

   A. Medulloblastoma
   B. Pineocytoma
   C. PNET
   D. ATRT

4. Subtypes of pediatric embryonal tumors include the following EXCEPT

   A. Medulloblastoma
   B. Typical teratoid rhabdoid tumor
   C. Primitive neuroectodermal tumor
   D. Pineoblastoma

5. The following factors are associated with neurocognitive decline after pediatric central nervous system (CNS) radiation treatment EXCEPT

   A. Higher radiation dose
   B. Tumor histology
   C. Larger target volume
   D. Younger age

6. A typical dose fractionation schedule used for pediatric LOW-grade astrocytoma is

   A. 45 Gy in 25 fractions
   B. 50.4 Gy in 28 fractions
   C. 60 Gy in 30 fractions
   D. 66 Gy in 33 fractions

7. Radiation dose for neuroblastoma subclinical disease is usually on the order of

   A. 10 Gy
   B. 15 Gy
   C. 20 Gy
   D. 35 Gy

8. In terms of pediatric rhabdomyosarcoma, the general risk of distant metastases is

   A. 5%
   B. 10%
   C. 15%
   D. 20%

9. Beckwith–Weidemann syndrome is associated with what percentage risk of pediatric tumors?

   A. 1%
   B. 10%
   C. 25%
   D. 50%

10. Which of the following risk factors is NOT consistent with average risk medulloblastoma

    A. Patient age greater than 3 years old
    B. Less than 1.5-cm^2 residual tumor after resection
    C. No evidence of dissemination
    D. Not anaphasic histology

11. The most common site of pediatric rhabdomyosarcoma is

    A. Orbit
    B. Head and neck
    C. Extremity
    D. Genitourinary

12. In terms of pediatric rhabdomyosarcoma, the general risk of lymph node metastases is

    A. 5%
    B. 10%
    C. 15%
    D. 20%

13. The third most diagnosed pediatric malignancy is

    A. Neuroblastoma
    B. Wilms' tumor
    C. Leukemia
    D. Brain tumors

14. Five-year survival for high-risk neuroblastoma is approximately

    A. 10%
    B. 20%
    C. 30%
    D. 40%

15. Five-year survival for low-risk neuroblastoma is approximately

    A. 100%
    B. 90%
    C. 80%
    D. 60%

16. Risk stratification of neuroblastoma is dependent on the following EXCEPT

    A. INSS stage
    B. N-myc amplification
    C. Age
    D. Tumor grade

17. Favorable histology Wilms' tumor is treated with the following RT dose approach

    A. No radiation therapy for stages I to III
    B. No radiation therapy for stage I, 10.8 Gy for stages II to III
    C. No radiation therapy for stages I to II, 10.8 Gy for stage III
    D. 10.8 Gy for stages I to III

18. The following are subtypes of pediatric kidney cancers EXCEPT

    A. Anaplastic Wilms' tumor
    B. Clear cell sarcoma of the kidney
    C. Favorable histology Wilms' tumor
    D. Rhabdosarcoma of the kidney

19. The dose fractionation considered to be most appropriate for the definitive radiation therapy of Ewing's sarcoma is

    A. 36 Gy in 20 fractions
    B. 45 Gy in 25 fractions
    C. 55.8 Gy in 31 fractions
    D. 59.4 Gy in 33 fractions

20. The utilization of whole lung irradiation is commonly associated with which pediatric tumor with lung metastases?

    A. Astrocytoma
    B. Rhabdosarcoma
    C. Wilms' tumor
    D. Ewing's sarcoma

Chapter 1: Answers

1. A
Orbital rhabdomyosarcoma (RMS) is considered to be stage I disease. Other stage I RMS scenarios include head and neck (nonparameningeal), GU (nonprostate/bladder), as well as the liver/biliary tract.

2. A
Staging is based on the INSS system:
   Stage 1—Localized tumor and complete gross excision. With or without positive surgical margins. Ipsilateral nodes negative (unless positive nodes are attached to and removed with the primary tumor)

3. B
The list of embryonal tumors include:
   Medulloblastoma
   PNET
   ATRT

4. B
This embryonal group of tumors includes medulloblastoma, ATRT, PNET, and pineoblastoma.

5. B
Factors associated with neurocognitive decline include younger age at RT, larger target volume (especially craniospinal volume), and higher radiation dose.

6. B
The usual dose is 50.4 to 54 Gy in 1.8-Gy fractions with no dose response has been observed in randomized trials.

7. C
Dose to the primary neuroblastoma is 21.6 Gy in 1.8-Gy fractions to subclinical disease with a boost of 14.4 Gy to gross residual disease.

8. C
Lymph node involvement at diagnosis is overall 15%, but depends on the location of the primary. Lymph node involvement is rare in orbital primaries, but occurs in approximately 25% of extremity, trunk, and paratesticular primaries). Overall, there is a 15% risk of metastatic disease at presentation.

9. B
Beckwith–Weidemann (Macrosomia, hemihypertrophy, macroglossia, ear pits, abdominal wall defects). Ten percent risk of childhood cancers including Wilms'.

10. D
Average risk medulloblastoma includes patients with each of the following features:
   Patient age greater than 3 years old
   Less than 1.5-cm^2 residual tumor after resection
   No evidence of dissemination
   Not anaplastic histology

11. D
Although rhabdomyosarcoma can occur anywhere in the body, common locations include:
   Genitourinary 30%
   Parameningeal 25%
   Extremity 13%
   Orbit 9%
   Head and neck (nonparameningeal) 7%
   Trunk 5%

12. C

Lymph node involvement at diagnosis is overall 15%, but depends on the location of the primary. Lymph node involvement is rare in orbital primaries, but occurs in approximately 25% of extremity, trunk, and paratesticular primaries. Overall, there is a 15% risk of metastatic disease at presentation.

13. A

Neuroblastoma is a malignant tumor arising from the sympathetic nervous system. It is the third most common malignancy in childhood, behind leukemia and brain tumors. It is the most common malignancy in children younger than 12 months of age.

14. C

For high risk patients (N-myc amplified (stage 2–4s) OR N-myc non-amp, >1-year old, stage 4), an expected 30% 5-year survival has been demonstrated.

15. B

For low-risk patients (All stage 1 or stage 2, N-myc non-amp, and <50% resection OR stage 4s, <1-year old, non-amp, FH), an expected 90% 5-year survival has been demonstrated.

16. D

Management of neuroblastoma is based on risk stratification into low-, intermediate-, and high-risk groups. Risk is stratified based on INSS stage, N-myc amplification, age, tumor histology, tumor ploidy, and extent of resection.

17. C

Wilms' tumor with favorable histology is managed by no radiation therapy for stages I to II, 10.8 Gy for stage III. All other patients with other histologies are treated with radiation therapy.

18. D

Histologic Classification of Renal tumors treated on Wilms' tumor protocols
   Favorable histology Wilms' tumor
   Anaplastic Wilms' tumor (focal or diffuse)
   Rhabdoid tumor of the kidney
   Clear cell sarcoma of the kidney

19. C

Definitive radiation dose for Ewing's sarcoma is 55.8 Gy in 1.8-Gy fractions. Postoperative doses are usually 45 to 50.4 Gy in 1.8-Gy fractions.

20. D

Whole lung irradiation is indicated in children with lung metastases at diagnosis of Ewing's sarcoma. A dose of 15 Gy in 1.5 Gy per fraction is usually used in this situation.

Recommended Reading

Ater JL, Zhou T, Holmes E, et al. Randomized study of two chemotherapy regimens for treatment of low-grade glioma in young children: a report from the Children's Oncology Group. *J Clin Oncol.* 2012;30(21):2641-2647.

Bernstein M, Kovar H, Paulussen M, et al. Ewing's sarcoma family of tumors: current management. *The Oncologist.* 2006;11(5):503–519.

Calaminus G, Bamberg M, Baranzelli MC, et al. Intracranial germ cell tumors: a comprehensive update of the European data. *Neuropediatrics.* 1994;25(1):26-32.

Calaminus G, Kortmann R, Worch J, et al. SIOP CNS GCT 96: final report of outcome of a prospective, multinational nonrandomized trial for children and adults with intracranial germinoma, comparing craniospinal irradiation alone with chemotherapy followed by focal primary site irradiation for patients with localized disease. *Neuro Oncol.* 2013;15(6):788-796.

Fuller BG, Kapp DS, Cox R. Radiation therapy of pineal region tumors: 25 new cases and a review of 208 previously reported cases. *Int J Radiat Oncol Biol Phys.* 1994;28(1):229-245.

Lin LL, El Naqa I, Leonard JR, et al. Long-term outcome in children treated for craniopharyngioma with and without radiotherapy. *J Neurosurg Pediatr*. 2008;1(2):126-130.

Louis DN, Ohgaki H, Wiestler OD, et al. The 2007 WHO classification of tumours of the central nervous system. *Acta Neuropathol*. 2007;114(2):97-109.

Mansur DB. Multidisciplinary management of pediatric intracranial ependymoma. *CNS Oncol*. 2013;2(3):247-257.

Mansur DB, Rubin JB, Kidd EA, et al. Radiation therapy for pilocytic astrocytomas of childhood. *Int J Radiat Oncol Biol Phys*. 2011;79(3):829-834.

Muller K, Gnekow A, Falkenstein F, et al. Radiotherapy in pediatric pilocytic astrocytomas. A subgroup analysis within the prospective multicenter study HIT-LGG 1996 by the German Society of Pediatric Oncology and Hematology (GPOH). *Strahlenther Onkol*. 2013;189(8):647-655.

Ostrom QT, Gittleman H, Farah P, et al. CBTRUS statistical report: primary brain and central nervous system tumors diagnosed in the United States in 2006–2010. *Neuro Oncol*. 2013;15(suppl 2):ii1-ii56.

Packer RJ, Zhou T, Holmes E, Vezina G, Gajjar A. Survival and secondary tumors in children with medulloblastoma receiving radiotherapy and adjuvant chemotherapy: results of Children's Oncology Group trial A9961. *Neuro Oncol*. 2013;15(1):97-103.

Parham DM. Pathologic classification of rhabdomyosarcomas and correlations with molecular studies. *Mod Pathol*. 2001;14(5):506-514.

Gastrointestinal Malignancies

Suzanne Russo and Randall Kimple

2.1 Esophagus

Epidemiology and Risk Factors

- Esophageal cancer is the seventh leading cause of cancer death worldwide.
- Approximately 18,000 new cases of esophageal cancer occur in the United States each year.
- Approximately 15,000 deaths from esophageal cancer occur in the United States each year.
- The male-to-female ratio is 3 to 4:1 for esophageal cancer in the United States.
- Esophageal cancer occurs most commonly during the sixth and seventh decades of life, and is approximately 20 times more common in persons older than 65 years than in those younger than that age.
- In some regions (northern Iran, southern Russia, South Africa, and northern China), the incidence of esophageal carcinoma is estimated to be as high as 800 cases per 100,000 population. Within this population, 95% of esophageal cancers are of squamous cell histology and occur in the upper half of the esophagus.
- The epidemiology of esophageal carcinoma has changed over the past several decades in the United States. Before 1970, squamous cell carcinoma comprised 90% to 95% of esophageal cancer cases, the majority of tumors were located in the thoracic esophagus, and African American men with a long history of smoking and alcohol consumption were most affected. Over the last four decades, the incidence of adenocarcinoma of the distal esophagus and gastroesophageal junction (GEJ) has increased progressively, and currently comprises more than 70% of all the new cases of esophageal cancer.
- Tumor location:
  - Adenocarcinoma: distal: mid/proximal 75%:25%
  - Squamous cell: distal: mid/proximal 50%:50%
- Risk factors for esophageal cancer include:
  - Tobacco use (squamous > adenocarcinoma)
  - Excessive alcohol consumption (squamous > adenocarcinoma)
  - Caustic injury (squamous)
  - Tylosis (congenital hyperkeratosis) (squamous)
  - Prior history of head and neck cancer (squamous). Patients who have had one smoking-related cancer are at significant risk to develop another smoking-related cancer. In addition, infection with certain types of human papillomavirus (HPV) is linked to a number of cancers, including some head and neck cancers and is found in up to 1/3 of esophagus cancers from patients in parts of Asia and South Africa. Whether HPV plays a causative role in these cancers is unclear at this time. Of note, despite increasing incidence of HPV-related head and neck cancers, there is no evidence of HPV playing a causative role in esophageal cancers in patients from the United States.
  - Exposure to nitrosamines
  - Achalasia
  - Plummer–Vinson syndrome
  - High body mass index (BMI) (adenocarcinoma)

o Gastroesophageal reflux disease (GERD) (adenocarcinoma)
o Barrett's esophagus (adenocarcinoma). Barrett's esophagus is intestinal metaplasia of the esophageal epithelial lining and replacement with columnar epithelium. The malignant transformation rate is 0.5% per year for Barrett's.
o *Helicobacter pylori* infection, which can cause stomach cancer, has not been associated with esophageal cancer.

Prognosis

- Survival in patients with esophageal cancer depends on the stage of the disease.
  o AJCC Tumor Node Metastasis (TNM) stage 0—100% 5-year overall survival (OS)
  o AJCC TNM stage 1—80% 5-year OS
  o AJCC TNM stage 2A—40% 5-year OS
  o AJCC TNM stage 2B—30% 5-year OS
  o AJCC TNM stage 3—15% 5-year OS
  o AJCC TNM stage 4—0% 5-year OS
- Squamous cell carcinoma and adenocarcinoma appear to have equivalent survival rates.
- High initial standardized uptake value (SUV) on positron emission tomography (PET) is associated with poorer OS in patients receiving chemoradiation.
- The presence of fluorodeoxyglucose (FDG)-avid lymph nodes (LNs) is an independent adverse prognostic factor.
- A higher 5-year OS is reported for patients who had a pathologic complete response (pCR) following neoadjuvant chemoradiation (~48%).
- Overexpression and gene amplification of the human epidermal growth factor receptor 2 (HER-2) protein are associated with poor survival in esophageal cancer. In a study of 154 patients with esophageal adenocarcinoma, HER-2 positivity was seen in 12% of these patients and overexpression was seen in 14% of them.

Anatomy

- The anatomical regions of the esophagus include:
  o Cervical—from the cricoid cartilage to the thoracic inlet (~18 cm from incisors)
  o Upper Thoracic—thoracic inlet to tracheal bifurcation (~18–24 cm)
  o Mid Thoracic—tracheal bifurcation to just above the GEJ (~24–32 cm)
  o Lower Thoracic/GEJ—The GEJ is further stratified into subclassifications, which influence treatment management recommendations:
  o Siewert–Stein classification is anatomical classification of GEJ tumors.
    - Type I—adenocarcinoma of distal part of the esophagus (center within between 1 and 5 cm above the anatomic GEJ) (esophageal)
    - Type II—adenocarcinoma of the true cardia (between 1 cm above and 2 cm below the GEJ) (esophageal or gastric)
    - Type III—adenocarcinoma of the subcardial stomach (2–5 cm below GEJ) (gastric)
- The esophagus has an extensive, longitudinally continuous, submucosal lymphatic system. The esophagus contains little barrier to lymphatic spread, and lymphatics are interconnected making it possible for nodal involvement separate from the primary tumor.
  o The cervical esophagus drains to the cervical nodes.
  o The thoracic esophagus drains to the posterior mediastinal nodes.
  o The lower esophagus drains to the left gastric, celiac, and gastrohepatic nodes.

Presentation

- Dysphagia is the most common presenting symptom of esophageal cancer, usually for solids progressing to liquids.
- Weight loss is the second most common symptom occurring in more than 50% of people with esophageal carcinoma.

- Hematemesis (bleeding from the tumor).
- Pain is sometimes experienced in the retrosternal or epigastric areas, or in areas of symptomatic bone metastases.
- Hoarseness can be caused by invasion of the recurrent laryngeal nerve.
- Persistent cough or respiratory symptoms caused by aspiration or direct invasion of the tracheobronchial tree.
- Physical examinations in patients with esophageal cancer are typically normal unless there are metastases to neck nodes or the liver.

Diagnosis and Workup

- Physical exam, complete blood count (CBC), and chemistries
- Endoscopy ± barium swallow is indicated for any complaint of dysphagia in an adult
- Esophagogastroduodenoscopy allows direct visualization and biopsies of the tumor
- Endoscopic ultrasound (EUS) to assess depth of penetration and LN involvement
- For dysplasia or cancer limited to the mucosa or submucosa (T1a) by endoscopic ultrasonography, endoscopic mucosal resection (EMR) can be considered for diagnosis and staging
- Bronchoscopy to rule out the presence of a fistula in midesophageal cancers
- CT of the chest and abdomen is recommended for staging
- For early-stage esophageal cancer, PET/CT is optional, but for locoregional esophageal cancer, PET/CT is recommended. PET/CT staging detects up to 20% metastases not seen on CT
- For locally advanced (T3/T4) adenocarcinoma of the GEJ infiltrating into the cardia or Siewart type III tumors, laparoscopy is recommended to improve accuracy of staging
- Bone scan if alkaline phosphatase is elevated
- PFTs to assess operability
- Nutritional status should be evaluated in patients with dysphagia—Albumin and total protein
- Liver function studies should be performed in alcoholic patients

Staging

The American Joint Cancer Committee/Union for International Cancer Control (AJCC/UICC) 2010 TNM classification for esophageal cancer is outlined. Esophageal tumors with epicenters within 5 cm of the GEJ that also extend into the esophagus are classified and staged according to the AJCC/UICC esophageal scheme. Tumors with an epicenter in the stomach that are more than 5 cm from the esophagogastric junction or those within 5 cm of the esophagogastric junction without extension into the esophagus are staged as gastric cancers.

- Tis—Carcinoma in situ/high-grade dysplasia
- T1—Lamina propria or submucosa
  - o T1a—Lamina propria or muscularis mucosa
  - o T1b—Submucosa
- T2—Muscularis propria
- T3—Adventitia
- T4—Adjacent structures
  - o T4a—Pleura, pericardium, diaphragm, or adjacent peritoneum
  - o T4b—Other adjacent structures (aorta, vertebral body, trachea)
- N0—No regional LN metastasis
  - o N1—One to two regional LNs (N1 is site dependent)
  - o N2—Three to six regional LNs
  - o N3—More than six regional LNs
- M0—No distant metastasis
  - o M1—Distant metastasis (M1a and M1b are site dependent)

Stage Classification

Stage IA	T1	N0	M0
Stage IB	T2	N0	M0
Stage IIA	T3	N0	M0
Stage IIB	T1,T2	N1	M0
Stage IIIA	T4a	N0	M0
	T3	N1	M0
	T1,T2	N2	M0
Stage IIIB	T3	N2	M0
Stage IIIC	T4a	N1,N2	M0
	T4b	Any N	M0
	Any T	N3	M0
Stage IV	Any T	Any N	M1

Treatment Overview

- Treatment of esophageal cancer varies by disease stage.
- Tis, T1aN0M0, and select patients with T1bN0M0 by endoscopic ultrasonography may be considered for endoscopic therapy, such as EMR or endoscopic submucosal dissection (ESD).
- T1b and any N, surgery may be the initial treatment, but for primary tumors greater than T1b or if there is any suspicion of nodal involvement on ultrasonography, trimodality treatment is recommended.
- Trimodality (chemoradiation followed by surgery) is supported by level 1 evidence.
  - 15% to 30% will have a pCR
  - pCR is associated with a 3-year survival rate of approximately 50%, compared to 27% (<pCR)
- Preoperative chemotherapy followed by surgery is another option but the increase in 2-year OS is less than 6%, compared with approximately 13% with trimodality therapy.
- Stage IV disease is treated with chemotherapy, palliative measures, and supportive care.

Surgery

- Surgery remains the cornerstone treatment for esophageal cancer. Any esophageal cancer patient who is a surgical candidate should be staged appropriately and evaluated for surgery.
- Contraindications to surgery include:
  - Metastasis to N2 nodes (cervical or supraclavicular LNs) or presence of distant metastases; treatment of esophageal cancer with celiac axis LN involvement remains controversial
  - Invasion of adjacent structures (recurrent laryngeal nerve, tracheobronchial tree)
  - Severe comorbid illness(es)
  - FEV-1 <1.2 L and LVEF <0.4 are relative contraindications
- EMR is an experimental approach to patients with T1a disease or high-grade dysplasia. This should be performed at centers with high volume/expertise.
- Esophagectomy
  - Transhiatal esophagectomy uses an abdominal and a cervical incision with blunt mediastinal dissection through the esophageal hiatus.

- Advantages:
  - Avoids chest incision and associated prolonged discomfort that can result in compromised respiratory function.
  - The gastrointestinal tract is anastomosed using the stomach.
- Disadvantage:
  - Poor mediastinal exposure and nodal sampling
  - Radial margins possibly inadequate by blunt dissection
- Transthoracic esophagectomy uses or an abdominal and a right thoracic incision.
  *Retrospective prospective studies show no difference in survival between techniques.
- Video-assisted thoracoscopy (VATS) for thoracic mobilization of the esophagus can be used to reduce the size of the chest incision.
- Laparoscopy can be used to mobilize the gastric conduit and reduce the size of the abdominal incision.
- Minimally invasive techniques have been associated with a shorter hospital stay, less postoperative discomfort, and faster recovery time compared to open surgery.
  - EMR is used for high-grade dysplasia and mucosa-limited cancers only. A population-based study of 1,618 patients with grade Tis, T1a, or T1b demonstrated OS and CSS times with EMR comparable to open surgery.
- Surgery alone—3-year survival rate of 6% to 35%; median survival—13 to 19 months.
- Local recurrence rate—approximately 40%
- Operative mortality—4% to 10%
  - Respiratory complications (15%–20%)—atelectasis, pleural effusion, and pneumonia
  - Cardiac complications (15%–20%)—cardiac arrhythmias and myocardial infarction
  - Septic complications (10%)—wound infection, anastomotic leak, and pneumonia
    *Intrathoracic leak can lead to sepsis and death

Chemotherapy Alone

- Postoperative continuance of chemotherapy started preoperatively may be beneficial.
- Neoadjuvant chemotherapy alone offers limited benefit.
  - **INT 0113** (Kelsen, *N Engl J Med.* 1998; doi:10.1056/NEJM199812313392704)
    - Phase III
    - 467 patients; resectable—T1–2NxM0 squamous cell and adenocarcinoma
    - Surgery alone versus 5-fluorouracil (FU)/cisplatin × 3 followed by surgery

	MS (Months)	4-y OS	cCR/pCR
Surgery alone	16	23%	–
Chemo then surgery	15	26%	12%/2.5%

  - **Medical Research Council** (*Lancet.* 2002; doi:10.1016/S0140-6736(02)08651-8; Allum, *J Clin Oncol.* 2008; doi:10.1200/JCO.2009.22.2083)
    - Phase III
    - 802 patients; resectable squamous cell and adenocarcinoma
    - Surgery alone versus 5-FU/cisplatin × 2 followed by surgery

	Complete Resection rate	2-y OS	5-y OS	*Pre-Op XRT Given
Surgery alone	54%	34%	17%	9%
Chemo then surgery	60%	43%	23%	9%

*Addition of radiation before surgery.

○ **MAGIC** (Cunningham, *N Engl J Med.* 2006; doi:10.1056/NEJMoa055531)
  *Perioperioperative chemotherapy improves survival over surgery alone
  ▪ European randomized trial demonstrated survival benefit associated with of preoperative and postoperative epirubicin, cisplatin, and 5-FU (ECF)
  ▪ Included patients with distal esophageal adenocarcinoma; All greater than stage II

	5-y OS	MS (Months)	PFS (Months)
Surgery alone	23%	20 mo	13 mo
Perioperative chemotherapy	36%	24 mo	19 mo
P-value		.009	<.001

Radiation Alone

- 3-year OS—0%. (Control Arm RTOG 85-01)
- Postoperative radiation associated with increased local control, but no survival benefit.
- **Preoperative Radiation Versus Surgery Alone** (Arnott, *Cochrane Database Syst Rev.* 2005; doi:10.1002/14651858.CD001799)
  ○ Meta-analysis. Five randomized trials; mostly SCC
  ○ 1,147 patients
  ○ Median follow-up—9 years
  ○ Trend survival benefit (HR 0.89, $P = .06$) with preoperative radiation (~3%–4%)

Chemoradiation

- There is no survival benefit associated with postoperative chemoradiation.
- Chemotherapy and radiation therapy (RT) for esophageal cancer are delivered preoperatively to reduce the primary tumor facilitating higher curative resection rates, and to treat subclinical regional metastases.

Neoadjuvant Chemoradiation Versus Surgery Alone
- **Walsh** (*N Engl J Med.* 1996; doi:10.1056/NEJM199608153350702)
  *Neoadjuvant chemoradiation followed by surgery improves OS over surgery alone.
  ○ Phase III
  ○ 113 operable patients
  ○ Adenocarcinoma only
  ○ Surgery alone versus 40 Gy (15 fx) with concurrent 5-FU/cisplatin (2 cycles) followed by surgery
  ○ pCR—25% for patients receiving neoadjuvant chemoradiation
  ○ Criticized for small sample size, no CT staging, short follow-up, poor outcome in surgery alone arm compared to historical controls
  ○ 11 patients withdrew from chemoradiation arm; 1 for surgery arm

	MS (Months)	3-y OS
Surgery alone	11	6%
Neoadjuvant CRT and surgery	16	32%

- **EORTC** (Bossett, *N Engl J Med.* 1997; doi:10.1056/NEJM199707173370304)
  *Neoadjuvant chemoradiation followed by surgery offers improved cancer-specific and disease-free survival but does not improve OS over surgery alone.
  ○ Phase III
  ○ 282 operable patients; T1–3N0M0 and T1–2N1M0 patients

o Squamous only
o Surgery alone versus 37 Gy (10 fx, split course 2 weeks apart) with concurrent 5-FU/cisplatin (2 cycles) followed by surgery
o pCR—26% for patients receiving neoadjuvant chemoradiation
o Neoadjuvant chemoradiation associated with a higher rate of postoperative death

	MS (Months)	3-y CSS	3-y DFS	3-y OS	Post-Op Death
Surgery alone	18.6	14%	17%	36%	5%
Neoadjuvant CRT + surgery	18.6	33%	21%	36%	17%

- **Urba** (*J Clin Oncol.* 2001; 19(2):305–313)
  *Neoadjuvant chemoradiation followed by surgery resulted in a nonsignificant OS benefit over surgery alone.
  o Phase III
  o 100 operable patients; Stages I to III
  o Squamous (25%) and adenocarcinoma (75%)
  o Surgery alone versus 45 Gy (150-cGy BID, no elective nodal radiation) with concurrent 5-FU/cisplatin/vinblastine (2 cycles) followed by transhiatal esophagectomy
  o 94% had surgery 3 weeks after treatment
  o pCR—28% for patients receiving neoadjuvant chemoradiation associated with better prognosis
  o Worse outcome for squamous histology

	MS (Months)	LR	3-y OS
Surgery alone	18	19%	15%
Neoadjuvant CRT and surgery	17	42%	30%
P-value	–		.15

- **Bates** (*J Clin Oncol.* 1996;14(1):156–163)
  o Phase II
  o 35 operable patients; Stages I to III; poor accrual—closed early
  o Squamous (80%) and adenocarcinoma (20%)
  o Surgery alone versus 45 Gy (25 fx) with concurrent 5-FU/cisplatin (2 cycles) followed by Ivor-Lewis esophagectomy
  o pCR—51% for patients receiving neoadjuvant chemoradiation
  o Preesophagectomy endoscopy with negative biopsy did not correlate with surgical pathology findings from esophagectomy in 41%

	MS (Months)
All patients	25.8
pCR patients	36.8
Non-pCR patients	12.9

- **Burmeister** (*Lancet Oncol.* 2005; doi:10.1016/S1470-2045(05)70288-6)
  *Neoadjuvant chemoradiation results in improved OS compared to surgery alone.
  - Phase III
  - 256 operable patients; T1–3, N0–1; poor accrual—closed early
  - Squamous and adenocarcinoma
  - Surgery alone versus 35 Gy (15 fx) with concurrent 5-FU/cisplatin then surgery
  - pCR patients—13% had 49% 5-year OS

	R0 Rate	3-y DFS	3-y OS
Surgery alone	60%	30%	35%
Neoadjuvant CRT and surgery	80%	35%	35%

- **CALGB 9781** (Tepper, *J Clin Oncol.* 2008; doi:10.1200/JCO.2007.12.9593)
  *Neoadjuvant chemoradiation results in improved OS compared to surgery alone.
  - Phase III
  - 56 operable patients; Stages I to III; poor accrual—closed early
  - Squamous and adenocarcinoma (61%)
  - Surgery alone versus 50.4 Gy (28 fx) concurrent 5-FU/cisplatin (2 cycles) then surgery
  - pCR—40% for patients receiving neoadjuvant chemoradiation

	MS	5-y OS
Surgery alone	1.8 y	16%
Neoadjuvant CRT and surgery	4.5 y	39%
P-value	.02	.005

- **Federation Francophone Cancerologie Digestive (FFCD) 9101** (Mariette, *J Clin Oncol.* 2014; doi:10.1200/JCO.2013.53.6532)
  *Neoadjuvant chemoradiation results in improved outcomes compared to surgery alone.
  - Phase III
  - 195 patients; Stage I (19%), IIA (53%), and IIB (28%)
  - Squamous (23%), adenocarcinoma (75%), and large cell undifferentiated (2%)
  - Surgery alone versus 41.4 Gy (23 fx) with weekly carboplatin/paclitaxel then surgery
  - pCR—29% for patients receiving neoadjuvant chemoradiation
  - Closed: interim analysis deemed improbability of superiority of either arm

	R0 Resection Rate	3-y OS
Surgery alone	92.1%	53%
Neoadjuvant CRT and surgery	93.8%	47.5%

- **Chemoradiation Therapy for Oesophageal Cancer Followed by Surgery Study (CROSS)** (van Hagen et al., *N Engl J Med.* 2012; doi:10.1056/NEJMoa1112088)
  *Neoadjuvant chemoradiation improved outcomes compared to surgery alone.
  - Phase III
  - 368 patients; T1N1M0 or T2 to T3 N × M0
  - Squamous and adenocarcinoma
  - Surgery alone versus 45 Gy (25 fx) with concurrent weekly 5-FU/cisplatin (2 cycles) followed by surgery

o pCR—33% for patients receiving neoadjuvant chemoradiation
o An analysis of data from CROSS I and II showed overall recurrence rates were 35% for chemoradiation therapy (CRT) plus surgery and 58% for surgery alone. The rates of locoregional recurrence, peritoneal carcinomatosis, and hematogenous dissemination were all lower for patients receiving CRT (14% vs. 34%, 4% vs. 14%, and 29% vs. 35%, respectively)

	MS (Months)	R0 Resection Rate	5-y OS
Surgery alone	24	69%	16%
Neoadjuvant CRT and surgery	49.4	92%	39%

- **Gebski** (*Lancet Oncol.* 2007; doi:10.1016/S1470-2045(07)70039-6)
  *Neoadjuvant chemoradiation improves OS compared to surgery alone.
  o Meta-analysis (10 neoadjuvant chemoradiation or chemotherapy trials)
  o 2,933 patients (1,209 pre-op CRT vs. surgery alone; 1,724 pre-op chemo vs. surgery)
  o Hazard ratio of 0.9 ($P = .05$) associated with neoadjuvant chemotherapy alone
  o Hazard ratio of 0.81 ($P = .002$) associated with neoadjuvant chemoradiation
    ▪ Squamous cell HR 0.84
    ▪ Adenocarcinoma HR 0.75
  o 13% absolute survival advantage at 2 years with neoadjuvant chemoradiation
  o Chemo alone improved OS in adenocarcinoma but not squamous cell

Selective Esophagectomy RTOG 02-46 (Swisher, *JTCVS.* 2002; doi:10.1067/mtc.2002.119070; *Int J Radiat Oncol Biol Phys.* 2007; doi:10.1016/j.ijrobp.2007.07.195)
*Induction chemotherapy followed by definitive CRT with selective esophagectomy does not improve outcome (compared to historical controls) and increases toxicity.
  o Phase II
  o Squamous (27%) or adenocarcinoma (73%)
  o 43 patients; nonmetastatic resectable esophageal cancer; ≥T3 76%) and N1 (71%)
  o Induction 5-FU, cisplatin and paclitaxel (2 cycles), followed by concurrent chemoradiation (50.4 Gy/28 fx) and daily 5-FU with cisplatin over 5 days.
  o Salvage surgery for patients with residual or recurrent without metastases.
  o OS all patients
    ▪ 3 year—44%
    ▪ 5 year—37%
  o Clinical CR after neoadjuvant therapy—37%
    ▪ 5-year OS 53%
    ▪ 33% alive without surgery
    ▪ 13% alive with selective surgery
  o Clinical non-CR after neoadjuvant therapy—51%
    ▪ 21 patients underwent surgery
      – Residual disease (17 patients)
      – Recurrent disease (3 patients)
      – Choice (1 patient)
    ▪ Metastatic disease 3/21 patients
    ▪ 5-year OS 33%

Definitive Chemoradiation

- ***RTOG 85-01*** (Herskovic, *N Engl J Med.* 1992; doi:10.1056/NEJM199206113262403; Al-Sarraf, *J Clin Oncol.* 1998;16(4):1310–1317; Cooper, *JAMA.* 1999; doi:10.1001/jama.281.17.1623)
  *Definitive CRT yield results as good as trimodality therapy.

- o Phase III
- o 121 patients; Stage II/III patients—T1–3N0–1M0
- o Squamous cell and adenocarcinoma
- o Technique—Whole mediastinum 30 or 50 Gy, then boost
- o 64-Gy radiation alone versus 50 Gy (2 Gy/fx) with concurrent 5-FU/cisplatin (4 cycles)

	8-y OS	5-y OS	2-y OS	MS (mo)	LC
XRT	0%	0%	10%	9.3	36%
CRT	22%	27%	38%	14.1	57%
CRT expansion (69 patients)		14%		17.2	48%

No differences between squamous cell and adenocarcinomas

- **RTOG 94-05/INT 0123** (Minsky, *J Clin Oncol*. 2002;20(5):1167–1174)
*Higher radiation doses do not improve outcome; they increase complication rates.
  - o Phase III
  - o Squamous cell and adenocarcinoma
  - o 236 patients; Stage II/III patients—T1–4N0–1M0
  - o Technique—50.4 Gy (5-cm long and 2-cm radial margins) + 14.4-Gy boost (2-cm margin) with concurrent 5-FU/cisplatin (per RTOG 85-01)
  - o Closed after interim analysis showed 64.8-Gy arm doing worse.
  - o 7 of 11 deaths on 64.8-Gy arm occurred before 50.4 Gy

	2-y OS	MST
50.4 Gy	40%	18.1 mo
64.8 Gy	31%	13 mo

- **RTOG 01-13** (Ajani, *J Clin Oncol*. 2008; doi:10.1200/JCO.2008.16.6918)
*Induction chemotherapy followed by definitive CRT for inoperable esophageal Cancer did not meet 1-year survival endpoint and increased toxicity.
  - o Randomized phase II
  - o Non 5-Fu based versus 5-FU based chemotherapy followed by CRT
  - o 1-year OS for 5-FU arm 75.7%, both arms with excessive G3-4 toxicity
- **RTOG 04-36** (Suntharalingam, *J Clin Oncol*. 2014;32(3_suppl))
*The addition of cetuximab to paclitaxel/cisplatin and radiation does not improve OS for patients with inoperable esophageal cancer.
  - o Phase III
  - o 344 patients, T1N1M0; T2–4 Any N M0; Any T/N M1a
  - o Adenocarcinoma or squamous

	cCR Rate	2-y OS	2-y OS cCR	2-y OS Non-cCR	2-y OS Adenoca	2-y OS SCC
No cetuximab	56%	42%	58%	30%	41%	43%
cetuximab	59%	44%			43%	46%

Definitive Chemoradiation Versus Trimodality Therapy

- **Federation Francophone Cancerologie Digestive (FFCD) 9102** (Bedenne, *J Clin Oncol.* 2007; doi:10.1200/JCO.2005.04.7118)
  *Definitive chemoradiation with salvage esophagectomy
  - o Phase III
  - o 90% squamous cell
  - o 455 patients (259 randomized); Stage T3N0–1
  - o 46 Gy (23 fx) and concurrent 5-FU/cisplatin (2 cycles)—partial and complete clinical responder then randomized to surgery versus additional chemoradiation (20 Gy/10 fx) and concurrent 5-FU/cisplatin (3 cycles) for a total dose of 66 Gy
  - o For CRT alone—1.63 HR locoregional relapse ($P = .03$)
  - o 80% of recurrences within 2 years; 60% within 1 year
  - o Median survival for nonresponders—11 months

	MS (Months)	2-y OS	2-y LC
Trimodality 129 patients	18	34%	65%
CRT no surgery 130 patients	19	40%	57%

- **German** (Stahl, *J Clin Oncol.* 2009; doi:10.1200/JCO.2008.17.0506)
  *Definitive chemoradiation versus chemoradiation with planned esophagectomy
  - o Phase III, closed due to trend in improved 3-year OS with radiation cohort
  - o 172 patients; T3–4N0–1 staged by EUS (126 distal adenocarcinoma)
  - o 5-FU, leucovorin, etoposide, cisplatin (FLEP) then response assessment
    - ■ 76% assessed
    - ■ 37% responders
    - ■ 31% nonresponders
  - o Then randomized
    - ■ Concurrent chemoradiation (50 Gy/25 fx) with cisplatin/etoposide followed by surgery
    - ■ Additional concurrent chemoradiation (total dose 64.8 Gy) with cisplatin/etoposide
    - ■ Nonobstructed T3 had different boost (10-Gy EBRT then 4-Gy high dose rate [HDR] × 2- to 0.5-cm depth)
  - o 34% of patients developed metastases or refused surgery
  - o 82% R0 rate, 32% for nonresponders

	MS (Months)	3-y OS	3-y OS Responders	3-y OS Nonresponders	PFS
Trimodality	16	31%	58%	17.9%	64%
Definitive CRT	15	24%	55%	9.4%	41%

Brachytherapy

- **RTOG 92-07** (Gaspar, *Cancer.* 2000; doi:10.1002/(SICI)1097-0142(20000301) 88:5<988::AID-CNCR7>3.0.CO;2-U)
  *Brachytherapy boost not recommended
  - o Phase I/II
  - o 49 patients, Stage T1–2N0–1, 92% squamous cell

- ○ 50 Gy (25 fx) and concurrent 5-FU/cisplatin then
- ○ HDR 5 Gy × 3 LDR 20 Gy × 1
- ○ 24% G4 toxicity
  - ▪ 12% fistula
  - ▪ 10% death
- ○ MS 11 months
- ○ 3-year OS 29%
- ○ LD 63%

Radiation Technique

- Simulate patient with arms up using a wing board, alpha cradle, or vac-lock bag
- Use esophageal contrast to outline the esophagus, stomach, and small bowel
- Use three-dimensional conformal radiation treatment planning to optimize target dose, and achieve normal tissue dose limitations. Intensity-modulated RT (IMRT) may be used for tumors behind the heart
  - ○ Spinal cord ≤45 Gy
  - ○ Lungs 75% ≤20 Gy, 50% ≤5 Gy
  - ○ Heart 33% ≤50 Gy
  - ○ Liver 60% ≤30 Gy; ≤25-Gy mean dose
  - ○ Kidneys 66% one kidney ≤20 Gy
  - ○ Stomach—if stomach in field consider blocking at 45 Gy if feasible
- Target volume 3- to 4-cm proximal and distal margins; 1-cm circumferential radial margins (CRMs) for primary tumor and involved nodes with consideration of coverage of elective nodes if expansion does not result in excessive toxicity
- For proximal tumors, treat paraesophageal, supraclavicular, and upper mediastinal nodes
- For tumors below the carina treat paraesophageal, mediastinal nodes and include celiac axis and lesser curvature nodes for distal 1/3 esophageal tumors, including GEJ tumors
- Dose 1.8 to 2 Gy daily, five times weekly
  - ○ Preoperative dose 41.4 to 50.4 Gy
  - ○ Postoperative dose 45 to 50.4 Gy
  - ○ Definitive dose 50 to 50.4 Gy
  - ○ Higher doses (60–70 Gy) may be appropriate for cervical esophageal cancer if surgery not planned

Palliation

In patients with advanced disease or who are not candidates for surgery, palliation of dysphagia can be done using several treatment modalities:

- *Chemotherapy* as a single modality has limited use and can produce a short-lived response in a minority of patients. The 2006 Cochrane meta-analysis found no consistent benefit with any specific chemotherapy regimen.
- *RT* is successful in relieving dysphagia in approximately 50% of patients, and is typically combined with chemotherapy as definitive therapy in the absence of metastatic disease.
- *Endoluminal brachytherapy* using HDR is well-tolerated for superficial primary and recurrent esophageal cancer (Folkert, *Brachytherapy*, 2013).

	LC	18-Month OS
10 patients recurrent disease	11.1%	55.6 mo
4 patients unirradiated	75%	100%

- ○ Median dose of 12 Gy (range, 10–15 Gy) over 3 fractions in 3 weeks; prescribed to 7-mm median depth with mucosal dose limited to 8 to 10 Gy using a 12- to 14-mm applicator.

- o Median follow-up—15.4 months.
- o 6 (42.9%) patients had chronic Grade 1 adverse effects; 1 (7.1%) patient developed Grade 2 stricture. 1 (7.1%) patient Grade 3 developed tracheoesophageal fistula.
- **Laser therapy**
- Laser therapy (Nd:YAG laser) may provide temporary relief of dysphagia in up to 70% of patients. Multiple sessions are usually required to keep the esophageal lumen patent.
- **Photodynamic therapy**
- The photosensitizer porfimer (Photofrin) is FDA approved for palliation of patients with completely obstructing esophageal cancer or partially obstructing cancer that cannot be satisfactorily treated with Nd:YAG laser therapy. Intravenous injection of porfimer is followed 40 to 50 hours later with delivery of 630-nm wavelength laser light; a second laser light treatment may be given 96 to 120 hours after the injection.
- **Stents**
- Expandable metallic stents can be useful in patients with tracheoesophageal fistulas and are placed by endoscopy under fluoroscopic guidance.

Follow-Up

- History and physical exam every 3 to 6 months for 1 to 2 years, then every 6 months for 3 to 5 years, then annually thereafter.
- For locally advanced tumors FDG-PET before and after chemoradiation evaluating response to treatment is a strong predictor of survival.
- Following treatment FDG-PET should be considered at 4 to 6 months following treatment, and if normal, every 6 to 9 months for the first 2 years. Imaging should be based on symptoms 2 years following treatment.
- Other radiologic tests are reserved for symptom workup in the follow-up period.
- Endoscopy should be performed every 3 to 4 months for 2 years in patients undergoing chemoradiation without surgery, then every 6 months for 1 year after first normal exam. Endoscopy is recommended on an as-needed basis for patients undergoing esophagectomy.

2.2 Stomach

Epidemiology and Risk Factors

- It is the 15th most common cancer in the United States.
- There are about 24,500 cases of gastric cancer diagnosed in the United States per year.
- In the United States, the incidence in males is highest in African Americans, and in females the incidence is highest in Asians. In males and females, rates are lowest in Whites.
- Median age at diagnosis is 69 years.
- Gastric cancer is the fourth most common cause of cancer-related death in the world.
- Rates of gastric cancer have declined over the last 100 years. Decreases from:
  - o Refrigeration, increased consumption of fresh fruits and vegetables
  - o Decreased salt intake
  - o Decreased H. pylori infection with use of screening and antibiotics
- Geographic variation in the incidence gastric cancer exists.
  - o It is the most common cancer in Japan
  - o Highest rates: Asia and South America
  - o Highest death rates: Chile, Japan, South America, and Russia
  - o Lowest rates: North America
  - o Worldwide the male-to-female ratio is 1.5 to 2:1
- Tumor location
  - o GEJ, cardia, fundus approximately 35% (incidence of diffuse subtype increasing)
  - o Body approximately 25%
  - o Antrum and distal stomach approximately 40% (incidence of intestinal subtype increasing)
  - o 10% involving more than one part

- The most common histology of gastric tumors is adenocarcinoma (90%–95%)
  - Subclassification according to histology:
    - Tubular
    - Papillary
    - Mucinous
    - Signet-ring cells
    - Undifferentiated
  - Classification by gross appearance:
    - Ulcerative
    - Polypoid, scirrhous (diffuse linitis plastica)
    - Superficial spreading
    - Multicentric
    - Barrett ectopic adenocarcinoma
  - Borrmann's subtypes:
    - I—polypoid
    - II—ulcerating
    - III—infiltrating and ulcerating
    - IV—infiltrating (linitus plastica)
  - The Lauren system
    - Type I (intestinal) is EPIDEMIC and associated with environmental risk factors, a better prognosis, more than 40 years old, and no familial history. Intestinal, expansive, epidemic-type gastric cancer is associated with chronic atrophic gastritis, retained glandular structure, little invasiveness, and a sharp margin.
    - Type II (diffuse) is ENDEMIC and is not associated with environment or diet. It has a worse prognosis, more common in women and young patients. It is associated with genetic factors (such as CDH1), blood groups, and a family history of gastric cancer. Diffuse, infiltrative, endemic cancer, consists of scattered cell clusters with poor differentiation and usually has involved margins as it invades large areas of the stomach.
- The second most common is low grade B-cell gastric MALT lymphoma (mucosa associated lymphoid tissue).
  - More rare histologies include:
    - Gastrointestinal stromal tumors (2%)
    - Carcinoids (1%)
    - Adenoacanthomas (1%)
    - Squamous cell carcinomas (1%)
- Risk factors include:
  - H. pylori infection is the strongest risk factor for gastric cancer
  - Diet rich in salted, smoked, or pickled foods
  - Tobacco use
  - Obesity
  - Previous gastric surgery
  - Gastric ulcers
  - Pernicious anemia
  - Chronic atrophic gastritis
  - Radiation exposure
  - Genetic factors in 10% of cases
    - Germline truncating mutations of the E-cadherin gene (CDH1)
    - Hereditary nonpolyposis colorectal cancer
    - Li–Fraumeni syndrome
    - Familial adenomatous polyposis
    - Peutz–Jeghers syndrome

Prognosis

- Survival in patients with gastric cancer depends on the stage of the disease.
  - AJCC TNM stage IA—71% 5-year OS
  - AJCC TNM stage IIA—46% 5-year OS
  - AJCC TNM stage IIIA—20% 5-year OS
  - AJCC TNM stage IV—0% 5-year OS
- In the United States, approximately 25% present with localized disease, approximately 31% present with regional disease, and approximately 32% present with distant metastases.

Anatomy

- The stomach begins at the GEJ and ends at the duodenum.
- The stomach comprises three parts with distinct histologic features:
  - Cardia (upper) with predominantly mucin-secreting cells
  - Fundus (middle, largest part) with mucoid cells, chief cells, and parietal cells
  - Pylorus (distal, connects to duodenum) with mucus-producing and endocrine cells
- The stomach wall is made up of five layers. From the lumen out, the layers are:
  - Mucosa
  - Submucosa
  - Muscularis
  - Subserosa
  - Serosa
- A peritoneum covers the anterior surface of the stomach.
- The GEJ has no serosa.
- Primary lymphatic drainage is along the celiac axis with additional drainage along the splenic hilum, suprapancreatic nodal groups, porta hepatis, and gastroduodenal areas.
- Pattern of lymphatic spread related to tumor location:
- Stomach supplied by celiac artery via three branches:
  - Left gastric—upper right stomach
  - Common hepatic → Right Gastric—lower right stomach
  - Right Gastroepiploic lower area of greater curvature
  - Splenic artery → Left Gastroepiploic—upper area of greater curvature
  - Short Gastrics—fundus

Presentation

- Early stage gastric cancer is typically asymptomatic.
- Patients with more advanced disease complain of:
  - Indigestion
  - Postprandial fullness
  - Dysphagia
  - Nausea or vomiting
  - Loss of appetite
  - Melena
  - Hematemesis
  - Weight loss

Diagnosis and Workup

- Physical exam is usually normal, except for patients presenting with late stage gastric cancer. Physical findings may include:
  - Weight loss/cachexia
  - Anemia

- o   Melena
- o   Enlarged stomach
- o   Hepatomegaly
- o   Periumbilical metastasis (Sister Mary Joseph nodule)
- o   Enlarged left supraclavicular nodes (Virchow nodes)
- o   Axillary adenopathy (Irish node)
- o   Ovarian metastases (Kruckenberg tumor)
- o   Paraneoplastic syndromes:
  - ■   Dermatomyositis
  - ■   Acanthosis nigricans
  - ■   Circinate erythemas
- • Workup for suspected gastric cancer includes:
- o   CBC, chemistries, liver, and renal function
- o   CEA (elevated in 33%)
- o   H. pylori
- o   Upper endoscopy and biopsy (endoscopic resection for early stage cancers)
- o   Endoscopic ultrasound if no evidence of M1 disease is found for:
  - ■   Depth of penetration
  - ■   LN involvement
- o   Chest/abdomen/pelvic CT with oral and IV contrast
- o   Bone scan if alkaline phosphatase elevated
- o   PET—CT evaluation not routine but may be useful if no evidence of M1 disease
- o   Laparoscopy to evaluate extent of disease and peritoneal disease (occult stage IV)
- o   Biopsy of metastatic disease should be considered
- o   CBC and comprehensive chemistry profile
- o   *HER2-neu* testing if metastatic adenocarcinoma is present

Staging

AJCC/UICC 2010 TNM classification for gastric cancer is outlined. Tumors with an epicenter in the stomach that are more than 5 cm from the esophagogastric junction or those within 5 cm of the esophagogastric junction without extension into the esophagus are staged as gastric cancers.

- • T0—No evidence of primary tumor
- • Tis—Carcinoma in situ, intraepithelial tumor without invasion of lamina propria
- • T1—Tumor invades lamina propria, muscularis mucosa, or submucosa
  - o   T1a—Tumor invades lamina propria or muscularis mucosa
  - o   T1b—Tumor invades submucosa
- • T2—Tumor invades muscularis propria
- • T3—Tumor penetrates subserosal connective tissue without invasion of visceral peritoneum or adjacent structures
- • T4—Tumor invades serosa (visceral peritoneum) or adjacent structures
  - o   T4a—Tumor invades serosa (visceral peritoneum)
  - o   T4b—Tumor invades adjacent structures
- • N0—No regional LN metastases
  - o   N1—Metastases in 1 to 2 regional LNs
  - o   N2—Metastases in 3 to 6 regional LNs
  - o   N3—Metastases in 7 or more regional LNs
  - o   N3a—Metastases in 7 to 15 regional LNs
  - o   N3b—Metastases in 16 or more regional LNs

- M0—No distant metastasis
  o M1—Distant metastasis

Stage Classification

Stage IA	T1	N0	M0
Stage IB	T2	N0	M0
	T1	N1	M0
Stage IIA	T3	N0	M0
	T2	N1	M0
	T1	N2	M0
Stage IIB	T4a	N0	M0
	T3	N1	M0
	T2	N2	M0
	T1	N3	M0
Stage IIIA	T4a	N1	M0
	T3	N2	M0
	T2	N3	M0
Stage IIIB	T4b	N0–1	M0
	T4a	N2	M0
	T3	N3	M0
Stage IIIC	T4b	N2–3	M0
	T4a	N3	M0
	T3	N3	M0
Stage IV	Any T	Any N	M1

Treatment Overview

Surgery

- 50% to 60% are surgical candidates.
- Select T1a gastric cancers may undergo endoscopic resection:
  o Well-differentiated, nonulcerated
  o ≤2 cm, confined to the mucosa
- Radical gastrectomy has historically been used for resectable stages IB to III disease to achieve negative margins due to the extensive lymphatic network around the stomach and the propensity for this tumor to extend microscopically. A subtotal gastrectomy is used for distal gastric tumors and may be performed if a 5-cm proximal margin can be achieved for nondiffuse type tumors (8 cm for diffuse-type cancers).
- D0 Dissection: Limited surgery
- D1 Dissection: Resection of tumor and first echelon LNs
- D2 Dissection: Resection of tumor, first and second echelon nodes (perigastric, celiac, splenic, hepatic artery, cardiac LNs, + distal pancreatectomy and splenectomy)

- D2 LN dissection is standard of care as it provides greater staging information, and may provide a survival benefit but extent of the LN dissection is somewhat controversial. D1 gastrectomy is associated with less anastomotic leaks, a lower postoperative complication rate, a lower reoperation rate, decreased length of hospital stay, and a lower 30-day mortality rate with similar 5-year survival rates to D2 resections.
- Randomized trials of D2 dissections:

	n	5-y OS (%)		Op Mortality (%)		Complications (%)	
		D1	D2	D1	D2	D1	D2
MRC	400	35	33	6.5	13	28	46
Dutch	711	45	47	4	10	25	43 SS
S. Africa	43	78	76	0	0		
Hong Kong	55	58	32	0	0		
Japanese 9501	523	69	70			20.9	28.1 NSS
Italian	162					10	16 NSS
Taiwanese	221	54	60D3*				

- *Meta-analysis* (McCullogh et al., *Cochran Databases Syst Rev.* 2004; doi:10.1002/bjs.4839) D2 dissection carries increased mortality risks associated with spleen and pancreas resection and no evidence of OS benefit, but possible benefit in T3 + tumors.

Adjuvant Therapy

- Stage T1N0 or higher should undergo surgery with preoperative and postoperative chemotherapy.
- Stage IB or higher treated without preoperative chemotherapy should receive adjuvant chemoradiation.

Chemotherapy

- In HER-2 negative disease, combination regimens using platinum–fluoropyrimidine doublet are used; triplet regimens are controversial, but the addition of an anthracycline (epirubicin) has demonstrated benefit.
- In HER-2 positive disease, chemotherapy with trastuzumab plus cisplatin and 5-FU or capecitabine is recommended.
- Second-line chemotherapy includes irinotecan and docetaxel or paclitaxel.

Neoadjuvant Chemotherapy

- Neoadjuvant chemotherapy has several theoretical advantages:
  o Increase resectability
  o Early treatment of subclinical metastases
  o Greater tolerability prior to surgery
  o Measures in vivo chemotherapy sensitivity
- A Japanese trial did not demonstrate a survival benefit with neoadjuvant chemotherapy.

Adjuvant Chemotherapy

- Randomized clinical trials comparing adjuvant combination chemotherapy to surgery alone did not demonstrate a consistent survival benefit.

- *Meta-analyses:* No benefit to adjuvant chemotherapy
  - Earle (*Eur J* Cancer. 1999; doi:10.1016/S0959-8049(99)00076-3) of 20 randomized trials, adjuvant systemic chemotherapy was associated with a survival benefit (OR 0.80; 95% CI). In subgroup analysis patients with node-positive disease demonstrated the greatest benefit.
  - JCO 11:1441, 1993   13 trials   no benefit
  - Ann Oncol 11: 837, 2000   11 trials   no benefit

Perioperative (Neoadjuvant and Adjuvant) Chemotherapy

- MAGIC Trial (Cunningham, *N Engl J Med.* 2006; doi:10.1056/NEJMoa055531)
  *Perioperioperative chemotherapy improves survival over surgery alone.
- European randomized trial demonstrated survival benefit associated with preoperative ECF and 3 cycles of postoperative ECF compared with surgery alone.
- Benefit was similar to that demonstrated in the U.S. adjuvant chemoradiation trial (INT 0116).
- Included patients with distal esophageal adenocarcinoma; all greater than stage II.

	5-y OS	MS (Months)	PFS (Months)
Surgery alone	23%	20 mo	13 mo
Perioperative chemotherapy	36%	24 mo	19 mo
P-value		.009	<.001

Intraoperative Radiation

- **NCI** (Sindelar, et al., *Arch Surg.* 1993; doi:10.1001/archsurg.1993.01420160040005)
  *IORT did not improve local control (LC) and had similar complication rates.
  - 60 patients randomized, 19 patients excluded due to inoperability
  - Randomized to IORT (20 Gy; 11–15-MeV electrons) versus two control arms
    - Gastrectomy alone for lesions confined to stomach (stages I/II)
    - Resection and postoperative XRT (50 Gy/25 fx) for tumors extending beyond the gastric wall (stages III/IV)

	MS (Months)	LRFS (%)
IORT	21	92
Control	25	44

Preoperative Chemoradiation (No Phase III Data)

- **RTOG 99-04** (Ajani et al., *J Clin Oncol.* 2005;23(16S):4019)
  *Pre-op CRT induces 26% path CR
  - Multi-institution phase II study evaluating neoadjuvant CRT
  - 2 cycles induction 5-FU + Leu then concurrent CRT (5-FU/paclitaxel)
  - Surgery attempted 5 to 6 weeks after CRT; 50% D2
  - MS 22.1 months
  - pCR rate of 26%
  - R0 rate of 77%
  - DM 30%; 19% LF

Adjuvant Radiation

- **British Stomach Cancer Group** (Hallissey. *Lancet*. 1994 May 28; doi:10.1016/S0140-6736(94)92464-3) reported lower LR rates with postoperative radiation compared to surgery alone.

	LF	3-y OS	5-y OS
Surgery	27%	28%	20%
Surgery + RT	10%	22%	12%
Surgery + FAM	19%	30%	19%
P-value	<.01	NS	NS

Adjuvant Chemoradiation

- **Moertel** (*Lancet*. 1969; doi:10.1016/S0140-6736(69)92326-5) randomized advanced gastric cancer to 40-Gy postoperative radiation or 40 Gy with 5-FU. The CRT arm demonstrated improved survival.
- **Mayo Clinic** (Moertel, *JCO*, 1984;2(11):1249–1254) randomized to postoperative CRT (37.5 Gy/25 fx) with 5-FU or surgery alone, demonstrating improvement in OS associated with adjuvant CRT (23% vs. 4%).

	LF	5-y OS
Surgery alone	54%	4%
Surgery + CRT	39%	23%
Refused CRT		30%

- **The Gastrointestinal Tumor Study Group (GITSG)** (*Cancer*. 1990. doi:10.1002/1097-0142(19900401)65:7 <1478::AID-CNCR2820650705>3.0.CO;2–3) randomized to postoperative CRT (43.2 Gy) with 5-FU or chemotherapy alone, demonstrating improvement in OS associated with adjuvant CRT (18% vs. 6%)
- **Intergroup 0116** (Macdonald, *N Engl J Med*. 2001; doi:10.1056/NEJMoa010187; Smalley, *J Clin Oncol*. 2012; doi:10.1200/JCO.2011.36.7136)
  *Demonstrated OS benefit with postoperative CRT versus surgery alone.
  o Randomized phase III
  o 556 patients with resected stages Ib to IV, M0
  o Included gastric and GEJ tumors
  o Surgery alone versus surgery followed by 5-FU/leu (1 cycle) then CRT (45 Gy/25 fx) with 5-FU/leu (2 cycles) followed by 5-FU/leu (2 cycles)

	MS (Months)	DFS (Months)	3-y OS
Surgery alone	26	19	41%
Surgery + CRT	35	30	50%

- **CALGB 80101**(Interim toxicity analysis, Fuchs, *J Clin Oncol*. 2011;29(15_suppl):4003)
  o Randomization between INT 0116 CRT and Magic perioperative ECF.
  o 546 patients
  o Perioperative ECF did not improve survival over adjuvant CRT.
    ▪ MS 38 versus 37 months; Median DFS 28 versus 30 months
    ▪ 3-year OS 52 versus 50 month; 3-year DFS 47 versus 46 months
- **Dutch CRITICS** (Dikken, *BMC Cancer*. 2011; doi:10.1186/1471-2407-11-329)
  o Phase III
  o 3 cycles of preoperative epirubicin/cisplatin/capecitabine (ECC) then surgery

- o Randomized to adjuvant
  - ▪ 3 cycles ECC or
  - ▪ Concurrent CRT (45 Gy, cisplatin/capecitabine)
- **ARTIST** (Lee, *J Clin Oncol.* 2012; doi:10.1200/JCO.2011.39.1953)
  - o Phase III
  - o Randomized to Surgery, XP versus surgery, XP, XRT, XP
  - o 458 patients
  - o 3-year DFS
    - ▪ 70% XP
    - ▪ 80% XP, XRT, XP
  - o 3-year OS
    - ▪ 74% XP
    - ▪ 78% XP, XRT, XP
- CLASSIC (Bang, *Lancet.* 2012; doi:10.1016/S0140-6736(11)61873-4)
  - o Phase III
  - o 1035 patients
  - o Randomized to XELOX and surgery versus surgery alone
  - o 3-year DFS
    - ▪ 74% XELOX
    - ▪ 59% surgery alone

Phase III Trials for Gastric Cancer

	n	Treatment	Survival
INT 0116	556	Surgery, adj CRT vs. surgery alone	MS 36 mo vs. 27 mo
MAGIC	503	Perioperative ECF vs. surgery alone	5-y OS 36% vs. 23%
CALGB 80101	546	INT0116 vs. Perioperative ECF	MS 37 mo vs. 38 mo
ARTIST	458	Surgery, XP vs. surgery, XP, XRT, XP	3-y DFS 74.2% vs. 78.2% 3-y OS 70.1% vs. 80.1%
ACTS-GC	1059	Surgery alone vs. surgery and S-1	3-y RFS 53.1% vs. 65.4% 5-y OS 65.4% v 71.7%
CLASSIC	1035	XELOX and surgery vs. surgery alone	3-y DFS 74% vs. 59%
FNLCC	224	Perioperative chemo vs. surgery alone	5-y OS 38% vs. 24%
SAMIT	1495	Surgery, UFT vs. surgery, S-1 vs. surgery, T, UFT vs. surgery, T, S-1	3-y DFS 54% monotherapy vs. 52.7% sequential; 53% UFT vs. 58.2 S-1
ARTIST-II	1000	Surgery, XP vs. surgery, XP, XRT, XP	P
MAGIC B	1100	ECX/Bev vs. ECX	P
TOPGEAR	752	Preoperative vs. post-op chemo	P
CRITICS	788	ECX, surgery, ECX vs. ECX, surgery, chemo and CRT	P

CRT, chemoradiation therapy; ECF, epirubicin, cisplatin, and 5-FU; OS, overall survival.

Radiation Technique

- Simulate patient with arms up using a wing board, alpha cradle, or vac-lock bag.
- Use esophageal contract to outline the esophagus, stomach, and small bowel.
- Use three-dimensional conformal radiation treatment planning to optimize target dose, and achieve normal tissue dose limitations. IMRT may be used when normal tissue dose constraints cannot be met with 3D conformal treatment planning.
  - Spinal cord ≤45 Gy
  - Liver 60% ≤30 Gy; ≤25-Gy mean dose
  - Kidneys 66% one kidney ≤20 Gy
  - Heart 33% ≤40 Gy
- Use pretreatment diagnostic studies (EUS, UGI, PET, CT) and surgical clips (in postoperative patients) to identify tumor/gastric bed.
- The relative risk of nodal metastases is dependent on both site of origin and depth of invasion into the gastric wall.
  - For proximal cardia/GEJ tumors include 3 to 5 cm of distal esophagus and paraesophageal, nodes include perigastric celiac, splenic hilar, porta hepatic nodes.
  - For middle/fundus tumors include perigastric, suprapancreatic, celiac, splenic hilar, porta hepatic, and pancreaticoduodenal nodes.
  - For distal antrum/pylorus tumors include 3 to 5 cm of duodenal stump and perigastric, suprapancreatic, celiac, porta hepatic, and pancreaticoduodenal nodes.
  - If radiation is given preoperatively then include the first and second part of the duodenum for tumors extending to the GEJ.
- Dose 1.8-Gy daily, five times weekly, 25 to 28 fractions, 45 to 50.4 Gy, consider higher doses for positive surgical margins.

Palliation

Palliative Radiation

- Radiation provides relief from bleeding, obstruction, and pain in 50% to 75%
- Median duration of palliation is 4 to 18 months

Definitive Chemoradiation for Locally Advanced Unresectable

- **GITSG** (Schein, *Proc AACR* (Abstract). 1980; *Cancer*. 1982; doi:10.1002/1097-0142(19820501)49:9<1771::AID-CNCR2820490907>3.0.CO;2-M)
  - Randomized patients with locally unresectable nonmetastatic gastric cancer to 5-FU, methyl-CCNU versus CRT (50-Gy split course) with 5-FU to patients
  - 90 patients
  - Closed early due to excessive early deaths in the CRT arm. CRT was deemed too toxic as approximately 25% of the XRT patients died or deteriorated significantly within the first 10 weeks of treatment.
  - MS of CRT was inferior to chemotherapy alone (40 vs. 76 weeks).
  - The study was reanalyzed 4 years later, and 5-year OS was 18% for the CRT arm versus 6 % for the chemo alone arm. All long-term survivors had resection after CRT.
  - MS for all CRT patients was 40 weeks.
  - A total of 66 patients underwent eventual resection (7 pCR, 36 pPR).
- **Chemotherapy**
  - For metastatic gastric cancer, the National Comprehensive Cancer Network (NCCN) recommends palliative chemotherapy or entry into a clinical trial.
  - Platinum-based chemotherapy is considered first-line
  - Epirubicin/cisplatin/5-FU docetaxel/cisplatin/5-FU
  - Other active regimens
    - Irinotecan and cisplatin
    - Combinations with oxaliplatin and irinotecan
    - Angiogenesis inhibitor ramucirumab (Cyramza) recently approved second-line treatment of unresectable or metastatic gastric or GEJ adenocarcinoma following fluoropyrimidine or platinum

Follow-Up

- History and physical every 3 to 6 months for 1 to 2 years, then every 6 months for 3 to 5 years, then annually thereafter.
- Endoscopies and radiology as clinically indicated.
- Monitor for nutritional deficiency (B12) and iron in patients who undergo proximal gastrectomy; supplement as needed.

2.3   Pancreas

Epidemiology and Risk Factors

- Pancreatic cancer accounts for 3% of cancers in the United States.
- Pancreatic cancer is 13th in incidence but 8th as a cause of cancer death worldwide.
- There are approximately 46,000 new cases in the United States per year.
- Pancreatic cancer is the fourth leading cause of cancer deaths in the United States.
- The male to female ratio is 1:1.
- African American males have the highest incidence in the United States.
- 95% of all pancreatic carcinomas arise in exocrine pancreas.
- 75% of all pancreatic carcinomas occur within the head or neck of the pancreas:
  - 15% to 20% occur in the body of the pancreas;
  - 5% to 10% occur in the tail;
- 80% are adenocarcinoma of the pancreas
  - Other rare tumors include neuroendocrine, pancreatic lymphoma, adenosquamous carcinoma, mucinous carcinoma, cystadenocarcinoma, papillary cystic carcinoma, acinar cystadenocarcinoma
- Diabetes mellitus may be associated with a twofold increase in the risk.
- Less than 5% are associated with chronic pancreatitis; alcohol is not independent risk factor.
- 40% of pancreatic cancer cases are sporadic in nature.
- 30% are related to smoking; tobacco smokers are associated with approximately twofold greater risk than nonsmokers.
- 20% may be associated with dietary factors.
- 5% to 10% are hereditary:
  - Hereditary pancreatitis
  - Multiple endocrine neoplasia (MEN)
  - Hereditary nonpolyposis rectal cancer (HNPCC)
  - Familial adenomatous polyposis (FAP) and Gardner syndrome
  - Familial atypical multiple mole melanoma (FAMMM) syndrome
  - Von Hippel–Lindau syndrome (VHL)
  - Germline mutations in BRCA1 and BRCA2 genes.
- Pancreatic cancer is genetically complex and heterogeneous.
  - 80% to 95% KRAS2 gene mutations
  - 85% to 98% CDKN2 gene mutations, deletions, or hypermethylation
  - 50% p53 mutations
  - 55% Smad4 homozygous deletions or mutations

Prognosis

- Pancreatic carcinoma is usually fatal with MS for all patients in approximately 4 to 6 months.
  - 1-year survival rate approximately 24%
  - 5-year OS rate approximately 5%
  - Neuroendocrine tumors, cystic neoplasms, mucinous cystadenocarcinomas, intraductal papillary mucinous neoplasms (IPMNs)—better survival rates
- For the 20% of patients able to undergo a successful curative resection MS ranges from 12 to 19 months, and the 5-year survival rate is 15% to 20%.

- Predictors of long-term survival after surgery
  - Tumor diameter less than 3 cm
  - Absence of nodal involvement
  - Negative resection margins
- Smoking is the most significant reversible risk factor for pancreatic cancer.

Anatomy

- Four parts of the pancreas include:
  - Head (and uncinate process)
  - Neck
  - Body
  - Tail
- Pancreatic cancer first metastasizes to regional LNs, then liver and lungs.
- Nodal spread is related to location of primary tumor:
  - Head/Uncinate—peripancreatic, pancreaticoduodenal, hepatoduodenal ligament, porta hepatis, celiac axis
  - Body/Tail—peripancreatic, splenic artery, celiac axis, para-aortics
- Direct invasion of surrounding organs such as the duodenum, stomach, and colon is common.
- Peritoneal spread and ascites is common.
- Metastasis to bone is uncommon.

Presentation

The initial symptoms of pancreatic cancer are nonspecific and have a gradual onset.

- Anorexia
- Weight loss
- Malaise
- Nausea
- Fatigue
- Midepigastric pain with radiation of pain to mid- or lower back from retroperitoneal invasion of splanchnic nerve (1/3 no pain, 1/3 moderate pain, 1/3 severe pain at diagnosis)
- Significant weight loss
- Onset of diabetes mellitus within the previous year (Approximately 1% of cases of new-onset diabetes mellitus in adults are related to occult pancreatic cancer.)
- Painless obstructive jaundice
- Pruritus
- Depression
- Migratory thrombophlebitis (Trousseau sign)/venous thrombosis
- Palpable gallbladder (Courvoisier sign)
- Ascites or hepatomegaly from liver metastases
- Splenomegaly from portal vein obstruction
- Paraumbilical subcutaneous metastases (Sister Mary Joseph nodule or nodules)
- Metastatic mass in the rectal pouch (Blumer's shelf)
- Palpable metastatic cervical nodes—left clavicle (Virchow's node)

Diagnosis and Workup

- Physical examination may vary. Evaluate for
  - Midepigastric or back pain
  - Jaundice or icterus
  - Palpable abdominal mass

- o Hepatosplenomegaly
- o Sister Mary Joseph, Virchow, or Blumer's shelf nodes
- CBC, bilirubin (conjugated and total), gamma-glutamyltransferase (GGT), aspartate transaminase (AST) and Alanine Transaminase (ALT), Alk phos, serum albumin, total protein, coagulation studies
- Serum amylase and/or lipase levels: Elevated in less than 50% of patients with resectable pancreatic cancers and in only 25% of patients with unresectable tumors
- 75% to 85% have elevated CA 19-9
- 40% to 45% have elevated CEA
- Imaging studies
  - o CT (with CT guided biopsy if feasible). * Triple-phase spiral CT-scan findings are approximately 90% accurate for helping to determine the resectability potential of pancreatic carcinoma.
  - o Endoscopic ultrasonography (EUS, with EUS guided biopsy if feasible)
    - Equivalent to dual-phase, spiral CT for assessment of tumor resectability
    - Superior to CT for assessment of T stage
    - Inferior to CT for assessment of arterial involvement and distant metastases
    - EUS and CT are both poor at detecting occult nodal involvement
  - o Magnetic resonance imaging (MRI)
  - o Magnetic resonance cholangiopancreatography (MRCP)
  - o Endoscopic retrograde cholangiopancreatography (ERCP)
  - o PET-CT is useful to detect occult metastases
    - False-positive PET scans have been reported in pancreatitis.
    - PET scanning does not offer additional benefits to high-quality CT.
  - o Preoperative laporoscopic staging should be considered to avoid patients with liver or peritoneal metastases to undergo aggressive definitive therapy.

Staging

AJCC/UICC 2012 TNM classification for pancreatic cancer is outlined.
- T0—No evidence of primary tumor
- Tis—Carcinoma in situ
- T1—Tumor limited to the pancreas, 2 cm or smaller in greatest dimension
- T2—Tumor limited to the pancreas, larger than 2 cm in greatest dimension
- T3—Tumor extension beyond the pancreas (duodenum, bile duct, portal, or superior mesenteric vein) but not involving the celiac axis or superior mesenteric artery
- T4—Tumor involves the celiac axis or superior mesenteric arteries
- N0—No regional LN metastasis
  - o N1—regional LNs
- M0—No distant metastasis
  - o M1—Distant metastasis (M1a and M1b are site dependent)

Treatment Overview

Surgery

- Only 20% of patients are candidates for curative surgery at presentation.
- There is no benefit to subtotal resection (Haddock, *J Clin Oncol.* 2007; doi:10.1200/JCO.2006.10.2111).
- Invasion or encasement of greater than 50% of the superior mesenteric, celiac, and hepatic arteries are considered contraindications to surgery (T4 = unresectable).
- Invasion or encasement of the superior mesenteric or portal vein is no longer considered an absolute contraindication surgery as they can be partially resected or reconstructed.

Stage Classification

Stage IA	T1	N0	M0
Stage IB	T2	N0	M0
Stage IIA	T3	N0	M0
Stage IIB	T1–3	N1	M0
Stage III	T4	Any N	M0
Stage IV	Any T	Any N	M1

- Vascular reconstruction, which permits an attempt at surgical resection, has not been shown to improve survival.
- Curative resection options include the following:
  o Pancreaticoduodenectomy (Whipple procedure), with/without pylorus sparing
    - Removal of pancreatic head, duodenum, gallbladder, antrum of the stomach, with surgical drainage of distal pancreatic duct and biliary system through pancreaticojejunostomy
    - Controversy is the extent of lymphadenectomy that is necessary in a Whipple operation. Ratio of positive nodes to total nodes removed is a prognostic factor.
    - Overall mortality rate is 6.6%.
  o Total pancreatectomy
    - Indication for total pancreatectomy is tumor involves the neck of the pancreas.
    - Highest operative mortality rate is 8.3%.
    - Usually results in brittle diabetes.
  o Distal pancreatectomy
    - For tumors located in the body or tail
    - Removal of distal portion of the pancreas containing the tumor with oversewing of the distal pancreatic duct
    - Operative mortality rate 3.5%
- Selecting patients for surgery should be based on the probability of cure as determined by resection margins.

Adjuvant Chemotherapy

- **CONKO-001** (Oettle, *JAMA*. 2007; doi:10.1001/jama.2013.279201)
  *Adjuvant gemcitabine prolongs survival over surgery alone.
  o 3-year survival 36.5% versus 19.5%
  o 5-year survival 21% versus 9%
  o 10-year survival 12.2% versus 7.7%
- **ESPAC-Meta-analysis** (Neoptolemos, *Br J Cancer*. 2009; doi:10.1038/sj.bjc.6604838)
  *Adjuvant chemotherapy better than CRT
  o 822 patients
  o Adjuvant 5-FU/leu versus observation

	MS (Months)
observation	17
5-FU/leu	23

- **Meta-Analyses**

	n	Arm	MS (Months)	2-y OS	5-y OS
Stocken (2005)	348	Chemo	19	38%	19%
	338	No chemo	13.5	28%	12%
Boeck (2007)	482	Chemo	3	NR	3.1%
	469	No chemo	SS	NR	SS
Butturini (2008)	236	Chemo R0	20.8	42%	22%
	222	No chemo R0	13.8	27%	10%
	109	Chemo R1	15	29%	14%
	114	No chemo R1	13.2	31%	17%
			HR for death (95% CI)		
Lao (2013)	876	5-FU	0.62		
	670	No chemo			
	774	Gem	0.68		
	670	No chemo			
	774	Gem	1.1		
	876	5-FU			

Intraoperative Radiation

- **RTOG 85-05** (Tepper, *Int J Radiat Oncol Biol Phys.* 1991; doi:10.1016/0360-3016(91)90269-A)
  *No advantage of IORT over conventional therapy
  o 86 patients with locally unresected nonmetastatic pancreatic cancer
  o IORT dose 20 Gy
  o MS 9 months
  o 18 month actuarial survival 9%
  o After RTOG 85-05 unresectable patients were no longer offered IORT

- **NCI** (Sindelar, *Surgery.* 1988;103(2):247–256.)
  *IORT improves LC in resectable patients
  o 32 resected patients, 16 in each arm

	MS (Months)	LC
Surgery + IORT (20 Gy)	18	80%
Surgery + XRT (50 Gy)	12 NSS	0%

- **O'Conner** (*Int J Radiat Oncol Biol Phys.* 2005; doi:10.1016/j.ijrobp.2005.03.036)
  *No increase morbidity for IORT
  - Single institution retrospective analysis
  - 77 patients, 24 with unresectable disease
  - Included periampullary and pancreatic cancers
  - 3.7% operative mortality
  - IORT dose 17 Gy

	MS (Months)	5-y DSS
Periampullary (resected)	167	56%
Pancreatic resected	16	19%
Unresected (bypass)	11	0%

Adjuvant Chemoradiation

Conflicting data

- GITSG 91-73 (Kaiser and Ellenberg, *Arch Surg.* 1985; doi:10.1001/archsurg.1985.01390320023003)
  - Adjuvant CRT better than surgery alone
  - Randomized
  - 43 patients with resectable pancreatic cancer with R0 resections
    - No periampullary and cystadenomocarcinomas
    - 28% node positive
  - APPA 40-Gy split course (20 Gy/10 fx) → 2-week break → (20 Gy/10 fx) with bolus 5-FU first 3 days of each radiation cycle. 5-FU was then given for an additional 2 years.

	2-y DFS	2-y OS	5-y OS
Adjuvant CRT	48%	43%	14%
Surgery alone	14%	18%	6%

  - This trial was confirmed with another 30 patients (*Cancer*, 1987):
    - 2-year OS 46%
    - Local failure still occurred in 30% to 50%; hepatic failure in 40% to 50%
  - Criticisms: No QA, 1/3 did not complete all treatment; 5 did not get any treatment.
- **EORTC 40891** (Klinkenbijl, *Ann Surg.* 1999;230(6):776; Smeenk, *Ann Surg.* 2007; doi:10.1097/SLA.0b013e318156eef3)
  *No benefit to adjuvant CRT over surgery alone
- 218 patients with resectable pancreatic cancer, including
  - T1–2, not T3 primaries
  - Periampullary cancer
  - Positive margins
  - N1a
- Randomized to same regimen as GITSG but with CI 5-FU and no 5-FU × 2y

	2-y DFS	2-y OS	MS (Months)
Surgery alone	38%	41%	19
Adjuvant chemoradiation	37%	50%	24.5

Subset analysis of 60 patients with pancreatic head tumors

	2-y DFS NSS	2-y OS NSS	MST (Months) NSS	5-y OS SS
Surgery alone	23%	23%	12.6	10%
Adjuvant chemoradiation	37%	37%	17.1	20%

- Criticisms: No QA, included + margins and N1a, no 5-FU maintenance, 20% in CRT arm did not receive treatment due to post-op complications, inappropriate statistical design—if use one-sided log rank test then SS for OS (not powered to exclude a 10%–15% benefit); only 119 had true pancreatic cancers.
- **ESPAC-1** (Neoptolemos, *Lancet.* 2001; *N Engl J Med.* 2004; doi:10.1056/NEJMoa032295)
  *Adjuvant chemotherapy better than CRT
  o 2 × 2 study comparing
  o Adjuvant chemo (5-FU/Leu 5 days/month × 6 cycles)
  o Adjuvant CRT (40-Gy split course with 5-FU)
  o Adjuvant CRT followed by chemo
  o Surgery alone
  o 541 resected pancreatic cancer, including:
    ▪ Periampullary cancer
    ▪ Positive margins

	MS (Months)	5-y OS	P-Value
Adjuvant chemoradiation followed by chemo	15.9	10%	.05
Adjuvant chemoradiation	17.9	20%	
Adjuvant chemotherapy, no radiation	20.1	21%	.009
Surgery alone	15.5	8%	

- o Initially reported with 2 × 2 trial were two other trials allowing "background chemo"
- o Results were contradictory for randomized versus nonrandomized patients
- o For all patients receiving chemo had improved MS
- o For randomized patients—no benefit for chemotherapy
- o For all randomized/nonrandomized pts receiving CRT there was no MS benefit
- o Final results (2004) concluded that chemo beneficial while CRT was detrimental
- o Criticisms: No QA (~75% received correct radiation dose), 1/3 of pts in chemo alone group received radiation; 1/3 of CRT patients did not complete radiation; split-course radiation used; no restaging of patients after resection; progressive disease in 19%
- **SEER Data** (Hazard, *Cancer.* 2007; doi:10.1002/cncr.23047)
  o Meta-analysis
  o 3,008 patients

- o Pre- (23 patients) or post-op radiation versus surgery alone
- o RT improved OS in patients with T3 or N1 disease (not T1–2, N0)
- o RT improved CSS in patients with N1 disease only
- o No difference in OS for pre- versus post-op RT

	MS (Months)	2-y OS	5-y OS
Observation	12	32%	150%
RT	17	44%	13%

- **Mayo Clinic** (Corsini, *J Clin Oncol.* 2008; doi:10.1200/JCO.2007.15.8782)
  - o Retrospective review
  - o 472 patients, T1–3N0–1
  - o R0 resected cancers with adjuvant CRT (50.4 Gy with 5-FU) versus observation

	MS (Months)	2-y OS	5-y OS
Observation	19	28%	17%
CRT	25	50%	39%

- **Johns Hopkins** (Herman, *J Clin Oncol.* 2008; doi:10.1200/JCO.2007.15.8469)
  - o Retrospective review
  - o 616 patients
  - o R0 resected cancers with adjuvant CRT (5-FU based) versus observation

	MS (Months)	2-y OS	5-y OS
Observation	14	32%	15%
CRT	21	44%	20%

- **RTOG 97-04** (Regine, *JAMA.* 2008; doi:10.1001/jama.299.9.1019)
  *Gemcitabine to adjuvant 5-FU based CRT was associated with NSS survival benefit for patients with resected pancreatic cancer; most benefit was in pancreatic head tumors.
  - o Phase III
  - o 451 resected pancreatic cancers (388 pancreatic head tumors)
  - o 67% node positive
  - o 34% positive margins
  - o 1 cycle Gem versus 5-FU for 3 weeks prior to CRT (50.4/28 fx) concurrent 5-FU followed by Gem or 5-FU for 12 weeks after CRT

Pancreatic Head Subset

	MS (Months)	3-y OS	G4 Hematologic Toxicity
5-FU	16.9	21%	2%
Gem	20.6	32%	14%
P-value		.09	.001

*Radiation QA performed

- **Johns Hopkins-Mayo Clinic Collaborative Study** (Hsu, *Ann Surg Oncol.* 2010; doi:10.1245/s10434-009-0743-7)
  - ○ Retrospective review
  - ○ 794 JHU + 498 MC patients
  - ○ Matched pair analysis
  - ○ Resected cancers with adjuvant CRT (5-FU based) versus observation

	MS (Months)	2-y OS	5-y OS
Observation	15	35%	16%
CRT	21	45%	22%

*Improved survival with CRT when stratified by age, margin, node, and T stage

- **EORTC 40013-22012/FFCD-9203/GERCOR** (Van Laethem, *J Clin Oncol.* 2010 Oct 10;28(29):4450–4456. doi:10.1200/JCO.2010.30.3446)
  *Adjuvant gemcitabine-based CRT is feasible, well-tolerated, and not deleterious.
  - ○ Randomized phase II
  - ○ 90 resected pancreatic head cancers
  - ○ Gemcitabine alone (4 cycles) versus Gemcitabine (2 cycles) then CRT (50.4 Gy/28 fx) and concurrent weekly Gemcitabine

	MS (Months)	Median DFS (Months)	First LR
Gem alone	24	11	24%
CRT	24	312	11%

- **Yang** (*Arch Surg.* 2010)
  *Large, retrospective study supports the use of adjuvant CRT.
  - ○ 2,877 registry patients who underwent surgical resection with curative intent
  - ○ Approximately 50% no adjuvant therapy
  - ○ Approximately 25% received adjuvant CRT
  - ○ Approximately 10% received adjuvant chemo alone
  - ○ A significant survival benefit was found for the CRT patients

Neoadjuvant Therapy

- Spitz (*J Clin Oncol.* 1997;15(3):928–937) reported that preoperative and postoperative chemoradiation in patients having potentially curative pancreaticoduodenectomy for adenocarcinoma of the pancreatic head result in similar toxicity, patterns of failure, and survival.
- **Seer analysis** (Stessin, *Int J Radiat Oncol Biol Phys.* 2008; doi:10.1016/j.ijrobp.2008.02.065)
- 3,885 patients

	% Patients	MS (Months)
Neoadjuvant RT	2	23
Postoperative RT	38	17
Surgery alone	60	12

- Several trials conducted at MD Anderson demonstrate median survival up to 25 months using neoadjuvant CRT (gemcitabine based).

- **Evans** (*J Clin Oncol.* 2008; doi:10.1200/JCO.2007.15.8634)
  - o Phase II
  - o 86 patients
  - o Neoadjuvant CRT (30 Gy/10 fx including regional nodes) and weekly gemcitabine × 7
  - o 85% received surgery

	MS (Months)
All patients	22.7
Surgery	34
No surgery	7

- **Krishnan** (*Cancer.* 2007; doi:10.1002/cncr.22735)
  - o 247 patients
  - o Neoadjuvant CRT (30 Gy–10 fx or 50.4–28 fx) with gemcitabine or capecitabine
  - o 27 patients received induction gemcitabine prior to CRT

	MS (Months)
Induction Chemo/CRT	11.9
Neoadjuvant CRT	8.5

- Randomized phase II (Golcher, *Strahlenther Onkol.* 2015; doi:10.1007/s00066-014-0737-7) compared gemcitabine/cisplatin CRT to upfront surgery with both arms received adjuvant chemotherapy without significant differences detected.

	R0 Resection Rate	ypN0 Rate	MS (Months)
Upfront surgery	48%	30%	18.9
Neoadjuvant CRT	52%	39%	25

- Neoadjuvant chemotherapy alone is also an acceptable approach.
  - o Neoadjuvant gemcitabine results in less definitive pancreatic cancer surgery than gemcitabine/cisplatin (Palmer, *Ann Surg Oncol.* 2007; doi:10.1245/s10434-007-9384-x).
- **NEOPA** (NCT01900327) (Tachezy, *BMC Cancer.* 2014; doi:10.1186/1471-2407-14-411) is an ongoing phase III study randomizing patients to upfront surgery and gemcitabine CRT.
- **ALLIANCE A021101** (NCT01821612) is a single arm pilot study evaluating neoadjuvant FOLFIRINOX before CRT with capectabine followed by surgery and adjuvant gemcitabine (2 cycles) in patients with borderline resectable pancreatic cancer.

Chemotherapy Alone for Unresectable Pancreatic Caner

Several combinations of agents are used in the management of pancreatic carcinoma:
- FOLFIRINOX (LV5-FU [leucovorin/5-FU] plus oxaliplatin plus irinotecan) first-line treatment for patients with metastatic or locally advanced unresectable disease with good performance status (Conroy, *N Engl J Med.* 2011; doi:10.1056/NEJMoa1011923; European phase III trial—**ACCORD/PRODIGE**—Gem vs. FOLFIRINOX)
- Gemcitabine monotherapy: metastatic or locally advanced unresectable disease with poor performance status

- Gemcitabine, docetaxel, and capecitabine (GTX)
- Gemcitabine/Abraxane (albumin-bound paclitaxel) (Van Hoff, JCO, 2012; doi:10.1200/JCO.2011.36.5742 Phase III IMPACT for metastatic PC—Gem vs. Gem/abraxane)
- 5-FU/Leu (**ESPAC-3**, Neoptolemus, *JAMA*. 2012; doi:10.1001/jama.2012.7352; 5-FU/leu and gemcitabine equivalent in periampullary carcinoma)
- Erlotinib/gemcitabine
- Capecitabine monotherapy or capecitabine/erlotinib: second-line therapy if refractory to gemcitabine
- **ESPAC-4** (NCT01072981) compares gemcitabine/capecitabine to gemcitabine alone

Definitive Chemoradiation for Unresectable Pancreatic Cancer

- **GITSG 9273** (Moertel, *Cancer*. 1981;48(8):1705–1710)
  *CRT better than radiation alone; 60 Gy no better than 40 Gy
  o Phase III
  o 194 unresectable nonmetastatic pancreatic cancer
  o APPA 40-Gy split course (20 Gy/10 fx) → 2-week break → (20 Gy/10 fx) ± 20 Gy to reduced field with or without bolus 5-FU first 3 days of each radiation cycle. 5-FU was then given for an additional 2 years.
  o 5-FU increased MST from 6.3 to 10.4 months.

	MS (Months)	2-y OS	1-y OS
CRT (40 Gy)	8.3	10%	40%
CRT (60 Gy)	11.3	10%	
XRT alone (60 Gy)	5.5	1%	10%

- **GITSIG** (*JNCI*. 1988; doi:10.1093/jnci/80.10.751)
  *CRT better than chemo alone
  o Phase III
  o 48 unresectable non-metastatic pancreatic cancer
  o chemo alone (SMF) versus CRT with concurrent 5-FU then SMF

	MS (Months)	1-y OS
CRT	10.5	41%
SMF alone	8	19%

- **RTOG 88-01** (Komaki, *Cancer*. 1992; 69:2807–2812)
  *Dose escalation and whole liver radiation of no benefit
  o 61.2 Gy/34 fx to pancreas with 23.4 Gy/13 fx to liver with concurrent 5-FU
  o 73% had persistent or progressive disease
  o 31% liver progression
  o 27% abdominal progression
  o 8% extra-abdominal progression

- **ECOG E8282** (Cohen, *Int J Radiat Oncol Biol Phys*. 2005; doi:10.1016/j.ijrobp.2004.12.074)
  *Adding 5-FU and MMC to radiation increased toxicity without improving DFS or OS.
  o Phase III
  o 104 unresectable nonmetastatic pancreatic cancer
  o 59.4 Gy/33 fx with or without concurrent 5-FU + mitomycin C weeks 1 and 5

	Response	Median DFS (Months)	MS (Months)
Radiation alone	6%	5.0	7.1
CRT	9%	5.1	8.4

- **RTOG 98-12** (Rich, *Am J Clin Oncol*. 2004;27(1):51–56)
  *Weekly paclitaxel with concurrent radiation is toxic.
  - Phase II
  - 109 locally advanced nonmetastatic pancreatic cancer
  - 50.4 Gy/28 fx with concurrent weekly paclitaxel
  - MS 11.2 months
  - 1-year OS 43%
  - 2-year OS 13%
  - 40% Grade 3, 5% grade 4, and 1 toxic death
- **GERCOR** (Huguet, *J Clin Oncol*. 2007; doi:10.1200/JCO.2006.07.5663)
  *Adding 5-FU and MMC to radiation increased toxicity without improving DFS or OS.
  - 181 unresectable nonmetastatic pancreatic cancer
  - Gemcitabine or 5-FU based chemotherapy × 3 months, if no evidence of progression on reevaluation
    - Additional chemotherapy or
    - CRT

	Median PFS (Months)	MS (Months)
Chemo alone	7.5	11.7
CMT	10.8	15

Chemotherapy Alone Versus Chemoradiation for Unresectable Pancreatic Cancer

- While results of RTOG 97-04 cannot be directly compared to the results of CONKO-001, ESPAC-1, or ESPAC-3 due to differences in trial design and inclusion criteria, the MS in all four trials is similar.

	MS (Months)
RTOG 97-04 (Gemcitabine arm, radiation)	20.5
CONKO-001 (Gemcitabine arm, no radiation)	22.8
ESPAC-1 (Bolus 5-FU arm, no radiation)	20.1
ESPAC-3 (Gemcitabine and 5-FU/leu arms, no radiation)	23.6/23.0

- **FFCD-SFRO** (Chauffert, *Ann Oncol*. 2008; doi:10.1093/annonc/mdn281)
  *Gemzar alone better than CRT
  - Phase III
  - 119 patients with locally advanced nonmetastatic pancreatic cancer
  - CRT 60 Gy/30 fx with concurrent CI 5-FU and cisplatin weeks 1 and 5 versus induction Gemcitabine weekly × 7 weeks. Maintenance gemcitabine every 3 to 4 weeks given in both arms until disease progression or toxicity.

	MS (Months)	1-y OS	G3/4 Heme Tox
CRT	8.4	24%	10%
Gemcitabine alone	14.3	51%	17%

Radiation Technique

- Patients should undergo CT simulation with IV and oral contract.
- 3D conformal or IMRT with respiratory management techniques are used, especially if normal tissue dose constraints cannot be met with 3D conformal treatment planning.
- Presurgical imaging and surgical clips are used to determine the tumor bed in resected patients including high-risk peripancreatic nodes, anastomoses (pancreaticojejunostomy, hepaticojejunostomy, and gastrojejunostomy).
- CTV expansions should include areas at risk for microscopic disease; however, elective nodal radiation is controversial in the neoadjuvant setting.
- Tumor and involved nodes (with 1-cm margin) are used for treatment planning in the neoadjuvant setting.
- PTV expansion should take into account breathing and target motion as well as set up error (0.5–2 cm).
- Normal tissue dose constraints:
  - Spinal cord ≤45-Gy max
  - Liver
    - Adjuvant ≤25-Gy mean dose
    - Preoperative/Unresectable ≤30-Gy mean dose
  - Kidneys
    - Adjuvant 50% right and 65% left ≤18 Gy
    - Preoperative/Unresectable 70% both kidneys ≤18 Gy, if only one functional kidney 90% ≤18 Gy
  - Stomach, duodenum, jejunum
    - Adjuvant ≤55-Gy max, ≤10% each organ 50 to 54 Gy, <15% 45 to 50 Gy
    - Preoperative/Unresectable ≤55-Gy max, <30% each organ 45 to 55 Gy
- Dose
  - Adjuvant—45 Gy/25 fx ± 5- to 15-Gy boost to tumor bed or involved margins
  - Preoperative/Unresectable—45 to 54 Gy at 1.8 to 2.5 Gy/fx or 36 Gy at 2.4 Gy/fx
  - Palliation 25 to 36 Gy at 2.4 to 5 Gy/fx

Palliation

- Pain:
  - Narcotic analgesics
  - Neurolysis of the celiac ganglia
  - RT can palliate pain but does not affect survival
  - Endoscopic decompression
- Jaundice with pruritus or right upper quadrant pain or has developed cholangitis
  - Endoscopic placement of plastic or metal stent
  - Operative biliary decompression
- Duodenal obstruction secondary to pancreatic carcinoma
  - Gastrojejunostomy or an endoscopic procedure
  - Endoscopic stenting of duodenal obstruction is usually reserved for patients who are poor operative candidates

Follow-Up for Patients Undergoing Potentially Curative Treatment

- History and physical every 3 to 6 months for 2 years, then annually thereafter.
- CA19-9 every 3 to 6 months for 2 years, then annually thereafter.
- CT for symptom workup in the follow-up period.

2.4   Hepatobiliary

Epidemiology and Risk Factors

- Incidence: hepatocellular > gallbladder > extrahepatic cholangiocarcinoma > intrahepatic cholangiocarcinoma

Hepatocellular Carcinoma

- Occurs predominantly in patients with underlying chronic liver disease and cirrhosis
- Third leading cause of cancer deaths worldwide, more than 500,000 affected
- Worldwide, incidence in developing nations more than two times incidence in developed countries
- Incidence highest in Asia and Africa, where endemic high prevalence of hepatitis B and hepatitis C predisposes to chronic liver disease and hepatocellular carcinoma (HCC)
- Incidence in the United States approximately 25,000 cases/year
- Fastest growing cause of cancer mortality overall in the United States, approximately 15,000 cases/year
  - Second fastest growing cause of cancer deaths among women in the United States
  - Linked with hepatitis C epidemic in the United States
- Average age at diagnosis—65 years
  - Demographic shift to younger age at diagnosis due to alcoholic liver disease and viral hepatitis B and C acquired earlier in life
- Male: female ratio 3:1
- 48% Whites, 15% Hispanics, 14% African Americans, and 24% other (primarily Asians)
- Risk factors in the United States include:
  - Alcoholic cirrhosis
  - Hepatitis B (250 times more common with Hep B)
  - Hepatitis C
  - Hemochromatosis
  - Combination of hepatitis and alcohol significantly increases risk of cirrhosis and HCC
  - Obesity with nonalcoholic fatty liver disease (NAFLD) or nonalcoholic steatohepatitis (NASH) can progress to fibrosis, cirrhosis, and HCC
- Screening in high-risk patients with cirrhosis
  - CT and alpha-fetoprotein (AFP) every 6 to 12 months and serum AFP measurements
  - Screening results in increased rate of resectability (~30%–50%, nearly twice the rate of unscreened)
  - Elevated AFP values greater than 400 ng/mL are considered diagnostic of HCC with correlating clinical and radiologic findings; 75% to 91% specific
- Prevention
  - Hep B vaccine

Cholangiocarcinoma

- Approximately 2,500 cases/year
- Approximately 55% LN positive at diagnosis
- More than 90% are adenocarcinomas, 10% squamous cell
  - Cholangiocarcinomas can be further subcategorized into:
    - Intrahepatic—Least common
    - Extrahepatic (perihilar)
      - Include Klatskin tumors that at the bifurcation of right and left hepatic ducts
      - Distal extrahepatic
- Risk factors:
  - Long-standing inflammation
    - Primary sclerosing cholangitis (10%–20% lifetime risk)

- Intrahepatic cholangiocarcinoma may be associated with chronic ulcerative colitis without primary sclerosing cholangitis, a small subset of Crohn's disease, and chronic cholecystitis
  - Chronic cholangitis (cholecystectomy reduces risk)
  - High prevalence in Asians from endemic chronic parasitic infestation
    - Liver flukes (clonorchis sinensis and opisthorchis viverrini)
    - Other parasites, including Ascaris lumbricoides
  - Thorotrast
  - Congenital diseases of the biliary tree
    - Choledochal cysts
    - Caroli disease
  - Bile duct adenomas, biliary papillomatosis
  - Alpha-1-antitrypsin deficiency
  - Obesity
  - *Viral hepatitis, cirrhosis, and gallstones are not risk factors*
- Only approximately 10% are candidates for resection
- Male: female ratio 1:2.5
- Average age approximately 65 years
- Highest incidence in Native Americans (six times higher than that in non-Native Americans)

Gallbladder Cancer

- Highest incidence in India, Korea, Japan, Czech Republic, Slovakia, Spain, Columbia, Chile, Peru, Bolivia, and Ecuador
- Fifth most common GI cancer in the United States
- Most common biliary tract cancer (46%)
- Incidence dropped by more than 50% since 1973
- Three times more common than cholangiocarcinomas, approximately 5,000 cases/year
- Highest among American Indians/Alaska Natives and among White Hispanic
- 75% older than 64 years, median age at diagnosis 62 to 66 years
- Female-to-male approximately 2.5 to 3:1
- 50% with involved regional LN metastases at diagnosis
- Peritoneal dissemination more common with gallbladder primary
- Papillary histology is better than sclerosing or nodular
- Risk factors
  - Chronic inflammation
    - In >75%, the source of this chronic inflammation is cholesterol gallstones
    - Presence of gallstones increases risk four- to fivefold
    - Primary sclerosing
    - Cholangitis
    - Ulcerative colitis and Crohn's ileocolitis
    - Liver flukes
    - Chronic Salmonella typhi
    - Helicobacter infection
  - Calcification of the gallbladder (porcelain gallbladder)—10% to 25% incidence
  - Gallbladder polyps
  - Medications
    - Oral contraceptives
    - INH
    - Methyldopa
  - Chemical exposure
    - Pesticides (dichlorodiphenyltrichloroethane and benzene hexachloride)

- Rubber
- Vinyl chloride
- Heavy metals
  - o Occupational exposure
    - Textile
    - Petroleum
    - Paper mill
    - Shoemaking
    - Radiation exposure (radon in miners)
  - o Hereditary syndromes
    - Gardner syndrome
    - Neurofibromatosis type I
    - Hereditary nonpolyposis colon cancer
  - o Congenital defects
    - Anomalous pancreaticobiliary duct junctions
    - Choledochal cysts

Prognosis

Hepatocellular Carcinoma (HCC)

- In the past, HCC usually presented with advanced stage and right upper quadrant (RUQ) pain, weight loss, and decompensated liver disease, and was a universally fatal disease.
- Routine screening of patients with known cirrhosis, using CT and AFP, diagnoses patients earlier, and identifies a greater proportion who are amenable to potentially curative surgery.

Cholangiocarcinoma

- Tend to grow slowly and to infiltrate the walls of the ducts and spread along tissue planes with extension into the liver, porta hepatis, and celiac/pancreaticoduodenal lymphatics
- Most patients are not eligible for curative resection.
- OS is approximately 6 months.
- Many patients succumb to cholangitis (immediate antibiotics and biliary drainage).

Gallbladder Cancer

- Better than cholangiocarcinoma as more patients (~25%) undergo potentially curative resection but poor prognosis overall as usually present with advanced stage

Anatomy

- Vascular anatomy defines liver functional segments.
- Right and left lobes are divided by a line connecting the gallbladder fossa and the inferior vena cava.
  - o Right lobe divided into four segments (5, 6, 7, 8), each supplied by a branch of portal vein and drains into right hepatic vein
  - o Left lobe divided into three segments (2, 3, 4)
    - Segment 4 medial, adjacent to the middle hepatic vein
    - Segments 2 and 3 comprise left lateral segment to the left of the falciform ligament, drain via the left hepatic vein
- Caudate lobe (segment 1) is behind the portahepatis adjacent to the vena cava.
- Arterial supply:
  - o Hepatic artery supplies

- 30% of the blood flow to the normal liver parenchyma
- More than 90% to hepatic tumors
  - Portal vein
    - Is confluence of the splenic vein and the superior mesenteric vein
    - Supplies 70% to 85% of the blood into the liver
- Venous drainage:
  - Right hepatic vein
  - Middle hepatic vein
  - Left hepatic vein
  - 10 to 50 small hepatic veins drain directly into the vena cava
- Biliary anatomy is widely variable but typically follows hepatic arterial system.
  - Common bile duct branches off to form the cystic duct and becomes the hepatic duct
  - Hepatic duct divides into two to three additional ducts

Presentation

Hepatocellular Carcinoma

- HCC is usually discovered during routine screening or when symptomatic because of their size or location as tumors progress with local expansion, intrahepatic spread, and distant metastases.
- HCC with mass effect causes biliary obstruction.
  - Jaundice, most common
  - Clay-colored stools
  - Bilirubinuria (dark urine)
  - Pruritis
- Sometimes presents with hepatomegaly with or without RUQ tenderness and mass but usually small livers with cirrhosis.
- Signs of end-stage liver disease are common (ascites, coagulopathy, etc.).

Cholangiocarcinoma

- Presenting symptoms include:
  - Jaundice, most common
  - Clay-colored stools
  - Bilirubinuria (dark urine)
  - Pruritis
  - Weight loss approximately 30% at diagnosis
  - RUQ pain in advanced disease
- Hepatomegaly in 25%
- Courvoisier sign, if cholangiocarcinoma is distal to the cystic duct takeoff, there may be a palpable gallbladder

Gallbladder Cancer

- Presenting symptoms are usually not present until the later stages and include:
  - Abdominal pain
  - Fever
  - Nausea and vomiting
  - Bloating
  - Abdomen mass
  - Jaundice, anorexia, and weight loss with advanced disease
  - Courvoisier sign, palpable mass in the right upper
  - Periumbilical lymphadenopathy (Sister Mary Joseph nodes)
  - Left supraclavicular adenopathy (Virchow node)
  - Mass palpable on digital rectal examination (Blumer shelf)

Diagnosis and Workup

Hepatocellular Carcinoma

- Common abnormal laboratory values include:
  - Increased HBsAg/anti-HBc, anti-HCV—Viral hepatitis (current/past)
  - Increased iron saturation (>50%)—Underlying hemochromatosis
  - Low alpha-1-antitrypsin levels—Alpha-1-antitrypsine deficiency
  - Tumor/paraneoplastic phenomena
  - Increased AFP—Levels greater than 400 ng/mL considered diagnostic with appropriate imaging studies
  - Hypercalcemia—Ectopic parathyroid hormone production possible in 5% to 10% of patients with hepatocellular carcinoma
  - Thrombocytosis (normal/rapid increase in platelet count in patients with a history of thrombocytopenia)
- Laboratory studies include:
  - CBC
  - Electrolytes
  - Liver function tests
  - Coagulation studies
  - AFP
  - Hepatitis panel
  - Ammonia level if mental status changes
- Radiologic studies include:
  - Triple phase liver protocol CT or MRI with late arterial phase and portal venous phase for perfusion characteristics, extent and number of lesions, vascular anatomy, and extrahepatic disease
    - On CT, HCC appears as focal nodule with early enhancement on the arterial phase with rapid washout of contrast on the portal venous phase
    - MRI demonstrates high-signal intensity on T2 imaging associated with HCC
  - In patients with cirrhosis who are being considered for resection, survival following resection is correlated with the degree of portal hypertension, consider wedged hepatic vein pressure
  - PET-CT not adequate
  - Ultrasound can be difficult in the background of regenerative nodules in the cirrhotic liver. Findings on ultrasound should be confirmed with imaging and/or biopsy.
- Biopsy indicated for tumors larger than 2 cm with low AFP:
  - High-false negative biopsy rate for lesions less than 1 cm but ½ will be malignant so close follow-up with imaging is recommended.
  - For 1- to 2-cm lesions, there is an increased risk of HCC and biopsy should be performed.
  - If AFP elevated and imaging is consistent with HCC, biopsy may be omitted.
- Chest CT to evaluate for extrahepatic disease (primarily lung metastasis)
- Bone scan if clinically indicated

Cholangiocarcinoma and Gallbladder Cancer

- Extrahepatic cholestasis associate with elevated direct bilirubin levels, alkaline phosphatase and GGT
- AST, ALT, and tests of hepatic function (albumin, prothrombin time [PT]) usually normal in early disease
- Elevated PT and vitamin K malabsorption with prolonged obstruction
- CA 19-9 can be evaluated in pancreatic, bile duct malignancies and gallbladder cancer, as well as in benign cholestasis
- PSC patients only:
  - CA 19-9 >100 U/mL associate with 75% sensitivity and 80% specificity
  - Elevated CEA and CA 19-9—86% accuracy (CA 19-9 + (CEA × 40))
- *AFP not elevated in cholangiocarcinoma*

- Ultrasonography and/or CT, followed by some form of cholangiography:
  - ○ MRCP
  - ○ ERCP
  - ○ Percutaneous transhepatic cholangiography (PTC)
- Imaging studies include:
  - ○ Abdominal ultrasound—identifies mass in 50% to 75% of gallbladder cancer
  - ○ Triple phase protocol CT or MRI with late arterial phase and portal venous phase
- Cholangiography, via a percutaneous route, or ERCP may establish the diagnosis of gallbladder cancer by bile cytology
- PTC may allow access to the proximal biliary tree that has become obstructed and cytology can be obtained from drainage procedures
- Other methods to obtain tissue include CT or ultrasound needle aspiration if a mass lesion is present and endoscopic ultrasonographic (EUS) fine-needle aspiration
- Endoscopic ultrasonography can be useful to assess regional lymphadenopathy and depth of tumor invasion into the wall of the gallbladder
- Angiography may be used to confirm encasement of the portal vein or hepatic artery and may assist in preoperative planning for definitive resection

Staging

Hepatocellular Carcinoma

- Pathologic TNM is prognostic in patients undergoing resection, but not as useful in planning treatment, because it does not measure the severity of liver disease.
- AJCC/UICC 2010 TNM classification for hepatocellular carcinoma is outlined.
- T1—Solitary tumor without vascular invasion
- T2—Solitary tumor with vascular invasion or multiple tumors none greater than 5 cm
- T3a—Multiple tumors more than 5 cm
- T3b—Single tumor or multiple tumors of any size involving a major branch of the portal or hepatic vein
- T4—Tumors with direct invasion of adjacent organs other than gallbladder or with perforation of visceral peritoneum
- N0—No regional LN metastasis
  - ○ N1—regional lymph nodal metastases
- M0—No distant metastasis
  - ○ M1—Distant metastasis

Stage Classification

Stage I	T1	N0	M0
Stage II	T2	N0	M0
Stage IIIA	T3a	N0	M0
Stage IIIB	T3b	N0	M0
Stage IVA	Any T	N1	M0
Stage IVB	Any T	Any N	M1

- Child-Pugh-Turcotte score predicts perioperative survival, but does not incorporate size, number, and location of tumors, which influence resectability. The score uses five clinical measures of liver disease. Each measure is scored 1 to 3, with three indicating most severe.
- Scales that include tumor and liver disease characteristics include:

Measure	1 Point	2 Points	3 Points
Total bilirubin, μmol/L (mg/dL)	<34 (<2)	34–50 (2–3)	>50 (>3)
Serum albumin, g/dL	>3.5	2.8–3.5	<2.8
Prothrombin time (secs)	<4.0	4.0–6.0	>6.0
Ascites	None	Mild	Moderate to severe
Hepatic encephalopathy	None	Grade I–II (or suppressed with medication)	Grade III–IV (or refractory)

Points	Class	1-y OS	2-y OS
5–6	A	100%	85%
7–9	B	81%	57%
10–15	C	45%	35%

- ○ Barcelona Clinic Liver Cancer
  - ■ Stage 0—less than 2-cm tumors, normal bilirubin levels, normal portal pressure predict for safe resection and good survival
  - ■ Single tumors less than 5 cm or multiple tumors less than 3 cm are considered for resection if preserved liver function, or for transplantation if decompensated cirrhosis.
  - ■ Tumor exceeding these measurements are offered palliative therapy depending upon hepatic reserve resulting in 10% 3-year OS
- ○ Japan Integrated Staging System
- ○ Cancer of the Liver Italian Program (CLIP)

Cholangiocarcinoma

AJCC/UICC 2010 TNM classification for **intrahepatic bile duct tumors** is outlined.
- T1—Solitary tumor without vascular invasion
- T2a—Solitary tumor with vascular invasion or multiple tumors none greater than 5 cm
- T2b—Multiple tumors with or without vascular invasion
- T3—Tumor perforating the visceral peritoneum or involving local extrahepatic structures by direct invasion
- T4—Tumors with periductal invasion
- N0—No regional LN metastasis
  - ○ N1—Regional lymph nodal metastases
- M0—No distant metastasis
  - ○ M1—Distant metastasis

Stage Classification

Stage I	T1	N0	M0
Stage II	T2	N0	M0

(continued)

(continued)

Stage Classification

Stage III	T3	N0	M0
Stage IVA	T4	N0	M0
	Any T	N1	M0
Stage IVB	Any T	Any N	M1

AJCC/UICC 2010 TNM classification for ***perihilar bile duct tumors*** is outlined.
- Tis—Carcinoma in situ
- T1—Tumor confined to the bile duct with extension to muscle layer or fibrous tissue
- T2a—Tumor invading beyond the wall of the bile duct to surrounding adipose tissue
- T2b—Tumor invades adjacent hepatic parenchyma
- T3—Tumor invades unilateral branches of the portal vein or hepatic artery
- T4a—Tumor invades main portal vein or branches bilaterally; or common hepatic artery, or second order biliary radicals bilaterally; or unilateral second order biliary radicals with contralateral portal vein or hepatic artery involvement
- N0—No regional LN metastasis
  - N1—Regional nodes involved including cystic duct, common bile duct, hepatic artery, and portal vein
  - N2—Metastases to periaortic, superior mesenteric, and/or celiac artery LNs
- M0—No distant metastasis
  - M1—Distant metastasis (M1a and M1b are site dependent)

Stage Classification

Stage I	T1	N0	M0
Stage II	T2a–b	N0	M0
Stage IIIA	T3	N0	M0
Stage IIIB	T1–3	N1	M0
Stage IVA	T4	N0–1	M0
Stage IV	Any T	N2	M0
	Any T	Any N	M1

AJCC/UICC 2010 TNM classification for ***distal bile duct tumors*** is outlined.
- T1—Tumor confined to the bile duct
- T2—Tumor invades beyond the bile duct
- T3—Tumor invades the gallbladder, pancreas, duodenum, or other adjacent organs without involvement of celiac axis or superior mesenteric artery
- T4—Tumors involves celiac axis or superior mesenteric artery
- N0—No regional LN metastasis
  - N1—Regional lymph nodal metastases
- M0—No distant metastasis
  - M1—Distant metastasis

Stage Classification

Stage IA	T1	N0	M0
Stage IB	T2	N0	M0
Stage IIA	T3	N0	M0
Stage IIB	T1–3	N1	M0
Stage III	T4	Any N	M0
Stage IV	Any T	Any N	M1

Gallbladder Cancer

AJCC/UICC 2010 TNM classification for gallbladder cancer is outlined.
- Tis—Carcinoma in situ/high-grade dysplasia
- T1—Tumor invades Lamina propria or Muscularis propria
  - T1a—Lamina propria
  - T1b—Muscularis propria
- T2—Tumor invades perimuscular connective tissue, no extension beyond serosa or into liver
- T3—Tumor perforates the serosa (visceral peritoneum) and/or directly invades the liver and/or one other adjacent organ (stomach, duodenum, colon, pancreas, omentum, extrahepatic bile ducts)
- T4—Tumor invades main portal vein or two or more extrahepatic organs
- N0—No regional LN metastasis
  - N1—Regional nodes involved including cystic duct, common bile duct, hepatic artery, and portal vein
  - N2—Metastases to periaortic, pericaval, superior mesenteric, and/or celiac artery LNs
- M0—No distant metastasis
  - M1—Distant metastasis

Stage Classification

Stage I	T1	N0	M0
Stage II	T2	N0	M0
Stage IIIA	T3	N0	M0
Stage IIIB	T1–3	N1	M0
	T1,T2	N2	M0
Stage IIIB	T3	N2	M0
Stage IVA	T4	N0–1	M0
Stage IVB	Any T	N2	M0
	Any T	Any N	M1

Treatment Overview

Hepatocellular Carcinoma

Surgery

- Liver Transplantation
  - Indicated for single focus ≤5.5 cm, or up to 3 ≤4.5 cm (total diameter ≤8 cm)
  - A fraction of patients have access to transplantation, even in the developed world
  - Organ shortage remains a major limiting factor
  - Model for end-stage liver disease (MELD) score based on creatinine, bilirubin, and INR predicts death from cirrhosis
    - Highest meld score—highest risk of dying without transplantation
    - MELD scores are upgraded for stage 1 or 2 patients to reduce waitlist dropout
  - OS for transplant for appropriately chosen patients: 1-year OS 90%, 5-year OS 72.5%
  - Partial Hepatectomy
  - <15% to 30% of patients are candidates. Depends on degree of cirrhosis
  - Criteria for resection:
    - Childs-Pugh Class A, B
    - No portal HTN
    - Suitable tumor location
    - Adequate liver reserve
    - Suitable liver remnant—extent of resection tolerated based upon health of remnant liver
  - Resection of the liver is divided into two categories
    - Nonanatomic (wedge) resections—limited resections of a small portion of liver without respect to the vascular supply
    - Anatomic resections remove one or more of the eight segments of the liver
      - Right hepatic lobectomy—removal of segments 5 to 8
      - Extended right lobectomy (right trisegmentectomy)—segments 4 to 8
      - Left hepatectomy—segments 2 to 4
      - Left trisegmentectomy—segments 2, 3, 4, 5, and 8
      - Left lateral segmentectomy—segments 2 and 3
      - Caudate lobe can be removed as an isolated resection or as a component of one of the more extensive resections noted

Local Ablative Therapies

- Radiofrequency ablation, ≤3 cm not near vessels diaphragm bile duct organs
- Arterial directed therapies for 3 to 5 cm accessible for ablation
  - Bland embolization (TAE)
  - Transarterial chemoembolization (TACE)
  - TACE with drug eluting beads (DEB-TACE)
  - Arterial directed therapies contraindicated:
    - T bili >3 mg/dL
    - Near PV
    - Child-Pugh C
  - Radioembolization (yttrium-90 microspheres; Therasphere),
    - Therasphere, delivers low-dose brachytherapy to the tumor using 20 to 40 micrometer glass beads with radioactive yttrium delivered angiographically. Approximately 150 Gray over 10 to 12 days; max distance ~1 cm.

- Can also be used as a "bridge" to transplant
- Risk of radiation-induced liver disease (RILD) if T bili >2 mg/dL

Nonsurgical Therapies

- Unresectable patients greater than 5 cm can be considered for arterial directed or nonsurgical therapy
  - Sometimes tumor ablation can be offered to extend life or downstage to permit transplantation or resection
- HCC is minimally responsive to systemic chemotherapy
  - Doxorubicin-based regimens appear to have the greatest efficacy
    - RR 20% to 30%
    - Minimal effect on survival
  - Sorafenib (Llovet, *N Engl J Med*. 2008; doi:10.1056/NEJMoa0708857)
    - Increased time to disease progression (5.5 vs. 2.8 months placebo)
    - Disease control rate (43% vs. 32% placebo)
    - Sorafenib may follow arterially directed therapies in patients with adequate liver function once bilirubin returns to baseline if there is residual/recurrent disease not amenable to other local therapies
- RT
  - Majority of data comes from Childs-Pugh A patients, limited data for Childs-Pugh B patients or poor liver function
  - Safety for Childs-Pugh C cirrhosis is not established
  - All tumors irrespective of location may be amenable to external beam radiation
    - 3D conformal radiation
      - **Whole Liver**
      - **Borgelt** (*Int J Radiat Oncol Biol Phys*. 1981; doi:10.1016/0360-3016(81)90370-9) *Whole liver radiation relieves abdominal pain, nausea, vomiting, abdominal distention, ascites, and other symptoms.
      - **RTOG** (Russell, *Int J Radiat Oncol Biol Phys*. 1993; doi:10.1016/0360-3016(93)90428-X)
        - 1.5-cGy BID dose escalation 27, 30, 33 Gy
        - RILD: 0% at 27 and 30 Gy, 20% at 33 Gy
      - **High dose 3D-CRT** (Dawson, *Int J Radiat Oncol Biol Phys*. 2000, 2002)
        - Up to 90 Gy
        - Improved OS >70 Gy
        - 68% RR
        - DVH for RILD
          - Mean liver dose <31 Gy
        - TD50 39.8 Gy (HCC); 45.8-Gy liver metastases
      - **3D-CRT** (Mornex, *Int J Radiat Oncol Biol Phys*. 2006; doi:10.1016/j.ijrobp.2006.06.015)
        - Phase II
        - 25 patients with small volume HCC (1 nodule ≤5 cm or 2 ≤3 cm)
        - 66 Gy (33 fx) tolerated in Childs-Pugh A but not Childs-Pugh B
        - cCR 80%; cPR 12%
      - **Retrospective** (Seong, *Int J Radiat Oncol Biol Phys*. 2007)
        - 305 patients with definitive XRT

	MS (Months)	1-y OS (%)	2-y OS (%)	5-y OS (%)
XRT	11	45	24	6

    - IMRT
    - Stereotactic body radiation (SBRT)
      - **SBRT** (Seong, *J Clin Oncol*. 2008)

- 31 HCC and 10 IH cholangiocarcinoma
- Median dose 36 Gy (6 fx)
- Median OS—11.7 months, similar to Seong data
  - **SBRT Toxicity** (Osmundson, *Int J Radiat Oncol Biol Phys.* 2014; doi:10.1016/j.ijrobp.2014.11.028)
    - 96 patients central biliary tract tumors
      - 15 mm expansion of the portal vein from the splenic confluence to the first bifurcation of left and right portal veins
    - 53% primary liver; 47% metastatic
    - Median follow-up 27 months
    - Median biologic effective dose (BED)—85.5 Gy (37.5–151.2)
    - Median number of fractions—5 (range: 1–5)
      - −53.1%—5 fractions; 30.2%—3 fractions
    - 24.0% grade 2; 18.8% grade 3 hepatobiliary toxicity
    - Nondosimetric factors for grade 3 toxicity
      - Cholangiocarcinoma histology
      - Primary liver tumor
      - Biliary stent
    - Dosimetric factors for grade 3 toxicity
      - BED10 of 72 Gy (VBED1072) $\geq$21 cm^3
      - VBED1066 $\geq$24 cm^3
      - Mean BED10 (DmeanBED10) >14 Gy
      - VBED1072 and VBED1066 corresponding to V40 and V37.7 for 5 fractions and V33.8 and V32.0 for 3 fractions, respectively
  - SBRT can be considered as an alternative to ablation/embolization if contraindicated or failed in patients without extrahepatic disease
  - Appropriate for 1 to 3 tumors
  - Consider for larger lesions if sufficient uninvolved liver/adequate function
- Proton beam radiation may be appropriate in specific situations
- Palliative external beam radiation for symptom control for primary and metastatic HCC

Cholangiocarcinoma

Surgery

- Approximately 10% of patients present with early stage are candidates for curative resection.
  - Intrahepatic and Klatskin tumors require liver resection.
  - Approximately 15% of patients with proximal tumors are candidates.
  - OS is 40% for proximal tumors if negative margins.
  - Approximately 33% of patients with mid-ductal tumors are candidates.
  - Approximately 56% of patients with distal tumors are candidates.
- Reresection, ablation, or chemotherapy for intrahepatic cholangiocarcinomas with microscopic margins or residual disease
- Liver transplantation may be considered for patients with unresectable proximal tumors extending into liver or intrahepatic cholangiocarcinomas.
  - 53% 5-year OS overall
  - 80% 5-year OS for early stage
- Distal tumors require Whipple
- Periampullary tumors—better prognosis,
  - Long-term survival rate of 30% to 40%.
- High rates of tumor bed and regional nodal recurrence after curative surgery
- Regional node failure approximately 50%
- Metastases rate ~30% to 40%. Failures correlate with TNM stage

Radiation therapy

- Preoperative RT (45–50 Gy, 25–28 fx) + chemotherapy
  - 38% pCR rate with preoperative radiation and chemotherapy
- Several studies have shown an increase in median survival from 8 months with surgery alone to more than 19 months using adjuvant chemoradiation—no randomized studies.

Retrospective (Schoenthaler, *Ann Surg.* 1994;219(3):267–274)

	Number of Patients	MS (Months)
Surgery alone	62	6.5
Surgery + XRT (46 Gy)	45	11
Surgery + charged particles (60 Gy Eq)	22	14
Negative margins (all patients)		39
Microscopic residual (all patients)		19
Gross residual (all patients)		7

Todoroki (*Int J Radiat Oncol Biol Phys.* 2000;46(3):581–587)
  - 61 patients (28/47 microscopic and 13/14 gross residual got adjuvant radiation)
  - Surgery + adjuvant radiation with or without IORT boost

	LR (%)	5-y OS (%)
Surgery alone	69	13.5
Surgery + XRT	11 (all)	32 (all) 0 (XRT)
Surgery + IORT (20 Gy)		17
Surgery + XRT + IORT		39

Meta-analysis (Horgan, *J Clin Oncol.* 2012; doi:10.1200/JCO.2011.40.5381)
  - 6,712 patients with biliary cancers
  - Adjuvant therapy (chemo, radiation, CRT) compared with surgery alone
  - Nonsignificant improvement in OS with adjuvant therapy
  - Chemotherapy or chemoradiation better than radiation alone (SS)
  - Greatest benefit in LN+ disease or R1 resections
  - No differences between gallbladder or bile duct cancers

SWOG S0809 (Ben-Josef, *J Clin Oncol.* 2015; doi:10.1200/JCO.2014.60.2219)
  - 79 patients with pT2–4 or N+ biliary cancers (extrahepatic 68%; gallbladder 32%)
  - R0 resection—54 patients; R1 resection—25 patients
  - 86% completed adjuvant therapy (gemcitabine/capecitabine × 4) followed by concurrent capecitabine and radiation (45 Gy to regional lymphatics and 54–59.4 Gy to tumor bed)
  - 2-year survival 65% (67% for R0; 60% for R1)
  - Median OS 35 months (34 months for R0; 35 months for R1)

- o 17.5% local only relapse; 30% distant relapse; 11% combined relapse
- o The most common grade 3 to 4 adverse effects were neutropenia (44%), hand-foot syndrome (11%), diarrhea (8%), lymphopenia (8%), and leukopenia (6%). There was one death resulting from GI hemorrhage.
- Intraluminal brachytherapy and IORT are sometimes used to improve local control.

Unresectable disease—Retrospective—Intraluminal Brachy Boost (Alden, *Int J Radiat Oncol Biol Phys.* 1994; doi:10.1016/0360-3016(94)90115-5)

	MS (Months)
<45 Gy	4.5
>45–54 Gy (with brachy boost)	18
>54 Gy (with up to 25-Gy brachy boost)	24

Retrospective—Adjuvant CRT Gafoori (*Int J Radiat Oncol Biol Phys.* 2010; doi:10.1016/j.ijrobp.2010.06.018)
- o 37 patients
- o 1-year OS 59%; 2-year OS 22%
- o 1-year LC 90%; 2-year LC 71%

Borghero (*Ann Surg Oncol.* 2008. doi:10.1245/s10434-008-9998-7)
- o 65 patients extrahepatic bile duct with curative resection
- o 42 patient received adjuvant CRT

	LR (%)	5-y OS (%)
Surgery alone	38	36
Adjuvant CRT	37	42

Nelson (*Int J Radiat Oncol Biol Phys.* 2009; doi:10.1016/j.ijrobp.2008.07.008)
- o 33 patients with curative resection with adjuvant CRT
- o 12 patients with neoadjuvant radiation followed by surgery

	LR (%)	MS (Months)	5-y OS (%)	5-y DFSS (%)
Neoadjuvant RT			53	
Adjuvant CRT			23 NSS	
ALL	78	34	33	37

Dose Escalation (Crane, *Int J Radiat Oncol Biol Phys.* 2002;53(4):969–974)
- o 52 patients
- o Radiation with concurrent protracted venous infusion (PVI) 5-FU

	Median Time to LR (Months)
30 Gy	9
36–50.4 Gy	11
54–85 Gy	15

Retrospective Dose Response Analysis (Tao, *J Clin Oncol.* 2015; doi:10.1200/JCO.2015.61.3778)
- ○ 79 patients
- ○ Median follow-up 33 months
- ○ 89% received systemic therapy before radiation
- ○ 35 to 100 Gy (median, 58.05 Gy) in 3 to 30 fractions
- ○ Median biologic equivalent dose (BED) of 80.5 Gy (range, 43.75–180 Gy)
- ○ Median survival 30 months; 3-year survival 44%
- ○ Radiation dose—most important prognostic factor for local control and survival

BED	3-y Survival	3-y LC
>80.5 Gy	73%	78%
<80.5 Gy	38%	45%

Chemotherapy

- The most used agent is 5-FU (partial response rate ~12%).
- It is most often given as a radiation sensitizer.
- Gemcitabine and cisplatin are first-line chemotherapy in inoperable cholangiocarcinoma but do not appear to provide any local control or meaningful survival benefit when used without RT or surgery.
- Adjuvant TACE chemoembolization for intrahepatic cholangiocarcinoma has been used postattempted curative surgery.

Photodynamic therapy

- Photodynamic therapy (PDT) is an experimental local cancer therapy that uses IV administration of a photosensitizer (Porphyrin), which is then activated by light illumination at an appropriate wavelength.
- It improves biliary drainage and quality of life in patients with unresectable disease.
- One prospective, multicenter study showed a significant survival benefit with PDT.

Gallbladder Cancer

Surgery

- Complete surgical resection is the only curative therapy and includes cholecystectomy, hepatic resection, and regional lymphadenectomy.
- Bile duct excision may also be necessary, especially if jaundice is present.
- Approximately 25% are candidates for curative resection.
- Approximately 25% of T2 tumors have liver involvement.
- 5-year OS rates have increased 5% to 12% up to 38% and are thought to be related to more aggressive surgery and node dissection.
  - ○ **MS after surgery** (North et al. *Am Surg.* 1998;64(5):437)
    - ▪ 162 patients (some with post-op chemo and/or radiation)

	MS (Months)
Negative margins	67
Microscopic residual	9
Gross residual	4

- o **5-year OS associated with surgery** (Cubertafond, *Hepatogastroenterol.* 1999;46(27):1567–1571)
  - ▪ 724 patients

	5-y OS (%)
Tis	93
T1	18
T2	10
T3	0

- Nodal metastases outside of the regional area (porta hepatis, gastrohepatic ligament, retroduodenal area) are not resectable.
- Sometimes an incidental pathology finding after a cholecystectomy:
  - o If carcinoma in situ or only invasion of lamina propria (T1a) with negative margins—postoperative observation
  - o If ≥T1b or positive margins without metastatic disease—attempt to reresect with partial hepatic resection and regional lymphadenectomy (porta hepatis, gastrohepatic ligament, and retroduodenal LNs)
  - o If original surgery was laparoscopic, then port sites should be resected
  - o Because there is a high incidence of gallbladder cancer in porcelain gallbladder, open cholecystectomy should be performed
- Unresectable disease is usually limited to biopsy of the tumor and biliary decompression.
  No evidence-based clinical study exists to demonstrate clear benefit of any form of adjuvant therapy in gallbladder cancer.

Radiation therapy

- T1 or stage I disease confined to the mucosa are at low risk for LN metastases and adjuvant treatment is not warranted.
- Adequate surgical margins may be difficult to achieve and adjuvant RT (45–50.4 Gy) with or without concurrent chemotherapy (5-FU based) is sometimes used to control microscopic residual in the tumor bed and regional nodes.
- Interpretation of data from small, single institutional experiences over many years, with a variety of treatment methods used, is difficult:
  - o Patient selection bias
  - o Adjuvant radiation used in a variety of settings after curative resections with close or positive microscopic margins, gross macroscopic residual disease, and palliative debulking with bypass
  - o Lack of reporting of technical treatment data, histological grading, and extent

Retrospective DataDuke (Czito, *Int J Radiat Oncol Biol Phys.* 2005; doi:10.1016/j.ijrobp.2004.12.059)
  - o 22 patients; curative resection followed by CRT 45 Gy (25 fx) (5-FU based)
  - o Adjuvant radiation 20% with no difference in median OS (23.4 months)

	MS (Months)	5-y OS (%)	5-y DFS (%)	5-y LR (%)
Surgery alone	22.8	37	33	41

MSKCC (Duffy, *J Surg Oncol.* 2008; doi:10.1002/jso.21141)
- o 435 patients; 123 with curative resection
- o Adjuvant radiation 20% with no difference in median OS (23.4 months)

Seer Registry (Mojica, *J Surg Oncol.* 2007; doi:10.1002/jso.20831)
- o 3,187 cases resected gallbladder
- o Adjuvant radiation 17%

	MS (Months)
Surgery alone	8
Adjuvant radiation	14

*Survival benefit with radiation only for those with regional nodes or liver infiltration

Seer Registry (Wang, *J Clin Oncol.* 2008; doi:10.1200/JCO.2007.14.7934)
- • 4,180 cases resected gallbladder
- • Adjuvant radiation 18%
- • Survival benefit with radiation only for ≥T2N0 only

	MS (Months)
Surgery alone	8
Adjuvant radiation	15

Prospective Data
SWOG S0809 (Ben-Josef, *J Clin Oncol.* 2014; doi:10.1200/JCO.2014.60.2219)
- o Phase II
- o Extrahepatic cholangiocarcinoma and gallbladder cancer
- o Capecitabine/gemcitabine followed by concurrent capecitabine and radiation
- o Extrahepatic cholangiocarcinoma
  - ▪ 2-year OS 66%
  - ▪ DFS 51%
  - ▪ LF 11%

Retrospective—Unresectable Extrahepatic Cholagio (Gafoori, *Int J Radiat Oncol Biol Phys.* 2010; doi:10.1016/j.ijrobp.2010.06.018)
- o 37 patients
- o 1-year OS 59%; 2-year OS 22%
- o 1-year LC 90%; 2-year LC 71%

Meta-analysis (Horgan, *J Clin Oncol.* 2012; doi:10.1200/JCO.2011.40.5381)
- o 6,712 patients with biliary cancers
- o Adjuvant therapy (chemo, radiation, chemoradiation) compared with surgery alone
- o Nonsignificant improvement in OS with adjuvant therapy
- o Chemotherapy or chemoradiation better than radiation alone (SS)
- o Greatest benefit in LN+ disease or R1 resections
- o No differences between gallbladder or bile duct cancers
- • Adjuvant radiation after surgery with only microscopic residual disease remaining produces MS approximately 12 months (compared to 6–7 months without radiation)
- • Tumors beyond the mucosa AJCC stages T2 to T4 are candidates for adjuvant radiation following curative resection resulting in MS >16 months (compared to <6 months mean without radiation)

- RT (50.4 Gy) with or without concurrent chemotherapy (5-FU) in unresectable disease is to provide palliation of symptoms
- Gemcitabine and concurrent radiation associated with much toxicity in this setting

Chemotherapy

- Adjuvant chemotherapy can be given with single agent gemcitabine or 5-FU/capecitabine without clear evidence of benefit.
- Gemcitabine with or without cisplatin or capecitabine is used for unresectable, recurrent, or metastatic disease.
- Epidermal growth factor receptor (EGFR) is overexpressed in a vast majority of biliary tract cancers; trials using EGFR-targeting agents have been studied in the phase II setting with encouraging results but there is no phase III data.
- Selected patients with unresectable disease may be considered for surgical resection after response to chemotherapy, based on a data from a retrospective study demonstrating improved survival in a small number of patients who received gemcitabine/cisplatin followed by surgery.

Radiation Technique

Hepatocellular Carcinoma

- 3D-CRT/IMRT
  - Whole liver—21 Gy (3 Gy/fx)
  - Partial liver
- SBRT dose prescription
  - NTCP RILD ≤10%
  - Isocenter dose ≤90 Gy
- Normal tissue dose constraints:
  - Spinal cord ≤45-Gy max
  - Liver
    - Whole liver—≤30 Gy (3 Gy/fx)
    - 66% liver—≤50.4 Gy (1.8 Gy/fx)
    - 33% liver—≤28.4 Gy (1.8 Gy/fx)

Cholangiocarcinoma

- 3D-CRT or IMRT
  - 45 Gy (25 fx) then boost
  - XRT up to 60 Gy
  - Intraluminal brachytherapy—20 to 25 Gy
  - IORT—20 Gy
- Normal tissue dose constraints:
  - Spinal cord ≤45-Gy max
  - Kidneys 50% right and 65% left ≤18 Gy
  - Small bowel <10% 50 to 54 Gy, <15% 45 to 50 Gy
  - Liver
    - Whole liver—≤30 Gy (3 Gy/fx)
    - 66% liver—≤50.4 Gy (1.8 Gy/fx)
    - 33% liver—≤28.4 Gy (1.8 Gy/fx)

Gallbladder Cancer

- 3D-CRT or IMRT
- 45 to 50 Gy (25–28 fx)

- Normal tissue dose constraints:
  - Spinal cord ≤45-Gy max
  - Kidneys 50% right and 65% left ≤18 Gy
  - Small bowel <10% 50 to 54 Gy, <15% 45 to 50 Gy
  - Liver
    - Whole liver—≤ 30 Gy (3 Gy/fx)
    - 66% liver—≤ 50.4 Gy (1.8 Gy/fx)
    - 33% liver—≤ 28.4 Gy (1.8 Gy/fx)

Palliation

Hepatocellular Carcinoma

- Treatment focuses on pain control, ascites, edema, and encephalopathy management

Cholangiocarcinoma and Gallbladder Cancer

- Stents can be placed via ERCP or PTC to relieve biliary obstruction, pruritus, and improve quality of life.
  - Stents usually are used if the tumor is unresectable.
  - Debate exists about whether preoperative stenting is warranted, but most believe that it does not alter the outcome.
- Palliative surgical procedures may be considered if stenting cannot be accomplished.
  - Surgical bypass for tumors in the common bile duct should be performed.
- Celiac-plexus block via regional injection of alcohol or other sclerosing agent can relieve pain in the mid back associated with retroperitoneal spread.

Follow-Up

Hepatocellular Carcinoma

Imaging, H+P, and AFP every 3 to 6 months for 2 years, then every 6 to 12 months in patients treated with surgery or local therapy

Cholangiocarcinoma and Gallbladder Cancer

Consider CT, H+P, and tumor markers every 6 months for 2 years in resected patients.

2.5   Colorectal

Epidemiology and Risk Factors

- The majority of colorectal cancers occur in industrialized countries.
  - High incidence in the United States, Canada, Japan, parts of Europe, New Zealand, Israel, Australia
  - Lower incidence rates in Algeria and India
  - Recent rises in parts of the Japan, China (Shanghai), and Eastern Europe
- 93,090 new cases of colon cancer and 39,610 new cases of rectal cancer were reported in 2015.
  - Lifetime risk of developing a colorectal cancer is approximately 6% in the United States.
  - Incidence increases more after age 35 and rises rapidly after age 50.
    - Peak is in the seventh decade.
      - More than 90% of colon cancers occur after age 50.
      - NCCN recommends that all patients less than 70 years with colorectal cancer be tested for HNPCC.
  - There are approximately 49,700 deaths.
  - It is the third most common cancer in females and males.
  - The male:female ratio is 1.32:1.

- Both colon and rectal cancer incidences and mortality rates are decreasing in part due to screening and removal of polyps (3% per year in men and 2.2% per year in women).
- Approximately 75% are sporadic.
- Risk factors in approximately 25% of cases include:
  - Personal history of colorectal cancer or polyps
    - 30% synchronous lesions
    - Malignancy develops in 2% to 5%
  - Family history of colorectal cancer or polyps (15%–20%)
    - Relative risk increased in the first-degree relatives of affected.
    - Relative risk for offspring is 2.42.
    - If more than one family member is affected, relative risk increases to 4.25.
    - If first-degree family member is <45 years, the risk increase is higher.
  - Genetic predispositions
    - HNPCC (4%–7%)
      - Autosomal dominant—mismatch repair chromosomes 2, 3, 7
      - Revised Amsterdam criteria used for at-risk for HNPCC (all criteria met):
        - Three or more relatives who are diagnosed with an HNPCC-associated cancer (colorectal, endometrium, small bowel, ureter, or renal pelvis)
        - One affected person is a first-degree relative of the other two
        - One or more cases of cancer are diagnosed before age 50 years
        - At least two generations are affected
        - FAP has been excluded
        - Tumors have undergone a pathology review
    - FAP (1%)
      - Defect in adenomatous polyposis coli (APC) gene chromosome 5 q21
      - If left untreated, cancer develops in approximately 100% by age 40
    - Inflammatory bowel disease (IBD) (1%)
      - If dysplasia present risk is 30%
  - High-fat, low-fiber diet *(high fiber and calcium supplement may be protective)*
  - Tobacco
  - Alcohol intake >30 g per day (risk greater for rectal cancer; beer > wine)
  - Increased risk of proximal colon cancer after cholecystectomy (exposure to bile)
- Adenocarcinomas (98%)
  - Other histologies
    - Carcinoid (0.4%)
    - Lymphoma (1.3%)
    - Sarcoma (0.3%)
    - Squamous cell—transitional area from rectum to anus considered anal carcinomas
- Location
  - Cecum (20%)
  - Sigmoid (25%)
  - Rectum (20%)
  - Rectosigmoid junction (10%)
  - Left colon cancers are more common in males and right colon cancers are more common in females
- Approximately 10% of adenomas will become adenocarcinomas (takes up to 10 years) three classifications of adenomas:
  - Tubular
  - Tubulovillous
  - Villous

- Genetic pathways:
  o *K-ras* mutations and microsatellite instability identified in hyperplastic polyps that may also have malignant potential
  o DNA mismatch repair genes (*hMLH1, hMSH2, hPMS1, hPMS2,* and *hMSH6*) in approximately 90% of HNPCC and 15% of sporadic colon and rectal cancers
  o A separate carcinogenic pathway found in IBD as chronic inflammation may lead to genetic alterations
- Three pathways to colon and rectal carcinoma have been described:
  o *APC* gene adenoma-carcinoma pathway
  o HNPCC pathway
  o Ulcerative colitis dysplasia

Prognosis

- 8% of cancer deaths in men and 9% of cancer deaths in women in the United States
- Mortality rates are decreasing in both sexes
- Survival related to risk group stratification related to stage

Pooled analysis (Gunderson, *J Clin Oncol.* 2004; doi:10.1200/JCO.2004.08.173)
  o NCCTG, INT 0144, NSABP R01 and R02 trias
  o 3,791 patients
  o Increasing T and N stage negatively impact survival, but not N stage alone
  o Adjuvant therapy should be based on risk stratification groups
     ▪ Post-op chemotherapy improves OS for intermediate risk compared to surgery alone
     ▪ Post-op CRT improves DFS, OS, and LR for moderate-high and high risk compared to chemotherapy alone

Risk Group	5-y OS (%)	DFS (%)	LR (%)	DM (%)
Low T1–2N0	90	90	<5	10
Intermediate T1–2N1; T3N0	65–80	75	5–10	5–20
Moderately high T1–2N2; T3N1; T4N0	40–80	45–60	10–20	30–35
High T3N2; T4N+	25–60	30–35	15–20	>40

- 1- and 5-year mortality rates for colon and rectal cancer are 83% and 64%, respectively but with early detection the 5-year survival rate is 90%.
- Aspirin is for prevention.
- Aspirin prevents colon adenocarcinoma among patients with hereditary risk of colorectal cancer (Burn, *Lancet.* 2011; doi:10.1016/S0140-6736(11)61049-0).
- In a review of 51 randomized controlled trials, aspirin reduced the short-term incidence of cancer and risk of cancer death in patients with adenocarcinomas (Rothwell, *Lancet.* 2009; *Lancet.* 2010; doi:10.1016/S0140-6736(10)61543-7).
- 5-year survival rates are lower for Blacks (55%) than Whites (66%).
- Mortality rates are slightly higher in males than females.

Anatomy

- The large bowel starts at the cecum, which is not technically a part of the colon but if cancer develops in the cecum, it is treated like colon cancer.
- The colon is divided into four parts.
  - The ascending colon is on the right and continues upward to a bend at the hepatic flexure.
  - The transverse colon lies across the upper part of the abdomen and ends with a bend at the splenic flexure.
  - The descending colon starts at the splenic flexure on the left ending at the sigmoid colon.
  - The sigmoid colon is the end of the colon and connects to the rectum.
  - The rectum is about 15-cm long and ends at the sphincters comprising the dentate line, emptying into the anal canal.
- The colon and rectum are held by folds of mesenteries (fatty connective tissue with blood vessels, nerves, LNs, and lymphatics).
- The mesocolon is a mesentery that attaches the colon to the abdominal wall.
- The rectum is surrounded by a mesentery called the mesorectum.
- Layers:
  - Mucosa—includes the epithelium, lamina propria, and muscularis mucosa
  - Submucosa—connective tissue contains glands, blood, lymphatics, and nerves
  - Muscularis propria
  - Serosa—colon only; absent in the rectum
- The rectum is different than the rest of the colon; the outer layer is longitudinal muscle.
- The rectum contains three folds (valves of Houston):
  - Superior (at 10–12 cm on left)
  - Middle fold (at 8–10 cm on right)
  - Inferior (at 4–7 cm on left)

Presentation

- Many are asymptomatic discovered during digital or proctoscopic screening
- Bleeding 60%
- Change in bowel habits (43%)
  - Diarrhea
  - Caliber of the stool
  - Incomplete evacuation
  - Tenesmus
- Occult bleeding (26%): Detected via a fecal occult blood test (FOBT)
- Abdominal pain (20%)
- Back pain: Usually a late sign caused by a tumor invading or compressing nerve trunks
- Urinary symptoms
- Malaise (9%)
- Pelvic pain (5%)
- Peritonitis from perforation (3%)
- Jaundice, from liver metastases (<1%)

Diagnosis and Workup

- Screening for:
  - Asymptomatic, 50 to 75 years with no other risk factors
  - Change in bowel habits

- o Rectal and anal bleeding
- o Unclear abdominal pain
- o Unclear iron-deficiency anemia
- Screening options for the detection of adenomatous polyps and cancer for asymptomatic adults 50 to 75 years include:
  - o Flexible sigmoidoscopy (FSIG) every 5 years
  - o Fiberoptic flexible colonoscopy every 10 years
  - o Double-contrast barium enema (DCBE) every 5 years
  - o CT colonography every 5 years
- Other screening tests may include the following:
  - o Guaiac-based FOBT
  - o Stool DNA screening (SDNA)
  - o Fecal immunochemical test (FIT)
  - o Rigid proctoscopy
  - o Combined glucose-based FOBT and flexible sigmoidoscopy
- Screening for high-risk patients starts at age 40 and includes offering genetic counseling.
  - o Family history of colon and rectal cancer
  - o First-degree relative with adenoma aged younger than 60 years
  - o Genetic cancer syndromes
  - o HNPCC
  - o FAP
  - o Personal history of IBD
  - o Personal history of adenomas
  - o Personal history of colon or rectal cancer
    Screening intervals vary with risk factors
- Diagnostic workup includes:
  - o Physical examination with digital rectal exam (DRE)
    - ▪ Specific attention to the size and location of the rectal tumor
    - ▪ Enlarged LNs
    - ▪ Hepatomegaly
    - ▪ Examination includes the use of the following:
    - ▪ DRE—approximately 8 cm above the dentate line
      - – Size
      - – Ulceration
      - – Perirectal LNs
      - – Fixation to surrounding structures
      - – Sphincter function
  - o Rigid proctoscopy: location of the tumor in relation to the sphincters
  - o Endorectal ultrasonography to assess
    - ▪ Depth of invasion
    - ▪ Perirectal nodes
  - o Biopsy and histologic examination
  - o Full colonoscopy to in addition, evaluate the remainder of the colon
  - o CBC, chemistries, iver, and renal function tests
  - o CEA
  - o CT scan—chest, abdomen, and pelvis
  - o Endorectal or pelvic MRI
    PET scanning: Not routinely indicated

Staging

AJCC/UICC 2010 TNM classification for colorectal cancer is outlined.

- T0—No evidence of primary tumor
- Tis—Carcinoma in situ (mucosal); intraepithelial, or invasion of the lamina propria
- T1—Tumor invades submucosa
- T2—Tumor invades muscularis propria
- T3—Tumor invades through the muscularis propria into the subserosa or into nonperitonealized pericolic or perirectal tissue
- T4—Tumor directly invades organs/structures and/or perforates the visceral peritoneum
- N0—No regional LN metastasis
  - N1—Metastasis in 1 to 3 pericolic or perirectal LNs
  - N2—Metastasis in 4 or more pericolic or perirectal LNs
  - N3—Metastasis in any LN along the course of a named vascular trunk
- M0—No distant metastasis
  - M1—Distant metastasis

Historically, the Dukes Classification system was used:
- Dukes A—Limited to the rectal wall (Dukes A)
- Dukes B—Extends through the rectal wall into peri-rectal tissue
  - B1—Tumor penetration into muscularis propria
  - B2—Tumor penetration through muscularis propria
- Dukes C—metastases to regional LNs
  - C1—Limited to the rectal wall with nodal involvement
  - C2—Tumor penetrating through the rectal wall with nodal involvement
- Dukes—D distant metastases
  *Dukes and TNM systems do not include prognostic information such as histologic grade, vascular or perineural invasion, or DNA ploidy
  *The TNM staging of rectal cancer correlates with 5-year OS

Stage Classification

TNM				Dukes	5-y OS
Stage I	T1–2	N0	M0	A	>90%
Stage IIA	T3	N0	M0	B	60%–85%
Stage IIB	T4	N0	M0	B	
Stage IIIA	T1–2	N1	M0	C	55%–60%
Stage IIIB	T3–4	N1	M0	C	35%–42%
Stage IIIC	T1–4	N2	M0	C	25%–27%
Stage IV	Any T	Any N	M1	D	5%–7%

Treatment Overview

Surgery

Colon cancer

- Surgery for colon cancer involves removal of the mesentery that contains supplying and draining arteries, veins, and lymphatics.

- Adjuvant therapy for colon cancer depends on the stage of the tumor:
  - Stage III
    Routine use of adjuvant therapy not warranted for Stage II but could be considered for inadequately sampled nodes, T4 lesions, perforation, or poorly differentiated histology
- Chemotherapy for colon cancer may include:
  - 5-FU (Adrucil, 5-FU)
  - Folinic acid (Leucovorin)
  - Oxaliplatin (Eloxatin)
  - Capecitabine (Xeloda)
  - Irinotecan (Camptosar, CPT-11)
  - Raltitrexed (Tomudex)
- Targeted therapy may be given alone or combined with chemotherapy and may include:
  - Bevacizumab (Avastin)
  - Cetuximab (Erbitux)
  - Panitumumab (Vectibix)
- Adjuvant radiation is rarely warranted unless the tumor is inoperative or ruptured before or during surgery.

INT 0130 (Martenson, *J Clin Oncol.* 2004; doi:10.1200/JCO.2004.01.029)
  *No benefit to adjuvant CRT over chemotherapy alone in resected colon cancer
  *Higher toxicity rates associated with CRT compared to chemotherapy alone
  - Phase III
  - 224 patients, resected T3N1–2 or T4Nx
  - Randomized
    - Post-op chemotherapy (5-FU and levamisole)
    - Post-op chemoradiation (50.4 Gy/28 fx + 5-FU and levamisole)

	5-y OS (%)	5-y DFS (%)
Post-op Chemo	62	51
Post-op CRT	58	51

Rectal cancer

Surgery:
- Local excision for:
  - T1 only
  - Small (<3 cm in size)
  - <1/3 circumference
  - Exophytic/polypoid
  - Superficial and mobile (T1 and T2 lesions)
  - Low-grade tumors (well or moderately differentiated)
  - Located in low in the rectum (within 8 cm of the anal verge)
  - No palpable or radiologic evidence of enlarged mesenteric LNs
  - Likelihood of LN involvement 0% to 12%
    - Transanal endoscopic microsurgery (TEM) local excision uses a special proctoscope that distends the rectum with insufflated carbon dioxide and allows the passage of dissecting instruments for resection of lesions located higher in the rectum.
    TEM Transanal is not yet widely used due to significant learning curve/lack of availability.
- Surgery alone for locally advanced rectal cancer is associated with an LR rate of 30% to 50%. Techniques include:
  - Low Anterior Resection (LAR): Sphincter preserving; removal of tumor and mesorectum—need approximately 5-cm margin to sphincter for primary anastomosis
  - Abdomino-Perineal Resection (APR): Removal of tumor, mesorectum, levator muscles, and anus

o Total Mesorectal Excision (TME): En bloc sharp dissection of rectal mesentery to sacrum including all vessels
o Laparoscopic surgery for colorectal cancer offers the advantages of faster recovery time and less pain, compared with open surgery. However, data on oncologic outcome with laparoscopic rectal cancer resection has been lacking. (**COLOR II**, Bonjer, *N Engl J Med.* 2015; doi:10.1056/NEJMoa1414882)
- Factors influencing sphincter preservation in rectal cancer:
  o Surgeon training and volume
  o Neoadjuvant chemoRT
- Factors associated with difficult sphincter preservation:
  o Male sex
  o Morbid obesity
  o Preoperative incontinence
  o Direct involvement of anal sphincter muscles with carcinoma
  o Bulky tumors within 5 cm from the anal verge

Adjuvant Therapy

- Adjuvant therapy for rectal cancer includes both concurrent CRT and adjuvant chemotherapy.
- A total of approximately 6 months of perioperative therapy is recommended.

Chemotherapy

Dosing with concurrent radiation
- Continuous infusion (CI) 5-FU 225 mg/m^2 over 24 hours 5 or 7 days per week
- 5-FU 400-mg/m^2 IV bolus and leucovorin 20 mg/m^2 for 4 days during weeks 1 and 5 of XRT

Postoperative adjuvant chemotherapy
- Modified FOLFOX (5-FU, oxaliplatin, leucovorin)
- Infusional 5-FU/leucovorin
- Capecitabine
- Cpecitabine, oxaliplatin (CapeOx)

Radiation

- **Adjuvant Radiation With or Without Chemotherapy**
  *Post-op radiation alone inferior to post-op CRT
  *Post-op radiation improves LC and time to LR
  *Post-op radiation does not impact on DM or OS
  *Post-op radiation with CI 5-FU improves survival over bolus 5-FU
- **GITSG 71-75** (Holyoke, *N Engl J Med.* 1985; doi:10.1056/NEJM198506063122301; Thomas, *Radiother Oncol.* 1988; doi:10.1016/0167-8140(88)90219-8)
  *Adjuvant CRT better than surgery alone
  o Phase III
  o 227 patients; Dukes B2–C2
  o Chemo = bolus 5FU + CCNU
    ▪ Randomized to 4 arms
    ▪ Surgery alone
    ▪ Adjuvant radiation (44–48 Gy/22–24fx)
    ▪ Adjuvant CRT (40–44 Gy) + bolus 5-FU/CCNU
    ▪ Adjuvant chemotherapy (bolus 5-FU/CCNU)
      *Closed early
      *Not evaluated by intent to treat; 39% deviating from planned radiation

- **NCCTG 79-47-51** (Krook, *N Engl J Med.* 1991; doi:10.1056/NEJM199103143241101)
  *Post-op CRT better than post-op radiation alone
  o Phase III
  o 204 patients; T3–4 or N+ (Dukes B2-C)

	5-y OS (%)	10-y OS (%)	5-y DFS (%)	LR (%)	Toxicity (%)
Surgery alone	26	27	44	25	
Adj. XRT	33		50	20	16
Adj. Chemo	41		51	27	15
Adj. Chemo XRT	54	45	65	10	35

- ○ Randomized to:
  - Post-op radiation (46–50.4 Gy) alone
  - Post-op radiation (46–50.4 Gy) with concurrent 5-FU + 1 cycle semustine/5-FU before and after radiation

	5-y OS (%)	5-y LR (%)	RR (%)	DM (%)
Post-op XRT	48	25	63	46
Post-op CRT	58	14	42	29
P-value	.025	.036	.0016	.011

- **INT 0114** (Tepper, *J Clin Oncol.* 2002; doi:10.1200/JCO.2002.07.132)
  - ○ Phase III
  - ○ 1,695 patients; T3–4 N+
  - ○ Randomized to:
    - Post-op radiation (50.4–54 Gy) + bolus 5-FU
    - Post-op radiation (50.4–54 Gy) + bolus 5-FU leucovorin
    - Post-op radiation (50.4–54 Gy) + bolus 5-FU levamisole
    - Post-op radiation (50.4–54 Gy) + bolus 5-FU leucovorin levamisole

	7-y OS (%)	7-y DFS (%)
NSS for all regimens	~56	~50

*Increased toxicity with addition of levamisole
*Number of LNs examined associated with OS for N0 patients
*This study recommended a minimum of 14 nodes be examined but the absolute number is controversial.

- **NSABP R-01** (Fisher, *JNCI.* 1988; doi:10.1093/jnci/80.1.21)
  - *Post-op radiation improves LC and post-op chemo improves DFS + OS (in men only)
  - ○ Phase III
  - ○ 555 patients; Stages II to III, Duke's B to C
  - ○ Randomized to:
    - Surgery alone
    - Surgery with post-op radiation (46–47 Gy) + bolus 5-FU/leucovorin
    - Surgery with post-op chemotherapy (5-FU, semustine, vincristine–MOF)
    - Post-op radiation (50.4–54 Gy) + bolus 5-FU leucovorin levamisole

	LR (%)	DFS (%)	OS (%)
Surgery alone	25	30	43
Post-op chemo	16	42	53
Post-op XRT	16		

- **NSABP R-02** (Wolmark, *JNCI*, 2000;92(5):388–396)
  *Post-op radiation improves LC but not DFS + OS (no benefit to MOF in men):
  - Phase III
  - 594 patients; Stages II to III, Duke's B to C
  - Randomized to:
    - Surgery with post-op chemotherapy (5-FU/leu)
    - Surgery with post-op CRT (46–47 Gy) + bolus 5-FU/leu
    - Surgery with post-op chemotherapy (MOF)
    - Surgery with post-op CRT (MOF)

	5-y LR (%)
Radiation arms	8
Nonradiation arms	14

*No difference in OS or DFS

- **INT 0144** (O'Connell, *N Engl J Med*. 1994; doi:10.1056/NEJM199408253310803; Smalley, *J Clin Oncol*. 2006; doi:10.1200/JCO.2005.04.9544)
  *Protracted venous infusion during post-op CRT better than bolus
  *No benefit to semustine
  - Phase III
  - 660 patients; Stages II or III
  - Randomized to
    - Post-op radiation with bolus 5-FU ± semustine
    - Post-op radiation with PVI 5-FU ± semustine

	4-y OS (%)	4-y RFS (%)	DM (%)
PVI 5-FU regimens	70	63	40%
Bolus 5-FU regimens	60	53	31%

*PVI—more hand foot syndrome and diarrhea; Bolus—more heme toxicity

- **Preoperative Radiation Versus Surgery Alone**
  - *Improves rates of compliance, local control, sphincter preservation*
  - *Fewer early and late toxicities (smaller volume; APR scar not included)*
- **Stockholm I** (Cedermark, *Cancer*. 1990)
  - Phase III
  - 849 patients
  - AP/PA fields
  - Upper field border at L2
  - 25 Gy (5 fx)

	LR (%)	OS (%)	DFS (%)	Deaths in Elderly
Pre-Op XRT	12	30	72	8
Surgery alone	28	30	52	2
P-value	<.001		NS	

- **Stockholm II** (Cedermark, *Ann Surg Oncol.* 1996; Martling, *Cancer.* 2001; doi:10.1002/1097-0142(20010815)92:4<896::AID-CNCR1398>3.0.CO;2-R)
  - Phase III
  - 557 patients
  - Three- or four-field plans
  - Upper border mid L4
  - 25 Gy (5 fx)
  - No elderly patients

	LR (%)	OS (%)	OS (%)
Pre-op XRT and surgery	12	46	39 (all radiated patients ± surgery)
Surgery alone	25	39	36 (all patients without radiation)
P-value	<.001	.03	.02

- **Stockholm III** (Pettersson, *Br J Surg.* 2010; doi:10.1002/bjs.6914)
  - Phase III
  - 462 patients randomized to:
    - Short course pre-op radiation (25 Gy/5 fx) with immediate surgery
    - Short course pre-op radiation with surgery delayed 4 to 8 weeks
    - Long course pre-op radiation (50 Gy/25 fx)—surgery delayed 4 to 8 weeks
  - Short-course RT with immediate surgery had a more postoperative complications, but only if surgery was delayed beyond 10 days after the start of RT

	pCR (%)	Dworak G4 Regression (%)
Short course immediate surgery	1.7	1.7
Short course delayed surgery	11.8	10.1
Long course delayed surgery		

- **Swedish Study** (Pahlman, *N Engl J Med.* 1997; doi:10.1056/NEJM199704033361402; Folkesson, *J Clin Oncol.* 2005; doi:10.1200/JCO.2005.08.144)
  *This is the only pre-op short course radiation trial demonstrating improved OS:
  - Phase III
  - 1,168 patients less than 80 years old
  - Three- or four-field plans
  - Upper border mid L5
  - 25 Gy (5 fx)
  - Surgery 1 week after radiation with no increase in post-op morbidity

- o Late toxicity:
  - Increased bowel frequency—20 BM/week versus 10/week with surgery alone
  - Fecal incontinence—62% versus 27% with surgery alone
  - Impaired social life—30% versus 10% with surgery alone

	9-y CSS (%)	5-y OS (%)	5-y DFS (%)	LR (%)
Surgery alone	65	48	65	27
Pre-Op XRT	74	58	74	11
P-value	.004	.004	.002	<.001

- **Dutch TME** (Kapiteijn, *N Engl J Med.* 2001; doi:10.1056/NEJMoa010580; Peeters, *Ann Surg.* 2007; doi:10.1097/01.sla.0000257358.56863.ce)
  *Tumors extending beyond peritoneal reflection—no benefit from pre-op radiation
  - o Phase III
  - o 1,861 patients; Stages I to IV
    *included stage I patients unlikely to benefit—diminished difference
  - o Mandatory post-op radiation for surgery only arm if margins ≤1 mm
    *but only 47% with + margin received post-op radiation without effect on LC
  - o Pre-op radiation did not improve LC for + margins, only for narrow or—margins

	2-y LR (%)	5-y LR (%)	5-y Incontinence (%)	5-y OS (%)
Surgery Alone	2	6	33	65
Pre-Op XRT	9	11	62	65
P-value	.004	.004	.002	

- **Preoperative Versus Postoperative Radiation With or Without Chemotherapy**
- **Swedish Trial** (Pahlman, *Ann Surg.* 1990;211(2):187–195)
  - o Phase III
  - o 471 patients
    - 236 received pre-op radiation (25 Gy/5 fx) and surgery 1 week later
    - 235 received post-op radiation (60 Gy/30 fx)—only Aster-Coller B2, C1, C2
  - o 5-year survival NSS (~50%)

	LR (%)	5-y LR Probability (%)	Perioperative Complications (%)
Post-Op	21	26.8	18
Pre-Op	12	12.5	33
P-value	.02		<.01

- **MRC CR07/NCIC-CTG C0160** (Sebag-Montefiore, *Lancet*. 2009; doi:10.1016/S0140-6736(09)60484-0)
  *Pre-op radiation better than post-op radiation chemoradiation
  - Phase III
  - 1,350 patients with clinically resectable rectal cancer
  - Randomized to:
    - Pre-op short course radiation (25 Gy/5 fx) then TME
    - TME then selective post-op chemoradiation (45 Gy/25 fx) + 5-FU for involved CRM

	LR (%)	3-y DFS (%)	3-y OS
Pre-op XRT	4.4	77.5	
Post-op CRT	10.6	71.5	
P-value	.04	SS	NSS

- **German CAO/ARO/AIO-94** (Sauer, *N Engl J Med*. 2004; doi:10.1056/NEJMoa040694)
  *LC benefit but no survival benefit associated with pre-op radiation versus post-op CRT
  *Better compliance with pre-op CRT (92% vs. 54% post-op)
  *Better sphincter preservation with pre-op CRT
  - Phase III
  - 823 patients with T3/4 or N+ rectal cancer
  - Randomized to
    - Pre-op CRT (50.4 Gy/28 fx) + 5-FU (4 cycles total) + surgery
    - Surgery and post-op CRT (50.4 Gy/28 fx + 5.4 Gy/3 fx) + 5-FU (5 cycles)
      *5-FU bolus (days 1–5; weeks 1 + 5; 1,000 mg/m²/day)

	5-y LR (%)	5-y DM (%)	5-y DFS (%)	5-y OS (%)	Toxicity (%)	APR→LAR
Post-op	13	38	65	74	40	19
Pre-op	6	36	68	76	27	39
P-value	.006	.84	.32	.8	.001	.004

*pCR with pre-op CRT 8%
*18% post-op group overstaged and excluded

- **NSABP R-03** (Roh, *J Clin Oncol*. 2009; doi:10.1200/JCO.2009.22.0467)
  - Phase III—closed early
  - 267 patients (intended 900)
  - Randomized to
    - Pre-op CRT (50.4 Gy) + 5-FU/leu
    - Post-op CRT (50.4 Gy) + 5-FU/leu
  - pCR 15% for pre-op CRT

	5-y DFS (%)	5-y DM (%)	Sphincter Preservation (%)
Post-op	53.4	65.6	24.2
Pre-op	64.7	74.4	33.9
P-value	.11	.06	.13

- **Preoperative Radiation Versus Preoperative Chemoradiation**
  *Pre-op CRT improves pCR over pre-op radiation alone (15% vs. 5%).
  *Pre-op CRT improves LC over pre-op radiation alone (90% vs. 80%).
  *Pre-op CRT does not improve OS compared to pre-op radiation alone.
  *Pre-op CRT does not improve sphincter preservation compared to pre-op radiation alone.
- **Colorectal Cancer Collaborative Group** (*Lancet*. 2001;358:1291-1305; doi:10.1016/S0140-6736(01)06409-1)
  - o Meta-analysis of 22 randomized comparisons:
    - 6,350 pre-op radiation (14 trials)
    - 2,157 post-op radiation (8 trials)
    - No radiation

	OS (%)	Curative Resection (%)	LR (%)
Pre-op radiation	62 NSS	85	22.5
Post-op radiation			12.5
No radiation	63	86 NSS	

- **TROG 9801** (Ngan, *Dis Colon Rectum*. 2005; doi:10.1007/s10350-005-0032-x)
  *CRT with capecitabine equivalent outcome compared to PVI 5-FU
  - o Phase II; T3–4
  - o 82 patients
  - o Pre-op CRT (50.4 Gy) with CI 5-FU
  - o 4-year OS 82%
  - o 4-year DFS 69%
  - o 4-year LF 4%
- **EORTC 22921** (Bosset, *Eur J Cancer*. 2004; doi:10.1016/j.ejca.2003.09.032; *N Engl J Med*. 2006; doi:10.1056/NEJMoa060829)
  *Local control benefit from chemotherapy is similar whether it is pre-op or post-op.
  *Pre-op CRT produces more downstaging than radiation alone.
  - o Phase III
  - o 1,101 patients with clinically resectable rectal cancer
  - o Randomized to:
    - Pre-op radiation (45 Gy/25 fx)
    - Pre-op CRT (45 Gy/25 fx) + 5-FU/leu x 2 + TME
    - Pre-op radiation (45 Gy/25 fx) + TME + post-op 5-FU/leu (3–10 weeks after surgery × 4 cycles Q 3 weeks)
    - Pre-op CRT (45 Gy/25 fx) + 5-FU/leu × 2 + TME + post-op 5-FU/leu × 4

	LC (%) ($P = .02$)
Pre-op Chemo	91.3
Pre + Post Chemo	92.4
Post-op Chemo	90.4
XRT alone	82.9

*Pre-op chemo—82% completed all cycles versus 42.9% for post-op chemo
*NSS difference in 5-year OS between pre- and post-op chemo (64.8% vs. 65.8%)

- **FFCD 9203** (Gerard, *J Clin Oncol.* 2006; doi:10.1200/JCO.2006.06.7629)
  - Phase III
  - 733 patients with clinically resectable T3–4N0 rectal cancer
  - Randomized to:
    - Pre-op radiation (45 Gy/25 fx) + post-op 5-FU/leu × 4
    - Pre-op CRT (45 Gy/25 fx) + 5-FU/leu × 2 + post-op 5-FU/leu × 4

	5-y OS (%)	5-y LR (%)	pCR (%)	Sphincter Preservation (%)	Gr3–4 Toxicity (%)
XRT	67	16.5	3.6	52	2.7
CRT	67	8.1	11.4	52	14.6
P-value	NS	<.05	<.05	NS	<.05

*No difference in sphincter preservation

- **Polish** (Bujko, *Radio Oncol.* 2006; doi:10.1016/j.radonc.2006.04.012)
  *Pre-op CRT is equivalent to pre-op radiation alone for sphincter preservation.
  *10% have extension greater than 0.5 cm beyond negative margin after CRT.
  - Phase III
  - 312 patients with clinically T3–4 resectable rectal cancer
  - Randomized to:
    - Pre-op short course radiation (25 Gy/5 fx)
    - Pre-op CRT (50.4 Gy/25 fx) + 5-FU/leu × 2

	Sphincter Preservation (%)	Acute Radiation Toxicity (%)
XRT	61	3.2
CRT	58	18.2
P-value	.57	

- **TROG 0104** (Ngan, *J Clin Oncol.* 2012; doi:10.1200/JCO.2012.42.9597)
  - Phase III
  - 326 patients
  - Randomized
    - Pre-op 25 Gy (5 fx)
    - Pre-op 50.4 Gy (28 fx) with CI 5-FU

	3-y LR (%)	5-y OS (%)
Short-course	7.5	74
Standard fractionation	4.4 NSS	70 NSS

- **NSABP R-04** (Allegra, *J Clin Oncol.* 2014)
  *CRT with capecitabine equivalent outcome compared to PVI 5-FU
  - Phase III
  - 1,608 patients; Stages II or III
  - Randomized to:
    - Pre-op CRT (50.4 Gy) with capecitabine ± oxaliplatin
    - Pre-op CRT with PVI 5-FU ± oxaliplatin
  - CRT with PVI 5-FU or capecitabine resulted in outcomes and toxicity
  - NSS differences in LR, DFS, or OS with addition of oxaliplatin
  - Addition of oxaliplatin associated with SS more grade 3 to 4 diarrhea ($P < .0001$).
  - 3-year LC rates—87.4% to 88.2%
  - 3-year LC rates with R0 resection
    - 2% to 4 % (stage II)
    - 4% to 11% (stage III)
- **ACCORD 12/0405-Prodige 2** (Gerard, *JCO*, 2012; doi:10.1200/JCO.2012.42.8771)
  *Pre-op CRT with weekly oxaliplatin and 5-FU results in higher toxicity without additional therapeutic benefit.
- **German CAO/ARO/AIO-04** (Rödel, *Lancet Oncol.* 2012; 2015; doi:10.1016/S1470-2045(15)00159-X)
  *Improved pCR rate 3-year DFS with oxaliplatin without increased toxicity
  - Phase III
  - 1,236 patients
  - Pre-op CRT with weekly oxaliplatin and 5-FU
- **Dose Escalation, Endocavitary Boost, and Hyperfractionation**
- **PMH** (Wiltshire, *Int J Radiat Oncol Biol Phys.* 2006; doi:10.1016/j.ijrobp.2005.08.012)
  *Improved result with doses ≥46 Gy; no difference between 46 and 50 Gy.
  - Retrospective review of three phase II studies of pre-op CRT
  - 134 patients; T2N1–2 or T3–4N0–2
  - All patients received CI 5-FU
  - 121 patients underwent surgical resection

	pCR (%)	2-y LC (%)	2-y DFS (%)	2-y OS (%)
40 (20 fx)	15	72	62	72
46 (23 fx)	23	90	84	94
50 (25 fx)	33	89	78	92

- **Lyon R96.02** (Gerard, *J Clin Oncol.* 2004; doi:10.1200/JCO.2004.08.170; *J Clin Oncol.* 2007)
  *Dose escalation using endocavitary boost is feasible and well-tolerated.
  - Randomized
  - 88 patients; low rectal; T2–3Nx <2/3 circumference
  - Pre-op radiation (39 Gy/13 fx) ± endocavitary brachy boost of 85 Gy/3
  - No difference in morbidity, OS, or LR

	cCR (%)	pCR (%)	Sphincter Preservation (%)
XRT	20	10	44
XRT + EC	213	35	76

- **RTOG 00-12** (Mohiuddin, *J Clin Oncol.* 2006; doi:10.1200/JCO.2005.03.6095; *Int J Radiat Oncol Biol Phys.* 2013; doi:10.1016/j.ijrobp.2013.02.020)
  *No benefit to pre-op radiation with hyperfractionation and results in a higher rate of second cancers (five times the rate of standard fractionation)
  o Randomized phase II
  o 106 patients; T3–4N0–2
  o 46 Gy + 9.6-14.4 Gy boost (1.2 Gy BID) + CI 5-FU
  o 50.4 Gy with CI 5-FU/irinotecan
  o 102 patients underwent surgical resection

	pCR (%)	LR (%)	5-y DSS (%)	5-y OS (%)
Hyperfractionation	30	16	78	61
Standard fractionation	26	17	85	75

- **Induction Chemotherapy and Neoadjuvant Chemoradiation**
- **MSKCC** (Cercek, *K Natl Compr Canc Net.* 2014)
  o Retrospective
  o 300 high-risk rectal cancer patients
  o 61 received neoadjuvant FOLFOX (median 7 cycles)
  o 4 with cCRT declined CRT
  o 51 received CRT after FOLFOX
  o 49 underwent TME
  o 100% R0 resection
  o 27% pCR rate
  o 47% with tumor response >90%
- **MSKCC** (Garcia-Aguilar, *Ann Surg.* 2011; doi:10.1097/SLA.0b013e3182196e1f)
  o CRT without induction FOLFOX 18% pCR rate, whereas patients who received FOLFOX the following CRT
  o 25% pCR rate (2 cycles)
  o 30% pCR rate (4 cycles)
  o 38% pCR rate (6 cycles)
  o 80% received the prescribed regimen without interruption
- **Grupo Cancer de Recto Study GCR-3** (Fernandez-Martos, *Ann Oncol.* 2015; doi:10.1093/annonc/mdv223)
- Randomized phase II trial
- 108 patients; T3–4 or N+
- Pre-op CRT + capecitabine/oxaliplatin (CAPOX) + surgery + adjuvant CAPOX × 4
- Induction CAPOX + CRT and surgery

	pCR (%)	5-y OS (%)	5-y DFS (%)	5-y DM (%)	5-y LR (%)
Pre-op CRT + adjuvant CAPOX	13.5	78	64	2	21
Induction CAPOX + CRT	14.3 NSS	75 NSS	62 NSS	5 NSS	23 NSS

*Neoadjuvant approach associated with better toxicity profiles and improved compliance

- **Omission of Radiation**
  *Evidence surmounts supporting the feasibility of delivering chemotherapy in the neoadjuvant setting with selective use of pelvic radiation.
  *The rationale for early systemic chemotherapy is based on the fact that more patients with locally advanced rectal cancer develop distant metastases than local recurrences.

Study	#Patients/Inclusion Criteria	Treatment	R0 (%)	pCR (%)	LF (%)	DF (%)	OS (%)
Ischii	26/T3–4,N0–2	5-FU irinotecan	100	3.8	11.5	7.7	5-y 84
Cercek	6/T2–3N1	FOLFOX	100	33.3	0	16.7	NR
Uehara	32/MRI defined poor-risk Disease, T3anyN, T4N2, + CRM	CAPOX-bevacizumab	84	12.5	NR	NR	NR
Schrag	32/T3anyN,T2N15–12 cm from verge	FOLFOX-bevacizumab	100	25	0	12.5	4-y 91.6
Fernandez-Martos	28/T3, middle third, >2 mm from mesorectal fascia	CAPOX-bevacizumab	96	14.3	NR	NR	NR

- Ongoing Trials:
  - PROSPECT: Chemotherapy Alone or Chemotherapy Plus RT in Treating Patients With Locally Advanced Rectal Cancer Undergoing Surgery. *https://clinicaltrials.gov/ct2/show/NCT01515787*
  - Bevacizumab and Combination Chemotherapy in Rectal Cancer Until Surgery (BACCHUS). *https://clinicaltrials.gov/ct2/show/NCT01650428*
  - Neoadjuvant FOLFOX6 Chemotherapy With or Without Radiation in Rectal Cancer (FOWARC). *https://clinicaltrials.gov/ct2/show/NCT01211210*
- **MERCURY** (MRI and Rectal Cancer European Equivalence) (Taylor, *J Clin Oncol.* 2014; doi:10.1200/JCO.2012.45.3258)
  - Prospective observational study
  - 92% accuracy of MRI in predicting a curative resection
  - 374 patients with rectal cancer
  - MRI involvement of CRM was the only preoperative staging factor predictive of LR
- Despite demonstrating its value in preoperative evaluation of these patients, the clinical utility of MRI-based preoperative staging remains somewhat controversial.
  - **EXPERT-C** (Dewdney, *J Clin Oncol.* 2012; doi:10.1200/JCO.2011.39.6036) and **RAPIDO** (Nilsson, *BMC Cancer.* 2013. doi:10.1186/1471-2407-13-279) trials incorporate MRI risk stratification for selective use of radiation

Radiation Technique

- Three to four fields using 3D CRT treated prone with belly board and full bladder
- IMRT may be appropriate in certain cases for
  - Inability to meet normal tissue dose constraints (usually small bowel with extensive PAN adenopathy)
  - Reirradiation after recurrent disease
- Dose:
  - 45 Gy (1.8 Gy/fx) with boost to 50.4 Gy for pre-op patients
  - 45 Gy (1.8 Gy/fx) with boost to 50.4 Gy post-op or 54 Gy for high-risk patients
  - 45 Gy (1.8 Gy/fx) with boost to 54 Gy for inoperable patients

- Radiation field should include the tumor or tumor bed with 2- to 5-cm margin and include:
  - Presacral and internal iliac nodes for all patients
  - External iliac nodes for T4 tumors involving anterior structures
  - Scar with 1.5-cm margin and bolus for post-op APR patients
- IORT (10–20 Gy) should be considered for close or positive margins, T4 tumors or recurrent disease.
- PVI 5-FU or trice daily radiosensitizing capecitabine should be given concurrently.
- Female patients should be counseled regarding fertility options, and vaginal stenosis.
- Male patients should be counseled regarding fertility options.
- In patients with a limited number of lung or liver metastases, preoperative pelvic radiation can be considered in highly selective cases treated with curative intent and should not take the place of surgery.
- Normal tissue dose constraints:
  - Small bowel:
    - No more than 200 mL above 30 Gy
    - No more than 150 mL above 35 Gy
    - No more than 20 mL above 45 Gy
    - None above 50 Gy
  - Femoral heads:
    - No more than 50% above 30 Gy
    - No more than 35% above 40 Gy
    - No more than 5% above 44 Gy
  - Iliac crests:
    - No more than 50% above 30 Gy
    - No more than 35% above 40 Gy
    - No more than 5% above 50 Gy
  - External genitalia:
    - No more than 50% above 20 Gy
    - No more than 35% above 30 Gy
    - No more than 5% above 40 Gy
  - Bladder:
    - No more than 50% above 35 Gy
    - No more than 35% above 40 Gy
    - No more than 5% above 50 Gy
  - Large bowel:
    - No more than 200 mL above 30 Gy
    - No more than 150 mL above 35 Gy
    - No more than 20 mL above 45 Gy

Palliation

- Approximately 50% to 60% of patients with colorectal cancer will develop metastases.
- Approximately 80% to 90% of these will develop liver metastases.
- Management includes:
  - Palliative chemotherapy
    - FOLFOX
    - FOLFIRI
  - Palliative radiation for symptomatic sites of metastases
- If oligometastatic disease is in the liver:
  - Surgical resection—5-year DFS 20% and 5-year OS 38% for carefully chosen patients.
  - Carefully chosen patients with low volume favorable disease can be treated with neoadjuvant chemotherapy and convert to resectable disease (limited liver resection and standard rectal resection), with evaluation for resectability every 2 months during chemotherapy.

- o Liver-directed therapies are more controversial and include RFA, TACE, conformal CRT, and SBRT, usually resulting in increased time to progression.
- Oligometastatic disease in the lung can also be treated with resection or SBRT(controversial).
- Optimal candidates for aggressive treatment of oligometastatic disease include:
  *Prognosis following resection of pulmonary and liver metastases does not appear to be affected by synchronous versus metachronous presentation.
  - o Potential for R0 resection with curative intent
  - o The ability to preserve two contiguous hepatic segments
  - o Preservation of vascular inflow and outflow as well as biliary drainage
  - o The ability to preserve an adequate functional reserve

Follow-Up

- History/physical every 3 to 6 months for 2 years, then every 6 months for total of 5 years
- CEA every 3 to 6 months for 2 years, then every 6 months for total 5 years for T2 or higher
- CT CAP every year for 5 years for patients at high risk for recurrence
- Colonoscopy annually
  - o If adenoma repeat in 1 year
  - o If no adenoma repeat in 3 years then every 5 years

2.6 Anal Cancer

Epidemiology and Risk Factors

- Increasing incidence over the past several decades but remains uncommon
  - o Approximately 7,270 new cases in the United States per year
  - o Approximately 1,010 anal cancer deaths in the United States per year
- Approximately 4% of all lower GI cancers
- Average age at diagnosis approximately 60
- Approximately 60% occur in women
- Approximately 30% involve nodes at diagnosis
- Less than 10% of patients have distant metastases at the time of diagnosis
- 75% to 80% squamous cell carcinoma, arises near the squamocolumnar junction
  - o Keratinizing (basaloid)
  - o Nonkeratinizing (cloacogenic)
- Squamous cell carcinoma of perianal skin/anal verge generally treated as skin cancer
- Other histologies include:
  - o Adenocarcinoma
    - ■ Have higher local and distant failure rate
    - ■ Treat with definitive CRT and APR should be reserved for salvage
- Risk factors:
  - o HPV infection (HPV 16 and 18)
    - ■ 16 detected in approximately 85% to90% anal cancers
    - ■ History of anal warts (HPV)
    - ■ History of cervical, vaginal, or vulvar cancers
  - o AIDS especially if CD4 <200
    - ■ Not considered AIDS defining illness
  - o >10 sexual partners
  - o History of anal intercourse
  - o History of STDs
  - o Smoking
  - o Immunosuppression for transplant

Prognosis

- Anal cancer is usually curable.
- 5-year OS rate is 65.5% in the United States.
- 5-year OS rate is approximately 20% if LNs are involved.
- There is an improved survival if treatment is completed in <74 days (Allal, *Cancer*. 1997; doi:10.1002/(SICI)1097-0142(19970615)79:12<2329::AID-CNCR6>3.0.CO;2-G).
- Vaginal mucosa involvement predicts fistula formation with CRT.
- Prognostic factors for poor OS are:
  - Site (anal canal vs. perianal skin)
  - Size (size >5 cm)
  - Involved nodes
  - Male sex
  - HPV or p16 positivity are prognostic for improved OS
- In 2010, the U.S. FDA approved Gardasil vaccine to prevent anal cancer and precancerous lesions in males and females aged 9 to 26 years, in addition to cervical, vulvar, and vaginal cancer, and associated lesions caused by HPV types 6, 11, 16, and 18 in women.
- Routine screening for anal intraepithelial neoplasm (AIN) in high-risk populations (e.g., HIV) is controversial and randomized trials have not shown reduction in cancer incidence and mortality in these populations.

Anatomy

- The anal region comprises:
  - Anal margin
    - Starts at the anal verge and includes 5- to 6-cm radius of skin from the squamous mucocutaneous junction
    - Covered by epidermous and not squamous mucosa
  - Anal canal
    - Borders: Anorectal ring superiorly to anal verge inferiorly approximately 3 to 5 cm
    - The anorectal ring is a palpable ring formed by the junction of the upper internal sphincter, distal puborectalis, and deep portion of the external sphincter
    - Covered by squamous mucosa
    - The dentate line (or pectinate line) forms the bottom of the transition zone in which the columnar epithelium of the rectum transitions into the squamous epithelium of the lower anal canal
    - Lymphatic drainage:
      - Perianal skin, anal verge, canal distal to the dentate line → superficial inguinal nodes (with some communications to the femoral nodes and to the external iliac systems)
      - Around and above the dentate line → internal pudendal, hypogastric, and obturator nodes of the internal iliac systems
      - Proximal canal → perirectal and superior hemorrhoidal nodes of the inferior mesenteric system
- Disease may also spread by direct extension into surrounding tissues such as the rectovaginal septum or prostate.
- Hematogenous spread to the liver or lungs is less common (<10%).

Presentation

Symptoms of anal cancer can include:
- Anal discomfort
  - Tenesmus
  - Pain
- Change in bowel habits
- Mass near the anus
- Rectal bleeding
- Pruritis
- Less than 5% fecal incontinence due to sphincter destruction

Diagnosis and Workup

- Physical Exam should include:
  - Palpation of inguinal LNs
  - Inspection of the perineum
  - DRE
  - Anoscopy
  - Full pelvic exam with pap smear to rule out second primary and/or direct invasion
- CBC
  CEA not useful
- HIV if risk factors/CD4 count
- Proctoscopy with biopsy
- Biopsy or FNA if suspicious inguinal nodes on exam
- CXR or CT chest
- CT or MR of abd/pelvis
- Consider PET-CT for cT2–4N0 or any T, N+
- Transanal ultrasound to be considered especially if local excision considered

Staging

AJCC/UICC 2010 TNM classification for anal cancer is outlined.
- Tis—Carcinoma in situ (Bowen's disease, high-grade dysplasia, intraepithelial lesion (HSIL), anal intraepithelial neoplasia II to III (AIN II–III)
- T1—Tumor 2 cm or less in greatest dimension
- T2—Tumor more than 2 cm but not greater than 5 cm in greatest dimension
- T3—Tumor more than 5 cm in greatest dimension
- T4—Tumor invades adjacent structures (vagina, urethra bladder)
  Note: Direct invasion of the rectal wall, perirectal skin, subcutaneous tissue, or sphincter muscle is not classified as T4.
- N0—No regional LN metastasis
  - N1—Metastasis in perirectal node(s)
  - N2—Metastasis in unilateral internal iliac and/or inguinal nod(s)
  - N3—Metastasis in perirectal and inguinal nodes and/or bilateral internal iliac and/or inguinal nodes
- M0—No distant metastasis
  - M1—Distant metastasis (M1a and M1b are site dependent)

Stage Classification

Stage	T	N	M
Stage 0	Tis	N0	M0
Stage I	T1	N0	M0
Stage II	T2	N0	M0
	T3	N0	M0
Stage IIIA	T1–3	N1	M0
	T4	N0	M0
Stage IIIB	T4	N1	M0
	Any T	N2	M0
	Any T	N3	M0
Stage IV	Any T	Any N	M1

Treatment Overview

Surgery

- Historically all patients treated with abdominoperinoneal resection (APR—removes internal and external sphincters resulting in permanent colostomy)
  - 5-year OS 40% to 70%
  - LR rates high
- Early stage disease
  - Tis and precursor lesions (anal dysplasia or AIN)—ablation with minimally invasive methods such as infrared photocoagulation
  - T1N0—local excision results in greater than 90% LC if patients carefully selected
    - Properly staged
    - No involvement of anal sphincter
    - Small less than 2 cm
    - Moderately to well differentiated
    - Less than 40% circumferential involvement
    - Compliant patients only since close follow-up required

Mayo Clinic Data (Boman, *Cancer*. 1984;54(1):114–125)
- Retrospective
  - 188 patients
    - 13 patients with T1 lesions with minimal invasion treated with local excision
      - 5-year OS 71%
      - 1 required an APR for LR
    - 114 patients (not just T1) treated with APR alone
      - 40% LR

Interstitial Brachytherapy (James, *Br J Surg*. 1985; doi:10.1002/bjs.1800720411)
- Small, node-negative anal canal cancer
- LC for tumors less than 5 cm—64%
- LC for tumors greater than 5 cm—23%
- OS 60% for tumors less than 5 cm
- OS 30% for tumors greater than 5 cm
- 82% with LC retained normal anal function
- No direct comparison of brachytherapy to chemoradiation has been made
- Stages I to III—***Definitive CRT***
  - In the 1970s, neoadjuvant chemoradiation was pioneered at Wayne State University by Dr. Norman Nigro to reduce recurrence rate after APR.
    - The Nigro regimen consisted of:
      - 5-FU (1,000 mg/m^2/d CI days 1 to 4 and 29 to 32)
      - Mitomycin-C bolus (15 mg/m^2 on day 1)
      - Concurrent 30 Gy (2 Gy/fx), AP/PA to pelvis and inguinals

Wayne State (Leichman, *Am J Med*. 1985; doi:10.1016/0002-9343(85)90428-0)
*Established CRT is definitive treatment for anal cancer.
- 45 patients with ≥T2 (>2 cm)
- Nigro regimen
- Originally, all patients received an APR but 5/6 initial patients had a pCR; after this the APR was performed only for positive biopsy
- Posttreatment biopsy at 4 to 6 weeks
  - If residual tumor found then APR
    - All patients with positive biopsy had recurrence and died of cancer

- If biopsy negative then observe
  - No patient with negative biopsy had LR
  - 84% CR rate with CRT
  - 89% 4-year OS if negative biopsy

RTOG 83-14 (Sischy, *J Natl Cancer Inst.* 1989; doi:10.1093/jnci/81.11.850)
*Established CRT is definitive treatment for anal cancer.
- 79 patients with T1–4, N0
- Nigro regimen with MMC (**10 mg/m² day 2**) and 40.8 Gy (170 cGy/fx, 24 fx)
- Biopsy 6 to 8 weeks posttreatment
- APR if biopsy positive
- 10% positive biopsies

	1-y OS (%)	3-y OS (%)	3-y DFS (%)
CRT	97	73	61

CRT Versus Radiation Alone

- **ACT I—UKCCCR** (*Lancet.* 1996;348(9034):1049–1054. Northover, *Br J Cancer.* 2010; doi:10.1038/sj.bjc.6605605)
  *CRT is better than XRT alone.
  - 585 patients all stages including M1 but not T1N0
  - Randomized to:
    - Radiation (*n* = 279) or
    - CRT (*n* = 293)
    - Nigro regimen with MMC (**12 mg/m² day 1**) + 45 Gy (20–25 fx)
    - After a 6-week break, if >50% response
      - Boost RT 15Gy/6 fxs to primary
      - Or 25Gy Ir192 implant
  - If <50% response, APR considered

	3-y LC (%)	3-y OS (%)	3-y CSS (%)
XRT	39	58	38
CRT	61	65	39
P-value	<.0001	.25	.02

EORTC (Bartelink, *J Clin Oncol.* 1997;15(5):2040-2049)
*CRT decreases LR and colostomy rates compared to radiation alone
- 110 patients all stages excluding M1, T1–2N0
- Randomized to:
  - Radiation or
  - CRT
  - Nigro regimen with MMC (**15 mg/m² day 1**) and 45 Gy (25 fx)
  - Reevaluate after 6-week break
    *Used different definitions of LF and CR than the UKCCR trial.
    - cCR: boost RT 15Gy/6 fxs to primary with photons, electrons or brachytherapy
    - cPR: boost 20 Gy
    - APR considered if inadequate response

	5-y LC (%)	5-y OS (%)	Initial Complete Response Rate (%)	5-y Colostomy FS (%)	5-y EFS
XRT	55	64	54	47	43
CRT	68	69	80	72	61
P-value	.02	.02	.02	.002	.03

PMH (Cummings, *Int J Radiat Oncol Biol Phys.* 1991;21(5):1115–1125)
*Reported that time for tumor regression was 2 to 36 months; median time 3 months
*Did not recommend biopsy at 4 to 6 weeks
- Retrospective review; 7 studies
- 192 patients
- Treatment
  - RT alone
  - CRT with MMC/5-FU (uninterrupted and split)
  - CRT with 5-FU

	5-y CSS (%)	LC (%)	5-y RFS (%)
Radiation alone	68	56	50
CRT with 5-FU	64	60	62
CRT with 5-FU + MMC	78	86	86
P-value	.02	SS	.001

Can MMC Be Omitted?

RTOG 87-04 (Flam, *J Clin Oncol.* 1996;14(9):2527-2539)
*Mitomycin C should not be omitted—improves OS and colostomy-free survival.
- 291 patients all stages excluding M1, T1–2N0
- Randomized to CRT (45–50.4 Gy/25–28 fx):
  - With concurrent 5-FU (per Nigro 1,000 mg/m^2/d × 4 days on days 1–4 and 28–31) and no MMC, or
  - Nigro regimen with MMC (**10 mg/m^2 day 1 and 28**)
  - 12% patients had a treatment break for skin toxicity
  - Reevaluate after 4- to 6-week break
    - If biopsy positive, then 9 Gy with 5-FU and cisplatin
    - Postsalvage biopsies after another 6 weeks
      - 22 who underwent salvage, 4-year DFS—50%
      - APR considered if post salvage biopsy positive

	Positive Biopsy (%)	4-y LC (%)	4-y Colostomy FS	4-y DFS (%)	4-y OS (%)	Toxicity
CRT no MMC	15	86	59	51	7	7
CRT + MMC	7.7	92	71	73	75	23
P-value	NS	NS	.014	.003	NS	SS

Dose Escalation

RTOG 92-08 (John, *Cancer J Sci Am*. 1996;2(4):205–211)
*Dose escalate with treatment with break does not improve toxicity or survival
- Phase II
- 147 patients
- CRT with CI 5-FU and MMC (**10 mg/m² day 1 and 28**) with concurrent XRT 59/6 Gy with planned 2-week treatment break
  *Higher colostomy rate may be related to treatment break

	Skin Toxicity (%)	Colostomy Rate (%)
RTOG 87-04	6	7
RTOG 92-08	23	30

Replacing MMC With Cisplatin

RTOG 98-11 (Ajani, *JAMA*. 2008. doi:10.1001/jama.299.16.1914; Gunderson, *J Clin Oncol*. (Abstract) 2011; 29(4_suppl):367)
*Mitomycin C is superior to cisplatin.
*Criticism: Did delay in CRT 54 days negatively impact cisplatin arm?
- Phase III; 649 patients; T2–4 anal cancer
- Randomized to:
  - CRT with 5-FU (1,000 mg/m²/d × 4 days on days 1–4 and 29–32) + MMC (10 mg/m² on days 1, 29) or
  - **Induction** chemo with 5-FU 1000 mg/m²/d on days 1–4, 29–32, and cisplatin (75 mg/m² on days 1,29) followed by the same chemotherapy concurrent with CRT starting day 54
- Radiation: 30.6 Gy to bony pelvis then 14.4-Gy boost with superior border at inferior SI joints), then optional boost to 55 to 59 Gy for
  - T3–4,N+, or
  - T2 with residual disease after 45 Gy

	5-y LR Rate (%)	5-y DFS (%)	5-y DM (%)	5-y OS (%)	G3 Heme Toxicity (%)	5-y Colostomy Rate (%)
MMC arm	25	60	15	75	60	10
Cisplatin arm	33	54	19	70	42	19
P-value	.07	.17	.14	.10	.00004	.02

CALGB 9281 (Merepol, *J Clin Oncol*. 2008; doi:10.1200/JCO.2008.16.2339)
*No advantage for neoadjuvant chemotherapy in poor prognosis anal cancer
- Phase III
- 45 patients; T3–4 and/or N2–3
- 5-FU/cisplatin × 2 followed by CRT (45 Gy with concurrent 5-FU/MMC × 2- and 9-Gy boost ± 1 additional cycle 5-FU/cisplatin (total dose 54 Gy)
- Included 2-week planned treatment break

4-y OS (%)	4-y DFS (%)	4-y Colostomy Rate (%)
768	61	23

Treatment Breaks

Pooled Analysis of RTOG 87-06 and 98-11 (Ben-Josef, *J Clin Oncol.* 2010; doi:10.1200/JCO.2010.29.1351)

*Total treatment time, but not duration of RT, seems to have a detrimental effect on local failure and colostomy rate in anal cancer.

*Induction chemotherapy may contribute to local failure by increasing total treatment time.

*Age, sex, KPS, T stage, N stage, and radiation dose, but not radiation duration, were found to be statistically significant predictors of OS and colostomy-free survival.

ECOG E4292 (Chakravarthy, *Int J Radiat Oncol Biol Phys.* 2011; doi:10.1016/j.ijrobp.2011.02.042)

- Phase II; 33 patients
- 45 Gy to primary tumor and pelvic nodes, boost to primary and involved nodes to 59.4 Gy with planned 2-week treatment break after 36 Gy
- Concurrent chemotherapy 5-FU (1,000 mg/m^2/day on days 1–4 and cisplatin, 75 mg/m^2 on day 1) repeated after 36 Gy, when XRT resumed
- 5-year OS 69%

Objective Response Rate (CR +PR) (%)	Complete Clinical Response (%) All Patients	Complete Clinical Response in Patients Who Did Not Have Break (%)	Complete Clinical Response In Patients With Break (%)
97	78	92	68

ACT II—Second UKCCCR Trial: Chemoradiation and Maintenance Therapy for Anal Cancer (James, *ASCO.* (Abstract) 2009; Glynne-Jones, *ASCO.* (Abstract) 2012)

- Addressed two questions:
  - Does replacing MMC with cisplatin improve the CR rate?
  - Does adding 2 cycles of maintenance chemo (5-FU, cisplatin) reduce recurrence?
- Phase III; 940 pts
- All pts: 5-FU (1,000 mg/m^2/day on d1–4 and 29–32 and 50.4 Gy (28 fx_)
  - Randomization 1 (2 × 2 design)
    - MMC (**12 mg/m^2**, d1) or
    - Cisplatin (60 mg/m^2 on d1 and 29)
  - Randomization 2
    - 2 cycles of cisplatin and 5-FU weeks 11 and 14 or
    - No maintenance chemo
- 5-year follow-up suggests an equivalence between radiation with 5-FU and MMC and radiation with 5-FU and CDDP

Capecitabine (Glynne-Jones, *Int J Radiat Oncol Biol Phys.* 2008; doi:10.1016/j.ijrobp.2007.12.012)

- Phase II study
- 31 pts, all stages, HIV−
- CRT 50.4 Gy (28 fx) with MMC (12 mg/m^2 on day 1) and capecitabine 825-mg/m^2 PO BID on 5 days a week during radiation
- 81% completed planned radiation
- 68% received full chemo
- Response evaluation after 4 weeks by imaging and/or clinical exam
  - 77% CR
  - 16% PR
- Median f/u 14 months
  - 10% LR
  - Conclusion: effective and tolerated

IMRT

Duke (Kachnic, *Int J Radiat Oncol Biol Phys.* 2009; doi:10.1016/j.ijrobp.2010.09.030)
- Phase II trial of IMRT to reduce toxicity
- 29 patients
- Median dose 54 Gy with concurrent 5-FU/MMC

2-y OS (%)	LF (%)	G3 Diarrhea (%)	G3-4 Heme Tox (%)	Tx Break (%)
100	5	10	24	24

RTOG 05-29 Dose Painting (Kachnic, *Int J Radiat Oncol Biol Phys.* 2009; doi:10.1016/j.ijrobp.2010.09.030)
- Phase II trial of IMRT to reduce toxicity
- 63 patients
- T2 62%, 56% node negative
- T2+, N0–3, no mets
- Chemo: 5-FU (1,000 mg/m^2/day, 96 hour CI) and MMC (10 mg/m^2 IV bolus) on days 1 and 29 of RT
- T2 N0: 42 Gy delivered in 1.5 Gy daily fractions to elective nodal regions, with 50.4 Gy delivered in 1.8 Gy daily fractions to the primary anal tumor simultaneously
- T2 N1–3 and T3–4 N0–3: 45 Gy delivered in 1.5 Gy daily fractions to elective nodal regions, 50.4 Gy in 1.68-Gy daily fractions to nodes 3 cm or less, 54 Gy in 1.8-Gy daily fractions to primary tumor and nodes greater than 3 cm
- Patients were treated in prone position and most plans required seven to nine fields.
- 67% complete response at 8 weeks

	G2 (%)	G3/4 Tox (%)	> G3 Derm Tox (%)	Median TX Duration (Days)	Treatment Breaks (%)
RTOG 05-29	69	22	20	42.5	49
RTOG 98-11 (MMC arm)	81	36	47	49	61
P-value	.038	.014	<.001	<.001	.01

- Because of encouraging results, IMRT is deemed "usually appropriate" outside of a clinical trial setting although 75% of plans required revision after central review; of these 50% required rerevision of second submitted plan.
- **Special Populations: HIV+**
- **Hoffman** (*Int J Radiat Oncol Biol Phys.* 1999)
  o Retrospective
  o 17 HIV+ patients
- **Salvage APR after CRT**

	Hospitalizations (#)	Colostomy (#)
CD4 ≥200	0	0
CD4 <200	4	4

o   Biopsy at 6 weeks is not necessary, and can lead to fistula formation.
o   Reserve APR for salvage.
o   Regression continues for 3 to 12 months after CRT.

Ellenhorn (*Annals Surg Oncol.* 1994; doi:10.1007/BF02303552)
- Retrospective
- 38 pts treated with RT + 5-FU + MMC
- OS 5 years was 44% when salvage APR

Radiation Technique

- Dose
   o   The appropriate radiation dose for anal cancer has not been fully elucidated.
   o   A minimum dose is at least 45 Gy (25 fx) for T1N0.
   o   Conventionally, doses of radiation between 50.4 and 59.4 Gy are appropriate for more advanced:
      ▪   Two studies suggest that doses in excess of 55.8 Gy result in higher LC than lower doses (Rich, *Radiother Oncol.* 1993; doi:10.1016/0167-8140(93)90076-K; Fung, *Int J Radiat Oncol Biol Phys.* 1993).
      ▪   Increased radiation dose, however, did not increase LC when given with split-course in a phase II RTOG study, so a maximum dose of 59 Gy is considered standard.
   o   If the use of IMRT in RTOG 05-29 yields expected tumor control rates while minimizing toxicity, IMRT could be used to safely explore dose escalation.
- Split-course of radiation is not recommended.
   o   If there is significant skin breakdown, a treatment break of no more than 10 days is currently allowed by the most recent RTOG protocol.
- Technique
   o   3D conformal or IMRT should be used with CT for treatment planning.
   o   PET CT should be considered for treatment planning.
   o   Attempts should be made to limit dose to femoral heads.
   o   Sequential cone-downs:
      ▪   Inguinal nodes and pelvis, anus and perineum should be included in initial radiation field with superior border approximately L5-S1 treated to 30.6 Gy
      ▪   Superior border at bottom of SI joints for 14.4 Gy
      ▪   If inguinal nodes uninvolved, reduce field off inguinal nodes at 36 Gy
   o   For T2 lesions with persistent disease after 45 Gy, T3–4 lesions or N+, boost another 9 to 14 Gy to initially involved sites (total dose 54–59 Gy/30–32 fx).
   o   Treatment should take 6 to 7.5 weeks.
- Female patients should be counseled regarding fertility options, and vaginal stenosis.
- Male patients should be counseled regarding fertility options.
- Normal tissue dose constraints:
   o   Small bowel:
      ▪   No more than 200 mL above 30 Gy
      ▪   No more than 150 mL above 35 Gy
      ▪   No more than 20 mL above 45 Gy
      ▪   None above 50 Gy
   o   Femoral heads:
      ▪   No more than 50% above 30 Gy
      ▪   No more than 35% above 40 Gy
      ▪   No more than 5% above 44 Gy
   o   Iliac crests:
      ▪   No more than 50% above 30 Gy
      ▪   No more than 35% above 40 Gy

- No more than 5% above 50 Gy
  - External genitalia:
    - No more than 50% above 20 Gy
    - No more than 35% above 30 Gy
    - No more than 5% above 40 Gy
  - Bladder:
    - No more than 50% above 35 Gy
    - No more than 35% above 40 Gy
    - No more than 5% above 50 Gy
  - Large bowel:
    - No more than 200 mL above 30 Gy
    - No more than 150 mL above 35 Gy
    - No more than 20 mL above 45 Gy

Palliation

- Metastatic or recurrent anal cancer is difficult to treat, and usually requires chemotherapy.
  - Platinum
  - Doxorubicin
  - 5-FU or capecitabine
  - 5-FU, Taxol, Carboplatin
- Radiation is also employed to palliate specific locations causing symptoms.
- Diverting colostomy may be used for obstruction.
- Median survival rates for patients with distant metastases ranges from 8 to 34 months.

Follow-Up

- DRE, inguinal node palpation, anoscopy every 3 to 6 months for 5 years
- Chest/abdomen/pelvis annually for 3 years

Chapter 2: Practice Questions

1. Ideal dose fractionations for unresectable pancreatic cancer includes the following EXCEPT

   A. 40 Gy in 20 fractions
   B. 45 Gy in 25 fractions
   C. 50.4 Gy in 28 fractions
   D. 54 Gy in 30 fractions

2. Colorectal adenocarcinomas occur in what percentage of all colorectal cancers

   A. 60%
   B. 90%
   C. 95%
   D. 98%

3. The least frequent form of hepatobiliary cancer is

   A. Intrahepatic cholangiocarcinoma
   B. Extrahepatic cholangiocarcinoma
   C. Gallbladder
   D. Hepatocellular

4. Rates of gastric cancer have declined over the last 100 years due to the following EXCEPT

    A. Refrigeration
    B. Screening with imaging
    C. Decreased H. pylori infection
    D. Decrease salt intake

5. A gastric cancer patient with 20 regional lymph nodes is N-staged as

    A. N1
    B. N2
    C. N3a
    D. N3b

6. The lower esophagus directly drains into all of the following nodal areas EXCEPT

    A. Left gastric
    B. Celiac
    C. Gastrohepatic
    D. Posterior mediastinal

7. A patient with a 3-cm anal cancer with a unilateral inguinal node is staged as

    A. T1N1
    B. T2N1
    C. T1N2
    D. T2N2

8. A patient with five regional lymph nodes from esophageal cancer is N-staged as

    A. N1
    B. N2
    C. N3
    D. Number of lymph nodes is not relevant to N staging for this malignancy

9. All of the following are risk factors associated with anal cancer EXCEPT

    A. HPV 16/18
    B. AIDS
    C. Alcohol intake
    D. Smoking

10. Nodal drainage for anal cancers above the dentate line include the following EXCEPT

    A. Inguinal nodes
    B. Obturator nodes
    C. Hypogastric nodes
    D. Internal pudendal nodes

11. An esophageal cancer at 20 cm would be classified as

    A. Cervical
    B. Upper thoracic
    C. Mid thoracic
    D. Lower thoracic/GE junction

12. In terms of colorectal cancer, the following tumor location is least frequently observed

    A. Rectosigmoid junction
    B. Cecum
    C. Sigmoid
    D. Rectum

13. In terms of colorectal cancer, a patient with five positive lymph nodes has what N stage?

    A. N1
    B. N2
    C. N3
    D. The number of positive nodes is not relevant to colorectal staging

14. The majority of pancreatic cancers are located in

    A. Head of the pancreas
    B. Body of the pancreas
    C. Tail of the pancreas
    D. Equally among all three locations of the pancreas

15. The malignant transformation rate of Barrett's esophagus into adenocarcinoma is

    A. 0.5% per year
    B. 1.8% per year
    C. 3.2% per year
    D. 5% per year

16. The second most common histological subtype of gastric cancer is

    A. Lymphoma (MALT)
    B. Carcinoid
    C. Gastrointestinal stromal tumors (GIST)
    D. Squamous cell carcinoma

17. A patient with gastric cancer and invasion of the muscularis propria has the following T stage

    A. T1
    B. T2
    C. T3
    D. T4

18. All of the following are positive predictors of survival in pancreatic cancer EXCEPT

    A. Neurovascular invasion
    B. Tumor diameter less than 3 cm
    C. Negative nodal involvement
    D. Negative resection margins

19. In the Intergroup 0116 gastric trial assessing postoperative chemoradiation therapy versus surgery alone, median survival was improved by what amount?

    A. There was no statistically significant improvement.
    B. 4 months
    C. 9 months
    D. 12 months

20. The risk of developing distant metastases in low risk (T1–2N0) colorectal cancer is

    A. 0%
    B. 5%
    C. 10%
    D. 20%

Chapter 2: Answers

1. A

The following dose fractionations are used in pancreatic cancer:

Adjuvant—45 Gy/25 fx ± 5–15-Gy boost to tumor bed or involved margins

Preoperative/Unresectable—45–54 Gy at 1.8–2.5 Gy/fx or 36 Gy at 2.4 Gy/fx

Palliation—25–36 Gy at 2.4–5 Gy/fx

2. D

Adenocarcinomas occur in 98% of cases. Other histologies are less common:

Carcinoid (0.4%)

Lymphoma (1.3%)

Sarcoma (0.3%)

Squamous cell—transitional area from rectum to anus considered anal carcinomas

3. A

The incidence of hepatobiliary cancers from most to least frequent is: hepatocellular>gallbladder>extrahepatic cholangiocarcinoma>intrahepatic cholangiocarcinoma

4. B

Rates of gastric cancer have declined over the last 100 years. Decreases have occurred from:

refrigeration, increased consumption of fresh fruits and vegetables

decreased salt intake

decreased H. pylori infection with use of screening and antibiotics

5. D

The N staging of gastric cancer is as follows:

N0—No regional lymph node metastases

N1—Metastases in 1 to 2 regional lymph nodes

N2—Metastases in 3 to 6 regional lymph nodes

N3—Metastases in 7 or more regional lymph nodes

N3a—Metastases in 7 to 15 regional lymph nodes

N3b—Metastases in 16 or more regional lymph nodes

6. D

The esophagus has an extensive, longitudinally continuous, submucosal lymphatic system. The esophagus contains little barrier to lymphatic spread, and lymphatics are interconnected making it possible for nodal involvement separate from the primary tumor.

The cervical esophagus drains to the cervical nodes

The thoracic esophagus drains to the posterior mediastinal nodes

The lower esophagus drains to the left gastric, celiac and gastrohepatic nodes

7. D

This patient has T2 (Tumor more than 2 cm but not greater than 5 cm in greatest dimension) and N2 (metastasis in unilateral internal iliac and/or inguinal node(s)) disease.

8. B

N staging of esophageal cancer:

N0—No regional lymph node metastasis

N1—one to two regional lymph nodes (N1 is site dependent)

N2—three to six regional lymph nodes

N3—More than six regional lymph nodes

9. C

Risk factors for anal cancer:

HPV infection (HPV 16 and 18)

History of anal warts (HPV)

History of cervical, vaginal or vulvar cancers
AIDS especially if CD4 <200
>10 sexual partners
History of anal intercourse
History of STDs
Smoking
Immunosuppression for transplant

10. A
Lymphatic drainage of the anal canal:
Perianal skin, anal verge, canal distal to the dentate line superficial inguinal nodes (with some communications to the femoral nodes and to the external iliac systems)
Around and above the dentate line internal pudendal, hypogastric, and obturator nodes of the internal iliac systems
Proximal canal perirectal and superior hemorrhoidal nodes of the inferior mesenteric system

11. C
The anatomical regions of the esophagus include:
Cervical—from the cricoid cartilage to the thoracic inlet (~18 cm from incisors)
Upper Thoracic— thoracic inlet to tracheal bifurcation (~18–24 cm)
Mid Thoracic—tracheal bifurcation to just above the GE junction (~24–32 cm)
Lower Thoracic/GE Junction—beyond 32 cm

12. A
The location of colorectal tumors has been observed to have the following relative frequencies:
Cecum (20%)
Sigmoid (25%)
Rectum (20%)
Rectosigmoid junction (10%)
Left colon cancers are more common in males and right colon cancers are more common in females

13. B
N staging of colorectal cancer:
N0—No regional lymph node metastasis
N1—Metastasis in 1 to 3 pericolic or perirectal lymph nodes
N2—Metastasis in 4 or more pericolic or perirectal lymph nodes
N3—Metastasis in any lymph node along the course of a named vascular trunk

14. A
75% of all pancreatic carcinomas occur within the head or neck of the pancreas. 15% to 20% occur in the body of the pancreas. 5% to 10% occur in the tail.

15. A
Barrett's esophagus is intestinal metaplasia of the esophageal epithelial lining and replacement with columnar epithelium with a malignant transformation rate is 0.5% per year.

16. A
The second most common gastric tumors are MALT lymphomas. Other rare histologies include:
Gastrointestinal stromal tumors (2%)
Carcinoids (1%)
Adenoacanthomas (1%)
Squamous cell carcinomas (1%)

17. B
T staging for gastric cancer involves the following:
T1—Tumor invades lamina propria, muscularis mucosa, or submucosa
T2—Tumor invades muscularis propria
T3—Tumor penetrates subserosal connective tissue without invasion of visceral peritoneum or adjacent structures
T4—Tumor invades serosa (visceral peritoneum) or adjacent structures

18. A

Predictors of long-term survival after surgery

    Tumor diameter less than 3 cm

    Absence of nodal involvement

    Negative resection margins

19. C

The Intergroup 0116 trial assessing surgery alone versus surgery followed by 5-FU/leu (1 cycle) then CRT (45 Gy/25 fx) with 5-FU/leu (2 cycles) followed by 5-FU/leu (2 cycles) demonstrated a 9-month improvement in median survival and a 9% 3-year OS in favor of the postoperative chemoradiation arm.

20. C

The risk of developing distant metastases in low-risk colorectal cancer is approximately 10%. High-risk disease is associated with over a 40% risk.

Recommended Reading

Esophageal Cancer

Ajani JA, Winter K, Komaki R, et al. Phase II randomized trial of two nonoperative regimens of induction chemotherapy followed by chemoradiation in patients with localized carcinoma of the esophagus: RTOG 0113. *J Clin Oncol.* 2008;26(28):4551-4556.

Arnott SJ, Duncan W, Kerr GR, et al. Low dose preoperative radiotherapy for carcinoma of the oesophagus: results of a randomized clinical trial. *Radiother Oncol.* 1992;24(2):108-113.

Bedenne L, Michel P, Bouché O, et al. Chemoradiation followed by surgery compared with chemoradiation alone in squamous cancer of the esophagus: FFCD 9102. *J Clin Oncol.* 2007;25(10):1160-1168.

Bosset JF, Gignoux M, Triboulet JP, et al. Chemoradiotherapy followed by surgery compared with surgery alone in squamous-cell cancer of the esophagus. *N Engl J Med.* 1997;337(3):161-167. doi: 7/3/10.1056/NEJM199707173370304

Burmeister BH, Smithers BM, Gebski V, et al. Surgery alone versus chemoradiotherapy followed by surgery for resectable cancer of the oesophagus: a randomised controlled phase III trial. *Lancet Oncol.* 2005;6(9):659-668.

Fok M, Sham JS, Choy D, Cheng SW, Wong J. Postoperative radiotherapy for carcinoma of the esophagus: a prospective, randomized controlled study. *Surgery.* 1993;113(2):138-147.

Gignoux M, Roussel A, Paillot B, et al. The value of preoperative radiotherapy in esophageal cancer: results of a study of the E.O.R.T.C. *World J Surg.* 1987;11(4):426-432.

Kelsen DP, Winter KA, Gunderson LL, et al. Long-term results of RTOG trial 8911 (USA Intergroup 113): a random assignment trial comparison of chemotherapy followed by surgery compared with surgery alone for esophageal cancer. *J Clin Oncol.* 2007;25(24):3719-3725.

Launois B, Delarue D, Campion JP, Kerbaol M. Preoperative radiotherapy for carcinoma of the esophagus. *Surg Gynecol Obstet.* 1981;153(5):690-692.

Le Prise E, Etienne PL, Meunier B, et al. A randomized study of chemotherapy, radiation therapy, and surgery versus surgery for localized squamous cell carcinoma of the esophagus. *Cancer.* 1994;73(7):1779-1784.

Macdonald JS, Smalley SR, Benedetti J, et al. Chemoradiotherapy after surgery compared with surgery alone for adenocarcinoma of the stomach or gastroesophageal junction. *N Engl J Med.* 2001;345(10):725-730.

Medical Research Council Oesophageal Cancer Working Group. Surgical resection with or without preoperative chemotherapy in oesophageal cancer: a randomised controlled trial. Lancet. 2002;359(9319):1727-1733.

Minsky BD, Pajak TF, Ginsberg RJ, et al. INT 0123 (Radiation Therapy Oncology Group 94-05) phase III trial of combined-modality therapy for esophageal cancer: high-dose versus standard-dose radiation therapy. *J Clin Oncol.* 2002;20(5):1167-1174.

Nygaard K, Hagen S, Hansen HS, et al. Pre-operative radiotherapy prolongs survival in operable esophageal carcinoma: a randomized, multicenter study of pre-operative radiotherapy and chemotherapy. The second Scandinavian trial in esophageal cancer. *World J Surg.* 1992;16(6):1104-1109; discussion 1110.

Stahl M, Stuschke M, Lehmann N, et al. Chemoradiation with and without surgery in patients with locally advanced squamous cell carcinoma of the esophagus. *J Clin Oncol.* 2005;23(10):2310-2317.

Ténière P, Hay JM, Fingerhut A, Fagniez PL. Postoperative radiation therapy does not increase survival after curative resection for squamous cell carcinoma of the middle and lower esophagus as shown by a multicenter controlled trial. French University Association for Surgical Research. *Surg Gynecol Obstet.* 1991;173(2):123-130.

Tepper J, Krasna MJ, Niedzwiecki D, et al. Phase III trial of trimodality therapy with cisplatin, fluorouracil, radiotherapy, and surgery compared with surgery alone for esophageal cancer: CALGB 9781. *J Clin Oncol.* 2008;26(7):1086-1092.

Urba SG, Orringer MB, Turrisi A, Iannettoni M, Forastiere A, Strawderman M. Randomized trial of preoperative chemoradiation versus surgery alone in patients with locoregional esophageal carcinoma. *J Clin Oncol.* 2001;19(2):305-313.

Walsh TN, Noonan N, Hollywood D, Kelly A, Keeling N, Hennessy TP. A comparison of multimodal therapy and surgery for esophageal adenocarcinoma. *N Engl J Med.* 1996;335(7):462-467. doi: 10.1056/NEJM199608153350702

Wang M, Gu XZ, Yin WB, Huang GJ, Wang LJ, Zhang DW. Randomized clinical trial on the combination of preoperative irradiation and surgery in the treatment of esophageal carcinoma: report on 206 patients. *Int J Radiat Oncol Biol Phys.* 1989;16(2):325-327.

Gastric Cancer

Bamias A, Karina M, Papakostas P, et al. A randomized phase III study of adjuvant platinum/docetaxel chemotherapy with or without radiation therapy in patients with gastric cancer. *Cancer Chemother Pharmacol.* 2010;65(6):1009-1021.

Bonenkamp JJ, Hermans J, Sasako M, et al. Extended lymph-node dissection for gastric cancer. *N Engl J Med.* 1999;340(12):908-914.

Bozzetti F, Marubini E, Bonfanti G, et al. Subtotal versus total gastrectomy for gastric cancer: five-year survival rates in a multicenter randomized Italian trial. Italian Gastrointestinal Tumor Study Group. *Ann Surg.* 1999;230(2):170-178.

Cunningham D, Allum WH, Stenning SP, et al. Perioperative chemotherapy versus surgery alone for resectable gastroesophageal cancer. *N Engl J Med.* 2006;355(1):11-20. doi: 10.1056/NEJMoa055531

Cuschieri A, Weeden S, Fielding J, et al. Patient survival after D1 and D2 resections for gastric cancer: long-term results of the MRC randomized surgical trial. Surgical Co-operative Group. *Br J Cancer.* 1999;79(9–10):1522-1530.

Hartgrink HH, van de Velde CJ, Putter H, et al. Neo-adjuvant chemotherapy for operable gastric cancer: long term results of the Dutch randomised FAMTX trial. *Eur J Surg Oncol.* 2004;30(6):643-649.

Macdonald JS, Smalley SR, Benedetti J, et al. Chemoradiotherapy after surgery compared with surgery alone for adenocarcinoma of the stomach or gastroesophageal junction. *N Engl J Med.* 2001;345(10):725-730.

Robertson CS, Chung SC, Woods SD, et al. A prospective randomized trial comparing R1 subtotal gastrectomy with R3 total gastrectomy for antral cancer. *Ann Surg.* 1994;220(2):176-182.

Sasako M, Sano T, Yamamoto S, et al. D2 lymphadenectomy alone or with para-aortic nodal dissection for gastric cancer. *N Engl J Med.* 2008;359(5):453–462.

Stahl M, Walz MK, Stuschke M, et al. Phase III comparison of preoperative chemotherapy compared with chemoradiotherapy in patients with locally advanced adenocarcinoma of the esophagogastric junction. *J Clin Oncol.* 2009;27(6):851-856.

Van Cutsem E, Moiseyenko VM, Tjulandin S, et al. Phase III study of docetaxel and cisplatin plus fluorouracil compared with cisplatin and fluorouracil as first-line therapy for advanced gastric cancer: a report of the V325 Study Group. *J Clin Oncol.* 2006;24(31):4991-4997.

Webb A, Cunningham D, Scarffe JH, et al. Randomized trial comparing epirubicin, cisplatin, and fluorouracil versus fluorouracil, doxorubicin, and methotrexate in advanced esophagogastric cancer. *J Clin Oncol.* 1997;15(1):261-267.

Hepatocellular Cancer

Dawson LA, Eccles C, Craig T. Individualized image guided iso-NTCP based liver cancer SBRT. *Acta Oncol.* 2006;45(7):856-864.

Meng MB, Cui YL, Lu Y, et al. Transcatheter arterial chemoembolization in combination with radiotherapy for unresectable hepatocellular carcinoma: a systematic review and meta-analysis. *Radiother Oncol.* 2009;92(2):184-194.

Taguchi H, Sakuhara Y, Hige S, et al. Intercepting radiotherapy using a real-time tumor-tracking radiotherapy system for highly selected patients with hepatocellular carcinoma unresectable with other modalities. *Int J Radiat Oncol Biol Phys.* 2007;69(2):376-380.

Tse RV, Hawkins M, Lockwood G, et al. Phase I study of individualized stereotactic body radiotherapy for hepatocellular carcinoma and intrahepatic cholangiocarcinoma. *J Clin Oncol.* 2008;26(4):657-664.

Cholangiocarcinoma

Alden ME, Waterman FM, Topham AK, et al. Cholangiocarcinoma: clinical significance of tumor location along the extrahepatic bile duct. *Radiology.* 1995;197(2):511-516.

Bathe OF, Pacheco JT, Ossi PB, et al. Management of hilar bile duct carcinoma. *Hepatogastroenterology.* 2001;48(41):1289-1294.

Borghero Y, Crane CH, Szklaruk J, et al. Extrahepatic bile duct adenocarcinoma: patients at high-risk for local recurrence treated with surgery and adjuvant chemoradiation have an equivalent overall survival to patients with standard-risk treated with surgery alone. *Ann Surg Oncol.* 2008;15(11):3147-3156.

Cameron JL, Pitt HA, Zinner MJ, Kaufman SL, Coleman J. Management of proximal cholangiocarcinomas by surgical resection and radiotherapy. *Am J Surg.* 1990;159(1):91-97; discussion 97-98.

Flickinger JC, Epstein AH, Iwatsuki S, Carr BI, Starzl TE. Radiation therapy for primary carcinoma of the extrahepatic biliary system. An analysis of 63 cases. *Cancer.* 1991;68(2):289-294.

Gerhards MF, van Gulik TM, Bosma A, et al. Long-term survival after resection of proximal bile duct carcinoma (Klatskin tumors). *World J Surg.* 1999;23(1):91-96.

Gerhards MF, van Gulik TM, González González D, Rauws EA, Gouma DJ. Results of postoperative radiotherapy for resectable hilar cholangiocarcinoma. *World J Surg.* 2003;27(2):173-179.

González González D, Gouma DJ, Rauws EA, et al. Role of radiotherapy, in particular intraluminal brachytherapy, in the treatment of proximal bile duct carcinoma. *Ann Oncol.* 1999;10(suppl 4):215-220.

Heron DE, Stein DE, Eschelman DJ, et al. Cholangiocarcinoma: the impact of tumor location and treatment strategy on outcome. *Am J Clin Oncol.* 2003;26(4):422-428.

Jan YY, Yeh CN, Yeh TS, Chen TC. Prognostic analysis of surgical treatment of peripheral cholangiocarcinoma: two decades of experience at Chang Gung Memorial Hospital. *World J Gastroenterol.* 2005;11(12):1779-1784.

Kraybill WG, Lee H, Picus J, et al. Multidisciplinary treatment of biliary tract cancers. *J Surg Oncol.* 1994;55(4):239-245.

Kurisu K, Hishikawa Y, Miura T, et al. Radiotherapy of postoperative residual tumor of bile duct carcinoma. *Radiat Med.* 1991;9(2):82-84.

Mahe M, Romestaing P, Talon B, et al. Radiation therapy in extrahepatic bile duct carcinoma. *Radiother Oncol.* 1991;21(2):121-127.

Mogavero GT, Jones B, Cameron JL, Coleman J. Gastric and duodenal obstruction in patients with cholangiocarcinoma in the porta hepatis: increased prevalence after radiation therapy. *AJR Am J Roentgenol.* 1992;159(5):1001-1003.

Nakeeb A, Pitt HA, Sohn TA, et al. Cholangiocarcinoma: a spectrum of intrahepatic, perihilar, and distal tumors. *Ann Surg.* 1996;224(4):463–473; discussion 473-475.

Ove R, Kennedy A, Darwin P, Haluszka O. Postoperative endoscopic retrograde high dose-rate brachytherapy for cholangiocarcinoma. *Am J Clin Oncol.* 2000;23(6):559-561.

Pitt HA, Nakeeb A, Abrams RA, et al. Perihilar cholangiocarcinoma: postoperative radiotherapy does not improve survival. *Ann Surg.* 1995;221(6):788–797; discussion 797-798.

Reding R, Buard JL, Lebeau G, Launois B. Surgical management of 552 carcinomas of the extrahepatic bile ducts (gallbladder and periampullary tumors excluded): results of the French Surgical Association Survey. *Ann Surg.* 1991;213(3):236-241.

Sagawa N, Kondo S, Morikawa T, Okushiba S, Katoh H. Effectiveness of radiation therapy after surgery for hilar cholangiocarcinoma. *Surg Today.* 2005;35(7):548–552.

Schoenthaler R, Phillips TL, Castro J, Efird JT, Better A, Way LW. Carcinoma of the extrahepatic bile ducts: the University of California at San Francisco experience. *Ann Surg.* 1994;219(3):267-274.

Stein DE, Heron DE, Rosato EL, Anné PR, Topham AK. Positive microscopic margins alter outcome in lymph node-negative cholangiocarcinoma when resection is combined with adjuvant radiotherapy. *Am J Clin Oncol.* 2005;28(1):21-23.

Todoroki T, Kawamoto T, Koike N, Fukao K, Shoda J, Takahashi H. Treatment strategy for patients with middle and lower third bile duct cancer. *Br J Surg.* 2001;88(3):364-370.

Todoroki T, Ohara K, Kawamoto T, et al. Benefits of adjuvant radiotherapy after radical resection of locally advanced main hepatic duct carcinoma. *Int J Radiat Oncol Biol Phys.* 2000;46(3):581-587.

Válek V, Kysela P, Kala Z, Kiss I, Tomásek J, Petera J. Brachytherapy and percutaneous stenting in the treatment of cholangiocarcinoma: a prospective randomised study. *Eur J Radiol.* 2007;62(2):175-179.

Vallis KA, Benjamin IS, Munro AJ, et al. External beam and intraluminal radiotherapy for locally advanced bile duct cancer: role and tolerability. *Radiother Oncol.* 1996;41(1):61-66.

Valverde A, Bonhomme N, Farges O, Sauvanet A, Flejou JF, Belghiti J. Resection of intrahepatic cholangiocarcinoma: a Western experience. *J Hepatobiliary Pancreat Surg.* 1999;6(2):122-127.

Veeze-Kuijpers B, Meerwaldt JH, Lameris JS, van Blankenstein M, van Putten WL, Terpstra OT. The role of radiotherapy in the treatment of bile duct carcinoma. *Int J Radiat Oncol Biol Phys.* 1990;18(1):63-67.

Verbeek PC, Van Leeuwen DJ, Van Der Heyde MN, Gonzalez Gonzalez D. Does additive radiotherapy after hilar resection improve survival of cholangiocarcinoma? An analysis in sixty-four patients. *Ann Chir.* 1991;45(4):350-354.

Zlotecki RA, Jung LA, Vauthey JN, Vogel SB, Mendenhall WM. Carcinoma of the extrahepatic biliary tract: surgery and radiotherapy for curative and palliative intent. *Radiat Oncol Investig.* 1998;6(5):240-247.

Gallbladder Cancer

Czito BG, Hurwitz HI, Clough RW, et al. Adjuvant external-beam radiotherapy with concurrent chemotherapy after resection of primary gallbladder carcinoma: a 23-year experience. *Int J Radiat Oncol Biol Phys.* 2005;62(4):1030-1034.

Houry S, Haccart V, Huguier M, Schlienger M. Gallbladder carcinoma: role of radiation therapy. *Br J Surg.* 1989;76(5):448-450.

Mahe M, Stampfli C, Romestaing P, Salerno N, Gerard JP. Primary carcinoma of the gall-bladder: potential for external radiation therapy. *Radiother Oncol.* 1994;33(3):204-208.

Mojica P, Smith D, Ellenhorn J. Adjuvant radiation therapy is associated with improved survival for gallbladder carcinoma with regional metastatic disease. *J Surg Oncol.* 2007;96(1):8-13.

Takada T, Amano H, Yasuda H, et al. Is postoperative adjuvant chemotherapy useful for gallbladder carcinoma? A phase III multicenter prospective randomized controlled trial in patients with resected pancreaticobiliary carcinoma. *Cancer.* 2002;95(8):1685-1695.

Wang SJ, Lemieux A, Kalpathy-Cramer J, et al. Nomogram for predicting the benefit of adjuvant chemoradiotherapy for resected gallbladder cancer. *J Clin Oncol.* 2011;29(35):4627-4632.

Pancreatic Cancer

Bakkevold KE, Arnesjø B, Dahl O, Kambestad B. Adjuvant combination chemotherapy (AMF) following radical resection of carcinoma of the pancreas and papilla of Vater—results of a controlled, prospective, randomised multicentre study. *Eur J Cancer.* 1993;29A(5):698-703.

Ben-Josef E, Shields AF, Vaishampayan U, et al. Intensity-modulated radiotherapy (IMRT) and concurrent capecitabine for pancreatic cancer. *Int J Radiat Oncol Biol Phys.* 2004;59(2):454-459.

Berger AC, Garcia M Jr, Hoffman JP, et al. Postresection CA 19-9 predicts overall survival in patients with pancreatic cancer treated with adjuvant chemoradiation: a prospective validation by RTOG 9704. *J Clin Oncol.* 2008;26(36):5918-5922.

Burris HA 3rd, Moore MJ, Andersen J, et al. Improvements in survival and clinical benefit with gemcitabine as first-line therapy for patients with advanced pancreas cancer: a randomized trial. *J Clin Oncol.* 1997;15(6):2403-2413.

Butturini G, Stocken DD, Wente MN, et al. Influence of resection margins and treatment on survival in patients with pancreatic cancer: meta-analysis of randomized controlled trials. *Arch Surg.* 2008;143(1):75-83; discussion 83.

Chauffert B, Mornex F, Bonnetain F, et al. Phase III trial comparing intensive induction chemoradiotherapy (60 Gy, infusional 5-FU and intermittent cisplatin) followed by maintenance gemcitabine with gemcitabine alone for locally advanced unresectable pancreatic cancer. Definitive results of the 2000–01 FFCD/SFRO study. *Ann Oncol.* 2008;19(9):1592-1599.

Choti MA. Adjuvant therapy for pancreatic cancer—the debate continues. *N Engl J Med.* 2004;350(12):1249-1251.

Cohen SJ, Dobelbower R Jr, Lipsitz S, et al. A randomized phase III study of radiotherapy alone or with 5-fluorouracil and mitomycin-C in patients with locally advanced adenocarcinoma of the pancreas: Eastern Cooperative Oncology Group study E8282. *Int J Radiat Oncol Biol Phys.* 2005;62(5):1345-1350.

Corsini MM, Miller RC, Haddock MG, et al. Adjuvant radiotherapy and chemotherapy for pancreatic carcinoma: the Mayo Clinic experience (1975–2005). *J Clin Oncol.* 2008;26(21):3511-3516.

Crane CH, Abbruzzese JL, Evans DB, et al. Is the therapeutic index better with gemcitabine-based chemoradiation than with 5-fluorouracil-based chemoradiation in locally advanced pancreatic cancer? *Int J Radiat Oncol Biol Phys.* 2002;52(5):1293-1302.

Doi R, Imamura M, Hosotani R, et al. Surgery versus radiochemotherapy for resectable locally invasive pancreatic cancer: final results of a randomized multi-institutional trial. *Surg Today.* 2008;38(11):1021-1028.

Gastrointestinal Tumor Study Group. Further evidence of effective adjuvant combined radiation and chemotherapy following curative resection of pancreatic cancer. *Cancer.* 1987;59(12):2006-2010.

Gastrointestinal Tumor Study Group. Radiation therapy combined with Adriamycin or 5-fluorouracil for the treatment of locally unresectable pancreatic carcinoma. *Cancer.* 1985;56(11):2563-2568.

Gastrointestinal Tumor Study Group. Treatment of locally unresectable carcinoma of the pancreas: comparison of combined-modality therapy (chemotherapy plus radiotherapy) to chemotherapy alone. *J Natl Cancer Inst.* 1988;80(10):751-755.

Herman JM, Swartz MJ, Hsu CC, et al. Analysis of fluorouracil-based adjuvant chemotherapy and radiation after pancreaticoduodenectomy for ductal adenocarcinoma of the pancreas: results of a large, prospectively collected database at the Johns Hopkins Hospital. *J Clin Oncol.* 2008;26(21):3503-3510.

Hong TS, Ryan DP, Blaszkowsky LS, et al. Phase I study of preoperative short-course chemoradiation with proton beam therapy and capecitabine for resectable pancreatic ductal adenocarcinoma of the head. *Int J Radiat Oncol Biol Phys.* 2011;79(1):151-157.

Kalser MH, Ellenberg SS. Pancreatic cancer. Adjuvant combined radiation and chemotherapy following curative resection. *Arch Surg.* 1985;120(8):899-903.

Klaassen DJ, MacIntyre JM, Catton GE, Engstrom PF, Moertel CG. Treatment of locally unresectable cancer of the stomach and pancreas: a randomized comparison of 5-fluorouracil alone with radiation plus concurrent and maintenance 5-fluorouracil—an Eastern Cooperative Oncology Group study. *J Clin Oncol.* 1985;3(3):373-378.

Klinkenbijl JH, Jeekel J, Sahmoud T, et al. Adjuvant radiotherapy and 5-fluorouracil after curative resection of cancer of the pancreas and periampullary region: phase III trial of the EORTC gastrointestinal tract cancer cooperative group. *Ann Surg.* 1999;230(6):776–782; discussion 782-784.

Koshy MC, Landry JC, Cavanaugh SX, et al. A challenge to the therapeutic nihilism of ESPAC-1. *Int J Radiat Oncol Biol Phys.* 2005;61(4):965-966.

Kosuge T, Kiuchi T, Mukai K, et al. A multicenter randomized controlled trial to evaluate the effect of adjuvant cisplatin and 5-fluorouracil therapy after curative resection in cases of pancreatic cancer. *Jpn J Clin Oncol.* 2006;36(3):159-165.

Krishnan S, Rana V, Janjan NA, et al. Induction chemotherapy selects patients with locally advanced, unresectable pancreatic cancer for optimal benefit from consolidative chemoradiation therapy. *Cancer.* 2007;110(1):47-55.

Loehrer PJ Sr, Feng Y, Cardenes H, et al. Gemcitabine alone versus gemcitabine plus radiotherapy in patients with locally advanced pancreatic cancer: an Eastern Cooperative Oncology Group trial. *J Clin Oncol.* 2011;29(31):4105-4112.

McGinn CJ, Zalupski MM, Shureiqi I, et al. Phase I trial of radiation dose escalation with concurrent weekly full-dose gemcitabine in patients with advanced pancreatic cancer. *J Clin Oncol.* 2001;19(22):4202-4208.

Moertel CG, Childs DS Jr, Reitemeier RJ, et al. Combined 5-fluorouracil and supervoltage radiation therapy of locally unresectable gastrointestinal cancer. *Lancet.* 1969;2(7626):865-867.

Moertel CG, Frytak S, Hahn RG, et al. Therapy of locally unresectable pancreatic carcinoma: a randomized comparison of high dose (6000 rads) radiation alone, moderate dose radiation (4000 rads + 5-fluorouracil), and high dose radiation + 5-fluorouracil: the Gastrointestinal Tumor Study Group. *Cancer.* 1981;48(8):1705-1710.

Moore MJ, Goldstein D, Hamm J, et al. Erlotinib plus gemcitabine compared with gemcitabine alone in patients with advanced pancreatic cancer: a phase III trial of the National Cancer Institute of Canada Clinical Trials Group. *J Clin Oncol.* 2007;25(15):1960-1966. Epub 2007 Apr 23.

Neoptolemos JP, Dunn JA, Stocken DD, et al. Adjuvant chemoradiotherapy and chemotherapy in resectable pancreatic cancer: a randomised controlled trial. *Lancet.* 2001;358(9293):1576-1585.

Neoptolemos JP, Stocken DD, Friess H, et al. A randomized trial of chemoradiotherapy and chemotherapy after resection of pancreatic cancer. *N Engl J Med.* 2004;350(12):1200-1210.

Oettle H, Post S, Neuhaus P, et al. Adjuvant chemotherapy with gemcitabine vs observation in patients undergoing curative-intent resection of pancreatic cancer: a randomized controlled trial. *JAMA.* 2007;297(3):267-277.

Picozzi VJ, Kozarek RA, Traverso LW. Interferon-based adjuvant chemoradiation therapy after pancreaticoduodenectomy for pancreatic adenocarcinoma. *Am J Surg.* 2003;185(5):476-480.

Philip PA. Locally advanced pancreatic cancer: where should we go from here? *J Clin Oncol.* 2011;29(31):4066-4068.

Regine WF, Winter KA, Abrams R, et al. Fluorouracil-based chemoradiation with either gemcitabine or fluorouracil chemotherapy after resection of pancreatic adenocarcinoma: 5-year analysis of the U.S. Intergroup/RTOG 9704 phase III trial. *Ann Surg Oncol.* 2011;18(5):1319-1326.

Regine WF, Winter KA, Abrams RA, et al. Fluorouracil vs gemcitabine chemotherapy before and after fluorouracil-based chemoradiation following resection of pancreatic adenocarcinoma: a randomized controlled trial. *JAMA.* 2008;299(9):1019-1026.

Rich T, Harris J, Abrams R, et al. Phase II study of external irradiation and weekly paclitaxel for nonmetastatic, unresectable pancreatic cancer: RTOG-98-12. *Am J Clin Oncol.* 2004;27(1):51-56.

Smeenk HG, van Eijck CH, Hop WC, et al. Long-term survival and metastatic pattern of pancreatic and periampullary cancer after adjuvant chemoradiation or observation: long-term results of EORTC trial 40891. *Ann Surg.* 2007;246(5):734-740.

Stocken DD, Büchler MW, Dervenis C, et al. Meta-analysis of randomised adjuvant therapy trials for pancreatic cancer. *Br J Cancer.* 2005;92(8):1372-1381.

Van Laethem JL, Hammel P, Mornex F, et al. Adjuvant gemcitabine alone versus gemcitabine-based chemoradiotherapy after curative resection for pancreatic cancer: a randomized EORTC-40013–22012/FFCD-9203/GERCOR phase II study. *J Clin Oncol.* 2010;28(29):4450-4456.

Colon Cancer

Amos EH, Mendenhall WM, McCarty PJ, et al. Postoperative radiotherapy for locally advanced colon cancer. *Ann Surg Oncol.* 1996;3(5):431-436.

Gastrointestinal Tumor Study Group. Adjuvant therapy with hepatic irradiation plus fluorouracil in colon carcinoma. *Int J Radiat Oncol Biol Phys.* 1991;21(5):1151-1156.

Gunderson LL, Nelson H, Martenson JA, et al. Locally advanced primary colorectal cancer: intraoperative electron and external beam irradiation ±5-FU. *Int J Radiat Oncol Biol Phys.* 1997;37(3):601-614.

Janjan NA. Postoperative radiotherapy for locally advanced colon cancer. *Ann Surg Oncol.* 1996;3(5):421-422.

Martenson JA Jr, Willett CG, Sargent DJ, et al. Phase III study of adjuvant chemotherapy and radiation therapy compared with chemotherapy alone in the surgical adjuvant treatment of colon cancer: results of intergroup protocol 0130. *J Clin Oncol.* 2004;22(16):3277-3283.

Schild SE, Gunderson LL, Haddock MG, et al. The treatment of locally advanced colon cancer. *Int J Radiat Oncol Biol Phys.* 1997;37(1):51-58.

Willett CG, Fung CY, Kaufman DS, Efird J, Shellito PC. Postoperative radiation therapy for high-risk colon carcinoma. *J Clin Oncol.* 1993;11(6):1112-1117.

Willett CG, Goldberg S, Shellito PC, et al. Does postoperative irradiation play a role in the adjuvant therapy of stage T4 colon cancer? *Cancer J Sci Am.* 1999;5(4):242-247.

Rectal Cancer

Aschele C, Cionini L, Lonardi S, et al. Primary tumor response to preoperative chemoradiation with or without oxaliplatin in locally advanced rectal cancer: pathologic results of the STAR-01 randomized phase III trial. *J Clin Oncol.* 2011;29(20):2773-2780.

Bentzen SM, Balslev I, Pedersen M, et al. Time to loco-regional recurrence after resection of Dukes' B and C colorectal cancer with or without adjuvant postoperative radiotherapy: a multivariate regression analysis. *Br J Cancer.* 1992;65(1):102-107.

Birgisson H, Påhlman L, Gunnarsson U, Glimelius B. Late gastrointestinal disorders after rectal cancer surgery with and without preoperative radiation therapy. *Br J Surg.* 2008;95(2):206-213.

Bosset JF, Collette L, Calais G, et al. Chemotherapy with preoperative radiotherapy in rectal cancer. *N Engl J Med.* 2006;355(11):1114-1123.

Cedermark B, Johansson H, Rutqvist LE, Wilking N. The Stockholm I trial of preoperative short term radiotherapy in operable rectal carcinoma: a prospective randomized trial. Stockholm Colorectal Cancer Study Group. *Cancer.* 1995;75(9):2269-2275.

Collette L, Bosset JF, den Dulk M, et al. Patients with curative resection of cT3-4 rectal cancer after preoperative radiotherapy or radiochemotherapy: does anybody benefit from adjuvant fluorouracil-based chemotherapy? A trial of the European Organisation for Research and Treatment of Cancer Radiation Oncology Group. *J Clin Oncol.* 2007;25(28):4379-4386.

Colorectal Cancer Collaborative Group. Adjuvant radiotherapy for rectal cancer: a systematic overview of 8,507 patients from 22 randomised trials. *Lancet.* 2001;358(9290):1291-1304.

Das P, Delclos ME, Skibber JM, et al. Hyperfractionated accelerated radiotherapy for rectal cancer in patients with prior pelvic irradiation. *Int J Radiat Oncol Biol Phys.* 2010;77(1):60-65.

De Caluwé L, Van Nieuwenhove Y, Ceelen WP. Preoperative chemoradiation versus radiation alone for stage II and III resectable rectal cancer. *Cochrane Database Syst Rev.* 2013;2:CD006041.

Dewdney A, Cunningham D, Tabernero J, et al. Multicenter randomized phase II clinical trial comparing neoadjuvant oxaliplatin, capecitabine, and preoperative radiotherapy with or without cetuximab followed by total mesorectal excision in patients with high-risk rectal cancer (EXPERT-C). *J Clin Oncol.* 2012;30(14):1620-1627.

Douglass HO Jr, Moertel CG, Mayer RJ, et al. Survival after postoperative combination treatment of rectal cancer. *N Engl J Med.* 1986;315(20):1294-1295.

Fernández-Martos C, Pericay C, Aparicio J, et al. Phase II, randomized study of concomitant chemoradiotherapy followed by surgery and adjuvant capecitabine plus oxaliplatin (CAPOX) compared with induction CAPOX followed by concomitant chemoradiotherapy and surgery in magnetic resonance imaging-defined, locally advanced rectal cancer: Grupo cancer de recto 3 study. *J Clin Oncol.* 2010;28(5):859-865.

Fisher B, Wolmark N, Rockette H, et al. Postoperative adjuvant chemotherapy or radiation therapy for rectal cancer: results from NSABP protocol R-01. *J Natl Cancer Inst.* 1988;80(1):21-29.

Folkesson J, Birgisson H, Pahlman L, et al. Swedish Rectal Cancer Trial: long lasting benefits from radiotherapy on survival and local recurrence rate. *J Clin Oncol.* 2005;23(24):5644-5650.

Frykholm GJ, Glimelius B, Påhlman L. Preoperative or postoperative irradiation in adenocarcinoma of the rectum: final treatment results of a randomized trial and an evaluation of late secondary effects. *Dis Colon Rectum.* 1993;36(6):564-572.

Gérard A, Buyse M, Nordlinger B, et al. Preoperative radiotherapy as adjuvant treatment in rectal cancer: final results of a randomized study of the European Organization for Research and Treatment of Cancer (EORTC). *Ann Surg.* 1988;208(5):606-614.

Gérard JP, Azria D, Gourgou-Bourgade S, et al. Clinical outcome of the ACCORD 12/0405 PRODIGE 2 randomized trial in rectal cancer. *J Clin Oncol.* 2012;30(36):4558-4565.

Gérard JP, Azria D, Gourgou-Bourgade S, et al. Comparison of two neoadjuvant chemoradiotherapy regimens for locally advanced rectal cancer: results of the phase III trial ACCORD 12/0405-Prodige 2. *J Clin Oncol.* 2010;28(10):1638-1644.

Gérard JP, Conroy T, Bonnetain F, et al. Preoperative radiotherapy with or without concurrent fluorouracil and leucovorin in T3-4 rectal cancers: results of FFCD 9203. *J Clin Oncol.* 2006;24(28):4620-4625.

Goldberg PA, Nicholls RJ, Porter NH, Love S, Grimsey JE. Long-term results of a randomised trial of short-course low-dose adjuvant pre-operative radiotherapy for rectal cancer: reduction in local treatment failure. *Eur J Cancer.* 1994;30A(11):1602-1606.

Guillem JG, Díaz-González JA, Minsky BD, et al. cT3N0 rectal cancer: potential overtreatment with preoperative chemoradiotherapy is warranted. *J Clin Oncol.* 2008;26(3):368-373.

Kapiteijn E, Marijnen CA, Nagtegaal ID, et al. Preoperative radiotherapy combined with total mesorectal excision for resectable rectal cancer. *N Engl J Med.* 2001;345(9):638-646.

Krook JE, Moertel CG, Gunderson LL, et al. Effective surgical adjuvant therapy for high-risk rectal carcinoma. *N Engl J Med.* 1991;324(11):709-715.

Lingareddy V, Ahmad NR, Mohiuddin M. Palliative reirradiation for recurrent rectal cancer. *Int J Radiat Oncol Biol Phys.* 1997;38(4):785-790.

Medical Research Council Rectal Cancer Working Party. Randomised trial of surgery alone versus surgery followed by radiotherapy for mobile cancer of the rectum. *Lancet.* 1996;348(9042):1610-1614.

Medical Research Council Rectal Cancer Working Party. Randomised trial of surgery alone versus radiotherapy followed by surgery for potentially operable locally advanced rectal cancer. *Lancet.* 1996;348(9042):1605-1610.

Mohiuddin M, Lingareddy V, Rakinic J, Marks G. Reirradiation for rectal cancer and surgical resection after ultra high doses. *Int J Radiat Oncol Biol Phys.* 1993;27(5):1159-1163.

Mohiuddin M, Marks G, Marks J. Long-term results of reirradiation for patients with recurrent rectal carcinoma. *Cancer.* 2002;95(5):1144-1150.

Ngan SY, Burmeister B, Fisher RJ, et al. Randomized trial of short-course radiotherapy versus long-course chemoradiation comparing rates of local recurrence in patients with T3 rectal cancer: Trans-Tasman Radiation Oncology Group trial 01.04. *J Clin Oncol.* 2012;30(31):3827-3833.

O'Connell MJ, Martenson JA, Wieand HS, et al. Improving adjuvant therapy for rectal cancer by combining protracted-infusion fluorouracil with radiation therapy after curative surgery. *N Engl J Med.* 1994;331(8):502-507.

Påhlman L, Glimelius B. Pre- or postoperative radiotherapy in rectal and rectosigmoid carcinoma: report from a randomized multicenter trial. *Ann Surg.* 1990;211(2):187-195.

Peeters KC, Marijnen CA, Nagtegaal ID. The TME trial after a median follow-up of 6 years: increased local control but no survival benefit in irradiated patients with resectable rectal carcinoma. *Ann Surg.* 2007;246(5):693-701.

Pettersson D, Cedermark B, Holm T, et al. Interim analysis of the Stockholm III trial of preoperative radiotherapy regimens for rectal cancer. *Br J Surg.* 2010;97(4):580-587.

Reis Neto JA, Quilici FA, Reis JA Jr. A comparison of nonoperative vs. preoperative radiotherapy in rectal carcinoma. A 10-year randomized trial. *Dis Colon Rectum.* 1989;32(8):702-710.

Roh MS, Colangelo LH, O'Connell MJ. Preoperative multimodality therapy improves disease-free survival in patients with carcinoma of the rectum: NSABP R-03. *J Clin Oncol.* 2009;27(31):5124-5130.

Sauer R, Becker H, Hohenberger W, et al. Preoperative versus postoperative chemoradiotherapy for rectal cancer. *N Engl J Med.* 2004;351(17):1731-1740.

Sauer R, Liersch T, Merkel S, et al. Preoperative versus postoperative chemoradiotherapy for locally advanced rectal cancer: results of the German CAO/ARO/AIO-94 randomized phase III trial after a median follow-up of 11 years. *J Clin Oncol.* 2012;30(16):1926-1933.

Sebag-Montefiore D, Stephens RJ, Steele R, et al. Preoperative radiotherapy versus selective postoperative chemoradiotherapy in patients with rectal cancer (MRC CR07 and NCIC-CTG C016): a multicentre, randomised trial. *Lancet.* 2009;373(9666):811-820.

Smalley SR, Benedetti JK, Williamson SK, et al. Phase III trial of fluorouracil-based chemotherapy regimens plus radiotherapy in postoperative adjuvant rectal cancer: GI INT 0144. *J Clin Oncol.* 2006;24(22):3542-3547.

Stockholm Rectal Cancer Study Group. Preoperative short-term radiation therapy in operable rectal carcinoma. A prospective randomized trial. *Cancer.* 1990;66(1):49-55.

Stockholm Colorectal Cancer Study Group. Randomized study on preoperative radiotherapy in rectal carcinoma. *Ann Surg Oncol.* 1996;3(5):423-430.

Swedish Rectal Cancer Trial. Improved survival with preoperative radiotherapy in resectable rectal cancer. *N Engl J Med.* 1997;336(14):980-987.

Swedish Rectal Cancer Trial. Initial report from a Swedish multicentre study examining the role of preoperative irradiation in the treatment of patients with resectable rectal carcinoma. *Br J Surg*. 1993;80(10):1333-1336.

Swedish Rectal Cancer Trial. Local recurrence rate in a randomised multicentre trial of preoperative radiotherapy compared with operation alone in resectable rectal carcinoma. *Eur J Surg*. 1996;162(5):397-402.

Tepper JE, O'Connell M, Niedzwiecki D, et al. Adjuvant therapy in rectal cancer: analysis of stage, sex, and local control—final report of intergroup 0114. *J Clin Oncol*. 2002;20(7):1744-1750.

Thomas PR, Lindblad AS. Adjuvant postoperative radiotherapy and chemotherapy in rectal carcinoma: a review of the Gastrointestinal Tumor Study Group experience. *Radiother Oncol*. 1988;13(4):245-252.

Valentini V, Morganti AG, Gambacorta MA, et al. Preoperative hyperfractionated chemoradiation for locally recurrent rectal cancer in patients previously irradiated to the pelvis: a multicentric phase II study. *Int J Radiat Oncol Biol Phys*. 2006;64(4):1129-1139.

van Gijn W, Marijnen CA, Nagtegaal ID, et al. Preoperative radiotherapy combined with total mesorectal excision for resectable rectal cancer: 12-year follow-up of the multicentre, randomised controlled TME trial. *Lancet Oncol*. 2011;12(6):575-582.

Wolmark N, Wieand HS, Hyams DM, et al. Randomized trial of postoperative adjuvant chemotherapy with or without radiotherapy for carcinoma of the rectum: National Surgical Adjuvant Breast and Bowel Project Protocol R-02. *J Natl Cancer Inst*. 2000;92(5):388-396.

Anal Cancer

Ajani JA, Winter KA, Gunderson LL, et al. Fluorouracil, mitomycin, and radiotherapy vs fluorouracil, cisplatin, and radiotherapy for carcinoma of the anal canal: a randomized controlled trial. *JAMA*. 2008;299(16):1914-1921.

Bartelink H, Roelofsen F, Eschwege F, et al. Concomitant radiotherapy and chemotherapy is superior to radiotherapy alone in the treatment of locally advanced anal cancer: results of a phase III randomized trial of the European Organization for Research and Treatment of Cancer Radiotherapy and Gastrointestinal Cooperative Groups. *J Clin Oncol*. 1997;15(5):2040-2049.

Flam M, John M, Pajak TF, et al. Role of mitomycin in combination with fluorouracil and radiotherapy, and of salvage chemoradiation in the definitive nonsurgical treatment of epidermoid carcinoma of the anal canal: results of a phase III randomized intergroup study. *J Clin Oncol*. 1996;14(9):2527-2539.

Northover J, Glynne-Jones R, Sebag-Montefiore D, et al. Chemoradiation for the treatment of epidermoid anal cancer: 13-year follow-up of the first randomised UKCCCR Anal Cancer Trial (ACT I). *Br J Cancer*. 2010;102(7):1123-1128.

UK Coordinating Committee on Cancer Research. Epidermoid anal cancer: results from the UKCCCR randomised trial of radiotherapy alone versus radiotherapy, 5-fluorouracil, and mitomycin. UKCCCR Anal Cancer Trial Working Party. *Lancet*. 1996;348(9034):1049-1054.

Gynecological Malignancies

Tracy Sherertz

3.1 Cervix

Epidemiology

- It is the #1 cause of cancer mortality in women in developing nations.
- Pap smear screening programs have decreased mortality by 70%.
- Risk factors include: Human papillomavirus (HPV) infection, smoking, immunosuppression (HIV/AIDS), early first intercourse, multiple sexual partners, history of venereal disease, high parity, prenatal exposure to diethyl stilbestrol (DES) (for clear cell histology).
- 90% to 95% are associated with HPV infection.
- HPV type 16 leads to highest risk of squamous cell carcinoma (SCC) and HPV type 18 leads to highest risk of adenocarcinoma.
- HPV 6 and 11 are associated with benign warts.

Pathology

- 80% to 90% of invasive tumors are SCC.
- 10% to 20% are adenocarcinomas.
- 1% to 2% are clear cell carcinomas.
- Invasive SCC originates in the squamocolumnar junction.

Presentation

- Abnormal vaginal bleeding or discharge
- Pelvic pain
- Dyspareunia
- Hydroureter, hydronephrosis
- Weight loss
- Anemia
- Palpable adenopathy in locally advanced disease

Diagnosis and Workup

- Full H&P with attention to gynecological history, abnormal bleeding and/or pelvic pain, and examination of abdomen and inguinal/supraclavicular regions

- Pelvic exam with speculum, bimanual palpation and rectovaginal exam. Examination under anesthesia (EUA) performed with Gynecological Oncologist
- PAP smear if not bleeding
- Colposcopy with 15× magnification; cold conization if no grossly visible tumor, biopsy if visible
- Complete blood count (CBC) with platelets, liver function tests (LFTs), and BUN/Cr; pregnancy test and HIV test as clinically indicated
- Cystoscopy, sigmoidoscopy, and/or barium enema for IIB, III, or IVA disease, or based on clinical symptoms
- Imaging (optional for ≤ IBI): chest x-ray (CXR), CT/PET, MRI for treatment-planning purposes
- International Federation of Gynecology and Obstetrics (FIGO) staging not allowing for: CT, MRI, PET, bone scan, lymphoangiography, or laparotomy

Staging

Stage IA1	≤3-mm depth, ≤7-mm spread
Stage IA2	>3 mm, ≤5-mm depth, ≤7-mm spread
Stage IB1	clinically visible, confined to cervix, ≤4 cm
Stage IB2	clinically visible, confined to cervix, >4 cm
Stage IIA1	≤4 cm, invades beyond uterus, no parametrial involvement
Stage IIA2	>4 cm, invades beyond uterus, no parametrial involvement
Stage IIB	parametrial involvement
Stage IIIA	lower 1/3 vagina invasion
Stage IIIB	pelvic sidewall involvement or hydronephrosis/non-fxt kidney
Stage IVA	invasion into bladder/rectal mucosa
Stage IVB	outside true pelvis, including PA nodes or other mets

Treatment Overview

- Types of hysterectomy (all take the uterus and cervix):
  - *Class I:* Total abdominal hysterectomy (TAH)—extrafascial removal of cervix, cuff, outside of pubocervical fascia
  - *Class II:* Modified radical hysterectomy (MRH)—uterus, paracervical tissues and upper 2 cm of vagina removed after dissection of the ureters to the point of their entry into the bladder. The uterine arteries are ligated and the parametria (medial to the ureters) and proximal uterosacral ligaments are resected.
  - *Class III:* Radical abdominal hysterectomy (RAH)—ureters, bladder and rectum are mobilized for en bloc removal of the uterus, cervix and upper 1/3rd of the vagina along with the paracervical and parametrial tissues. Uterine arteries are ligated at their origin, and the entire width of the parametria (to the pelvic side wall) is resected bilaterally. Maximal removal of uterosacral ligaments.

- Ovarian preservation and reduction in sexual function side effects are often the reason to prefer surgery over RT if both are options.

Radiation Therapy Technique

External Beam Radiation Therapy

- Small bowel contrast
- Prone in CT simulator if patient eligible for belly board, otherwise supine

Stage	Treatment Options
IA1 (≤3-mm depth, ≤7-mm spread)	1. Conization for fertility preservation (if no LVSI) 2. TAH (recommended if LVSI present) 3. Intracavitary brachy to 65 Gy
IA2 (>3 mm, ≤5-mm depth, ≤7-mm spread)	MRH Type II + PLND ± pelvicRT/chemoRT[a] 1. RT alone: 45-Gy pelvic EBRT + Brachy (dose to Pt A = 75 Gy) if inoperable 2. Radical trachelectomy + PLND for fertility preservation
IB1 (clinically visible, confined to cervix, ≤4 cm), and IIA1 (invades beyond uterus but no parametrial involvement, <4 cm)	1. Conization for fertility preservation (if no LVSI) 2. TAH (recommended if LVSI present) 3. Intracavitary brachy to 65 Gy
IB2 (confined to cervix, >4 cm) and IIA2 (invades beyond uterus, no parametrial involvement)	1. MRH Type II + PLND ± pelvicRT/chemoRT[a] 2. RT alone: 45-Gy pelvic EBRT + Brachy (dose to Pt A = 75 Gy) if inoperable 3. Radical trachelectomy + PLND for fertility preservation
IIB (invades beyond uterus, with parametrial involvement)	1. RH Type III + PLND ± pelvic RT/chemoRT[a] RT alone: 45-Gy pelvic EBRT + Brachy (dose to Pt A = 85 Gy) ± concurrent cisplatin 40-mg/m^2 weekly × 6
IIIA (lower 1/3 vagina invasion)	Definitive ChemoRT: 45-Gy pelvic + inguinal EBRT + Brachy (dose Pt A = 85 Gy) + cis 40-mg/m^2 weekly × 6, may need Syed for vaginal involvement
IIIB (pelvic sidewall involvement or hydronephrosis/nonfunctioning kidney)	Definitive ChemoRT: 45-Gy pelvic EBRT + sidewall boost (540 cGy) + Brachy (Pt A = 85 Gy) + cisplatin 40-mg/m^2 weekly × 6
IVA (invasion into bladder/rectal mucosa)	Definitive Chemoradiation: 45-Gy pelvic EBRT + Brachy (dose to Pt A = 85 Gy) + concurrent cisplatin 40-mg/m^2 weekly × 6
IVB (outside true pelvis)	
PA nodes	Pelvic + PA RT to 45 Gy, IMRT node boost to 60 Gy, w concurrent cisplatin 40-mg/m^2 weekly × 6 LND if nodes >2 cm.
Other mets	Chemotherapy alone
Extensive bleeding at presentation	Transfuse to Hgb >10, vaginal packing, 3 Gy × 3

[a] Post-op pelvic RT based on Sedlis + Peters criteria: Presence of LVSI, tumor >4 cm, >1/3.EBRT, external beam radiation therapy; IMRT, intensity-modulated radiation therapy; LVSI, lymphovascular space invasion; TAH, total abdominal hysterectomy.

- Radio-opaque vaginal marker, or place seeds within cervix and inferior extent of vaginal disease
- Four-field plan (assisted by node contouring)

- AP/PA:
  - Superior: L4/L5 (cover mid commons)
  - Inferior: obturator foramen and 4 cm below tumor
  - Lateral: 2-cm off pelvic brim
  - PA field: T12/L1, lateral at transverse proc.
- Laterals:
  - Same superior/inferior border as AP/PA fields
  - Anterior: ant-symphysis (include external iliacs, block a little bowel and genitalia)
  - Posterior: behind sacrum at least to S3, then block lower rectum
- Parametria boost—Stage II and above (if there is PM involvement)
  - Superior: bottom SI
  - Inferior: obturator foramen (same)
  - Medial: import brachy/EBRT isodoses and block at cumulative 65-Gy line (or place 6-cm midline block)
  - Lateral: 2 cm from pelvic brim (same)
- Add 4.5-cm midline block
  - Widen or narrow the block based on normal tissue tolerance and desired target coverage
- Energy—10 MV or higher
- Dose
  - Post-op: 50.40 Gy
  - Definitive: 45-Gy whole pelvis
  - Boost parametria to 50.4 to 60 Gy between implants if needed
- Total treatment time <8 weeks, 56 days

GEC-ESTRO Guidelines for Target Delineation

- Target volumes based on MRI, two-weighted images
  - GTV at diagnosis
  - GTV at brachy #1, brachy #2, and so on
  - HR-CTV to 85 Gy
    - Entire cervix
    - Residual disease at time of brachy
  - IR-CTV
    - HR-CTV + 1- to 1.5-cm margin, but not into bladder or bowel
    - Includes GTV at diagnosis
- Planning goal: Define the disease, define OARs, shape the dose accordingly
- No chemotherapy or EBRT on HDR days
- There is a movement away from 600-cGy fractions for HDR—may be able to lower dose based on volumetric planning

Tandem and Ovoid Brachytherapy

- General anesthesia or other sedation
- Dorsal lithotomy position
- EUA
  - Speculum—extent of disease and response to EBRT
  - Bimanual exam—extent (parametria, sidewall, vaginal involvement) + position of uterus
- Prep and drape the patient
- Foley (7 mL of 30% renografin soln in balloon)
- Insert Deaver retractors to visualize cervix
- Grasp anterior lip cervix with tenaculum

- Insert gold seeds at 6 + 12 o'clock of cervix
- Sound uterine canal, noting depth
- Dilate cervical os sequentially to 16 French (6 mm)
- Choose tandem length = sounding length −0.5 cm, max length above flange 8 cm; longer tandem = more dose to paracervical tissue
- Choose tandem curvature that conforms to uterus shape and balances sacral/bladder dose (sagittal view from CT sim helps)
- Place tandem through the os into the endometrium with flange flush against os (optional, place a smit sleeve to aid in subsequent outpatient fractions)
- Choose largest ovoids that will fit in fornix (r2 to reduce vag muc dose)
- Place ovoid over tandem and slide ovoids into vagina to maximum depth
- Squeeze ovoids to allow 3 to 4 cm separation, tighten wing nut
- Soak radio-opaque gauze in betadine (vs. clindamycin cream)
- Pack apparatus starting posteriorly
- Optional plain films to confirm placement: Goals: Tandem 1/3 distance between S1 and symphysis, tandem straight on AP and bisects ovoids on AP and lateral, flange flush to os, no packing above ovoids, ovoids at level of flange (can use scout CT films instead)
- DVT prophylaxis
- CT sim: (Optional) Use 30 mL of dilute contrast into bladder and 30-mL gastrograffin into rectum

ICRU 38 Guidelines

- *Pt A:* 2-cm cephalad and 2-cm lat from external os (parametria)—measured *from phlange*, receives ~85 Gy
- *Pt B:* 3-cm lateral to Pt A, fixed Pt even if Pt A is off-center (obturator nodes), measured *from midline*, gets 25% Pt A dose—55 Gy
- *Rectal Pt:* 0.5 cm from post vaginal packing, at level of ovoids
- *Bladder Pt:* posterior surface of Foley balloon
- *Vaginal Pt:* @ mid/lat point of ovoids on AP film

Dose Limits

- Rectum: 70-Gy Pt dose (4.1 Gy/fx), <65 Gy 2-mL EQD2
- Bladder: 75-Gy Pt dose (4.6 Gy/fx), <70 Gy 2-mL EQD2
- Upper vagina: 120 Gy
- Lower vagina: 90 Gy
- Uterus: 100 Gy
- Femoral heads: 50 Gy
- If HDR (for conversion, do BED calc with alpha/beta=10, then divide by 1.2 which is 2 Gy/fx conversion with 2/10):
- Ir-192, 10 Ci source, T½ = 74 days, 380 KeV

Outcomes

- Prognostic factors: age, race, socioeconomic status, Hgb level <10, tumor hypoxia, stage, extension to uterus
- IA1: Pelvic lymph node (LN): 1%
  PA LN: 0%
  5-year overall survival (OS): 95% to 98%
- IA2: Pelvic LN: 5%
  PA LN: 0%
  5-year OS: 90% to 95%

- IB1:   Pelvic LN: 15%
         PA LN: 5%
         5-year OS: 85%, LC 98%
- IB2:   Pelvic LN: 15%
         PA node: 5%
         5-year OS: 80% to 85%
         Concurrent chemo affords a 15% improvement in 5-year OS over extended field RT alone
         4-year OS: 85%
- IIA: Pelvic LN 30%
         PA LN: 10%
         5-year LC: 80%
         5-year OS: 70%
- IIB: Pelvic LN: 30%
         PA LN: 20%
         5-year LC: 80%
         5-year OS: 65%
- IIIA: Pelvic LN: 50%
         PA LN: 30%
         5-year LC: 70%
         5-year OS: 40% to 45%
- IIIB: Pelvic LN:50%
         PA LN: 30%
         5-year LC: 70%
         5-year OS: 40% to 45%
- IVA: Pelvic LN: 60%
         PA LN: 30%
         5-year LC: 25%
         5-year OS: 20%
- IVB: 5-year OS <10%

Data

- *Landoni:* Rad Hyst (64% req'd post-op RT) versus RT alone (70–90 Gy to Pt A) for <IIB:
  - No diff in OS (83%) EXCEPT ADENO, greater complications with surgery
  - If tumor >4 cm, 84% chance of XRT
- *GOG 109:* chemoRT versus Rt for high risk (+LNs, parametrium or margins)
  - Chemo was cis/5-FU
  - + OS benefit with the addition of chemotherapy
- *GOG 0724 (open):* post-op RT (+lns, parametria) with weekly cisplatin, randomized to ±4 cycles adjuvant carbo/taxol
- *Morris (RTOG 90-01):* IIB to IVA, bulky IB or IIA, or + LN, Pelvic + PA RT versus cisplatin/FU + pelvic RT, Dose to Pt A = 85 Gy in both arms
  - Improved LC, distant metastasis (DM), OS w/chemo
  - Advanced pts who cannot tolerate chemo should get PA+ pelvic RT (Rotman *RTOG* 79-20)
- *Keys (GOG 123):* Bulky IB
  - RT 75Gy versus cis/RT
  - Both followed by hysterectomy
  - Better OS in chemo arm (74% vs. 85%)

- *Whitney (GOG 85):* Stage IIB to IVA
  - o Standard pelvic RT (45 Gy + ICRT) randomized to HU versus cisplatin/5-FU
  - o 5-year OS: 47% versus 60%
- *Rose (GOG 120):* Stage IIB to IVA
  - o Pelvic RT to 41 to 51 Gy + 1 to 2 ICRT
  - o Randomized to cisplatin (40 mg/m^2) versus HU/cisplatin/5-FU versus HU
  - o Cisplatin-based had better OS/disease free survival (DFS)
- *Pearcey, NCIC:* RT versus RT+cis for advanced dz: no diff in PFS or OS

Post-Op Treatment

- *Intermediate risk* (Sedlis GOG 92)
  - o IB-IIA, RT to 46 to 50.4 Gy versus observation

LVI	Depth	Size
+	Deep	Any
+	Deep	>2 cm
+	Sup	>5 cm
−	Mid/deep	>4 cm

  - o Decreased LR from 28% to 15%
  - o Can offer concurrent chemotherapy for Sedlis criteria because LF was still high @ 15%
- *High risk* (Peters *RTOG* 91-12)
  - o IA2—IIA, RT (49.3 Gy) versus cis 70 to 75 q 3 weeks × 2, and 5-FU 1,000 1 to 4, + same RT
    - Positive margins
    - Parametrial involvement
    - Positive LNs
  - o OS benefit: 71% versus 81%
- NCCN high risk definition:
  - o +LN, +margins, lympho vascular invasion (LVI), deep stromal invasion, large primary tumor, +parametrium

Toxicity

- Radiation-related
  - o Gastrointestinal (GI) complications: SBO 5%
  - o Menopause/infertility
  - o Second malignancies
  - o More sexual dysfunction than surgery
  - o Fistula: 5%
  - o Femoral neck fracture: 5%
  - o Ovarian failure with 5 to 10 Gy
  - o Sterilization with 2 Gy
- Surgical
  - o Bladder dysfunction
  - o Infertility but not menopause
  - o Ureteral stricture/fistula

- o Lymphedema
- o Chronic constipation

Follow-Up

- Interval H&P every 3 to 6 months for 2 years, then every 6 to 12 months for 3 to 5 years, then annually
- Cervical/vaginal cytology annually, although likelihood of detecting asymptomatic recurrences by cytology alone is low
- Imaging (CXR, CT, PET/CT, MRI) as clinically indicated based on symptoms and exam
- Patient education regarding symptoms of recurrence, lifestyle modification (nutrition, smoking cessation, etc.)
- Patient education regarding sexual heath, use of vaginal dilator, and lubricants

3.2   Endometrium

Epidemiology

- Most common cause of cancer in women in developed countries
- Risk factors: Obesity, unopposed estrogen exposure, nulliparity, tamoxifen use, advanced age, lymphovascular space invasion (LVSI), lower uterine segment involvement, genetic factors including Lynch syndrome
- Depth of invasion correlated with risk of lymph node involvement
- Grade of invasion correlated with local recurrence risk
- Prognostic features: stage, grade, histology (clear cell/serous worse), depth of myometrial invasion, cervical involvement, LVSI

Pathology

- Endometrioid endometrial adenocarcinoma (estrogen-related): 75% of cases
- Papillary serous (UPSC), clear cell, and mucinous carcinomas (nonestrogen related): 20% of cases
- Leiyomyosarcoma/endometrial stromal sarcoma, uterine sarcoma, and adenosarcoma: ~5% of cases
- Papillary serous and clear cell histologies: behave more aggressively; often locally advanced at the time of diagnosis

Presentation

- Postmenopausal bleeding
- Pelvic pain
- Hydroureter/hydronephrosis in advanced disease

Diagnosis and Workup

- H+P including gynecological speculum exam with bimanual palpation and rectovaginal exam, noting extension to cervix, vagina, rectum, presence of lymphadenopathy, or ascites
- Endometrial biopsy in office, D+C if endometrial biopsy is negative
- Labs (CBC, complete metabolic profile [CMP], Ca-125, carcino embryonic antigen (CEA))
- Genetic counseling for family history
- CXR
- (Optional): EUA, cystoscopy/proctoscopy if suspicious, intravenous pyelogram (IVP), CXR, CTabd/pel

Staging

- Endometrial adenocarcinoma

Stage IA	<50% myometrial invasion
Stage IB	≥50% myometrial invasion
Stage II	Cervical stromal involvement
Stage IIIA	Extension to serosa or adnexa (direct involvement or mets)
Stage IIIB	Vaginal or parametrial involvement
Stage IIIC1	Pelvic lymph node involvement
Stage IIIC2	Para-aortic lymph node involvement
Stage IVA	Bowel or bladder mucosal involvement
Stage IVB	Distant mets (includes inguinal nodal involvement, peritoneal disease or lung/liver/bone mets)

- Leiyomyosarcoma/endometrial stromal sarcoma, uterine sarcoma, and adenosarcoma all with their own distinct (separate) staging systems

Treatment Overview

- All operable patients should have a TAH/bi-lateral oopherectomy (BSO) (or radical hysterectomy if cervical involvement) with peritoneal cytology.

Stage	Treatment Options
IA, G1-2	• Observation vs. *VCT* if adverse risk features present (*LVSI*, advanced age)
IB, G1	• Observation vs. VCT if adverse risk features present
IA, G3	• VCT or consider pelvic *EBRT* if adverse risk features present
IB, G2	• VCT or pelvic EBRT if adverse risk features present
IB, G3	• Pelvic EBRT or VCT if no adverse risk features present; consider VCT + chemotherapy if patient meets criteria for GOG 0429
II	• VCT if grade 1; pelvic RT + VCT for grade 2–3; consider chemotherapy for grade 3; consider VCT + chemotherapy if patient meets criteria for GOG 0249
III–IVA	• Surgery → Chemotherapy ± tumor-directed RT
Medically inoperable	• Tumor-directed EBRT 45 to 50.4 Gy ± Intracavitary brachytherapy boost 6 Gy × 3 fractions; consider boost to involved LNs to 60 Gy using IMRT

(continued)

(continued)

Stage	Treatment Options
Papillary/clear cell	• Surgery → Chemotherapy ± tumor-directed RT
Sarcoma/MMMTs	• Surgery. Consider chemotherapy for high-grade undifferentiated sarcoma or leiomyosarcoma; consider *post-op* RT for high-grade sarcomas, leiomyosarcomas, and carcinosarcomas; may improve local control but not OS

EBRT, external beam radiation therapy; IMRT, intensity-modulated radiation therapy; LVSI, lymphovascular space invasion; VCT, vaginal cuff brachytherapy.

Radiation Therapy Technique

- Pelvic external beam radiation therapy
  - Prone if patient good candidate for belly board
  - CT simulation with vaginal marker
  - Four field, at least 10-MV photons
  - Superior: L5-S1
  - Inferior: bottom of obturator foramen (include upper vagina)
  - Lateral: 2 cm beyond pelvic brim
  - Anterior: ant-symphysis, shield bowel (upper), and genitals
  - Posterior: behind sacrum to S3, then shield rectum
  - Dose: 45 Gy if planning IVRT, may go up to 50.4 Gy if not
  - Boost involved nodes to 60 Gy with intensity-modulated radiation therapy (IMRT)
- Whole abdominal radiation therapy
  - Supine, AP/PA versus 3DCRT, at least 10-MV photons
  - CT sim; optional 4D sim versus fluoro sim to assess diaphragm motion
  - Superior: 1 cm above diaphragm (assess via fluoro)
  - Inferior: ischial tuberosity
  - Lateral: peritoneal stripe
  - Dose: 30 Gy in 1.5-Gy fractions
  - Then drop border to L5-S1 and treat whole pelvic (WP) to 46.2 Gy in 1.8-Gy fractions
  - Block kidneys on PA from day 1
  - Block liver AP/PA after 22.5 Gy
  - If treating PALNs: upper border at top of T12 or where renal vessels cross aorta
- Intracavitary vaginal cuff brachytherapy
  - Use largest diameter vaginal cylinder to minimize mucosal surface dose.
  - Treat upper 3 to 5 cm of vagina; if IIIB, treat whole vagina.
  - *Many dose variations are acceptable for intracavitary vaginal cuff brachytherapy alone*:
    - 700 cGy × 3 fractions to 5 mm from the surface
  - If used as a boost for pelvic EBRT, reduce dose:
    - 500 cGy × 3 fractions to the vaginal surface
  - Length of vagina treated depends on stage and grade; average length of vagina is ~10 cm.

Outcomes

- I: 5-year OS: 90%
- II: 5-year OS: 80%

- IIIA: 5-year OS: 60%
- IIIB: 5-year OS: 40%
- IIIC: 5-year OS: 27% to 50%
- IVA: 5-year OS: 20%
- IVB: 5-year OS: 10% to 20%

Data

- *GOG 99* (Keys, *Gynecol Oncol*. 2004; doi:10.1016/j.ygyno.2004.01.009)
  - TAH versus TAH + Pelvic RT (50.4 Gy) for Int. Risk (IB, IC, II)
  - *Subgroup analysis:*
  - Risk factors: mod-poorly diff grade, LVI, outer 1/3 myometrial invasion
    - *High Intermediate Risk (HIR)*
      - >70 years with one other risk factor
      - >50 years with two other risk factors
      - Any age with all three risk factors
    - *Low Intermediate Risk (LIR): all others*
    - → RT reduced 4-year LRR for HIR pts 27% to 13%; for LIR pts 6% to 2%.
- *PORTEC trial* (Creutzberg, *Lancet*. 2000. doi:10.1016/j.ijrobp.2011.04.013)
  - (Old staging) IB (grade 2 or 3) and IC grade (1 or 2)
  - TAH versus TAH + Pelvic RT (46 Gy), no PLND
  - 5-year LR = 14% versus 4%, no diff in OS
- *Norwegian Radium Hospital* (Bergsjo, *Am J Obstet Gynecol*. 1966;95(4):496-507)
  - TAH + IVRT versus TAH + IVRT + EBRT (no PLND)
  - LR = 7% versus 2% (EBRT), no diff in OS
  - Trend toward improvement in OS for IC Grade 3
- *PORTEC2* (doi:10.1016/S0140-6736(09)62163-2): no surg staging, IC 1,2 and IB 3,II 1,2 (old staging)
  - VCT versus EBRT
  - VCT: 21 Gy/3 versus 46-Gy pelvic EBRT
  - LRR 5% versus 2%
  - Pelvic LN 3.8% versus 0.5% at 45 months
  - OS/DFS/DM same
  - Quality of life (QOL) better with VCT

Toxicity

- Acute side effects: fatigue, loose stools, diarrhea, skin irritation, vaginal irritation, rectal irritation, worsening of hemorrhoids, increased urinary frequency, and dysuria
- Long-term side effects: rectal bleeding, stricture formation, urinary frequency, atrophic vaginitis (bleeding)
- Potential complications:
  - Small bowel obstruction
  - Reduced bladder volume
  - Femoral head fractures or necrosis
  - Lower extremity edema
  - Vaginal narrowing/shortening and loss of natural lubrication
  - Incidence of major complications of 1% to 10%
- Complication rates:
  - Node dissection + Pelvic radiation: 5% to 12%
  - Pelvic radiation: 3% to 5%
  - Vaginal brachytherapy: 0% to 1%

Follow-Up

- Interval H&P every 3 to 6 months for 2 years, then every 6 months or annually
- Patient education regarding symptoms of recurrence, lifestyle modification (nutrition, weight loss, obesity prevention, exercise, smoking cessation, etc.)
- CA-125 optional
- Imaging (CXR, CT, PET/CT, MRI) as clinically indicated based on symptoms and exam
- Patient education regarding sexual heath, use of vaginal dilator, and lubricants
- Consideration of genetic counseling for patients <50 years, or with family history of endometrial and/or colorectal cancer

3.3   Vagina

Epidemiology

- Rare
- 1% to 2% gynecological cancers
- Incidence and mortality increase with age
- Risk factors:
  - *SCC: peak age 50 to 70 years*
    - Multiple lifetime sexual partners
    - Early age at first intercourse
    - Current smoker
    - Cervical intraepithelial neoplasia (CIN), VAIN, or Cis
    - VAIN associated with HPV, frequently multifocal
    - Immunosuppression
    - Pelvic RT
    - Increased incidence in younger women may be 2/2 HPV infection
  - *Clear cell adenocarcinoma: peak age second to third decade*
    - In utero exposure to DES

Pathology

- 80% to 90% squamous cell CA
- 5% to 15% clear cell adenoCA or other adenoCAs
- 5% melanoma, m. frequent in the lower 1/3rd
- 1% to 2% adult sarcomas, small cell, papillary serous, lymphoma
- Metastasis

Presentation

- Vaginal bleeding, discharge, dysuria, or pelvic pain
- Palpable mass (distal lesions occur more commonly on the posterior wall of the vaginal)
- Less commonly, abnormal Pap smear
- Risk of LN involvement by stage:
  - Stage I: 5%
  - Stage II: 25%
  - Stage III: 75%
  - Stage IV: 85%

Diagnosis and Workup

- H&P
- Labs: CBC, comprehensive metabolic profile including LFTs and alkaline phosphatase
- Pap smear
- EUA (with the gynecologic oncologist, speculum rotated for posterior wall, bimanual, and rectal exam) with directed biopsies of the cervix and vulva to rule/out primary cervical and/or vulvar CA
- If suspicious inguinal nodes, fine-needle aspiration (FNA) or excise
- Stage IIB to III disease:
  - Cystoscopy, especially if anterior wall is involved
  - Procto-sigmoidoscopy, especially if involving the posterior wall
- Imaging:
  - CXR + IVP
  - Pelvic CT and/or MRI (not to be used in staging)
    - Positive predictive value (PPV) of MRI for primary and metastatic tumors: 84%
    - Negative predictive value (NPV) 97%
    - Can help differentiate tumor from fibrotic tissue in recurrent disease

Staging

Stage I	Confined to vagina
Stage II	Paravaginal/parametrial extension
Stage III	Pelvic sidewall extension or pelvic/inguinal LN mets
Stage IVA	Invasion into bladder/rectal mucosa
Stage IVB	Distant mets

Treatment Overview

- Few studies because of rarity
- XRT often preferred over surgery since less morbid
- General indications for surgery:
  - Recurrence after XRT
  - Young pts with clear cell adenocarcinoma and/or to preserve ovarian function
- T1N0:
  - Surgery can preserve ovarian function
  - <5-mm invasion: intracavitary brachy alone
  - >5-mm invasion: intracavitary + interstitial brachytherapy
- T2 to T3
  - Pelvic EBRT + interstitial brachytherapy
- T4
  - Pelvic exenteration if high risk for fistula, or definitive RT as above
- Can add concurrent cisplatin for T3 to T4/N1, based on extrapolation from cervix

Radiation Therapy Technique

- Simulate supine in frog leg to minimize overlap of perineal tissues
- Vaginal markers/seeds at borders of tumor
- Target volumes:
  - AP/PA field borders
    - Sup: L5/S1, or L4/L5 if LN+
    - Inf: entire vagina and 3 cm below lowest extent of tumor
    - Lat: 2-cm lat to pelvic brim
  - If distal 1/3 involved, lateral borders need to include inguinal femoral nodes
    - Superolateral border: ant sup iliac spine
    - Lat border: greater trochanter
    - Inf: inguinal crease or 2.5 cm below ischium
  - Boost positive nodes up to 60 Gy
  - Inguinal nodes
    - IMRT
    - Anterior beam either lower energy or with supplemental e-beam
- Target dose:
  - In general:
    - Subclinical CTV = LQD2 dose: 60 to 65 Gy target entire vagina
    - Tumor CTV = LQD2 Dose: stage and site dependent, ~70 to 75 Gy to 80 to 85 Gy
- Brachytherapy
  - Largest diameter should be used to minimize the ratio of mucosal dose to tumor dose.
  - Upper 1/3 lesions are treated with intrauterine tandem and vaginal colpostats followed by treatment of the middle and lower 1/3 of the vagina with a cylinder.
  - If tumor has depth <0.5 cm, may use intracavitary applicator.
  - If tumor has depth >0.5 cm, use interstitial.
- Dose limitations
  - Upper vaginal mucosa tolerance: 120 Gy
  - Midvaginal mucosa tolerance: 80 to 90 Gy
  - Lower vaginal mucosa tolerance: 60 to 70 Gy
  - Vaginal doses of >50 to 60 Gy: significant risk of fibrosis and stenosis
  - Dilator recommended
  - Ovarian failure: 5 to 10 Gy
  - Sterilization: 2 to 3 Gy
  - Limit bladder ≤65 Gy, rectum ≤60 Gy

Outcomes

- 5-year OS:
  - Stage I: 75%
  - Stage II: 50%
  - Stage III: 30%
  - Stage IV: 20%

- Prognostic factors:
  - Stage
  - Age
  - Tumor size (>1/3 length)
  - Location (upper 1/3 better)
  - Histology (adenoCA)
  - Grade

- o Use of brachytherapy, RT dose >75 Gy
- o Shorter treatment time
- Definitive RT, Frank et al., *IJROBP*. 2005; doi:10.1016/j.ijrobp.2004.09.032
  - o 193 patients treated at a single institution 1970 to 2000
  - o 5-year DSS rates:
    - 85% for stage I
    - 78% for state II
    - 58% for stage III to IVA (P = .0013)
  - o 5-year DSS rates:
    - 82% for tumors <4 cm
    - 60% for tumors >4 cm (P = .0001)
  - o 5-year pelvic disease control rates:
    - 86% for stage I
    - 84% for stage II
    - 71% for stage III to IVA (P = .027)
  - o 5-year risk of complications:
    - 25% in current smokers
    - 18% in patients who claimed to have quit >6 months before XRT
    - 5% in patients who had no smoking history (P < .01)
- Role for chemotherapy is controversial.
- Concurrent chemoRT is reasonable for stages III to IV:
  - o This is based on extrapolating from cervical, vulvar, and anal literature.
  - o Many single institution studies have suggested improved control rates.

Toxicity

- Vaginal dryness/atrophy
- Pubic hair loss
- Vaginal stenosis/fibrosis (50%)
- Cystitis (50%)
- Proctitis (40%)
- Rectovaginal or vesicovaginal fistula (<5%)
- Vaginal necrosis (<5%–15%)
- Urethral stricture (rare)
- Bowel obstruction (rare)
- Vaginal dilators recommended to minimize stenosis

Follow-Up

- Interval H&P (including pelvic exam) every 3 months for 1 year, then every 4 months for 2nd year, then every 6 months for 3rd and 4th year, then annually after 5 years
- CXR annually
- Other imaging as clinically indicated

3.4 Vulva

Epidemiology

- 3% to 4% of all primary genital cancers
- Peak incidence seventh to eighth decades

- Mean age:
  - CIS: 44 years
  - Microinvasive carcinoma: 58 years
  - Invasive carcinoma: 61 years
- Incidence and mortality increase with age
- 70% from the labia majora/minora:
  - 10% to 15% clitoris
  - 5% perineum
  - <1% Bartholin's gland, vestibule
- Risk factors:
  - HPV 16, 18, 33
  - Vulvar intraepithelial neoplasia (VIN) (2%–5% progress to CA)
  - Bowen's disease (Cis)
  - Paget's disease
  - Erythroplasia
  - Chronic irritant vaginitis
  - Leukoplakia
  - Prior GU cancer
  - Employment in laundry and cleaning industry
  - Smoking

Pathology

- Keratinizing, differentiated, or simplex type
  - More common
  - Occurs in older women
  - Not related to HPV infection
  - Associated with vulvar dystrophies
- Classic, warty, or Bowenoid type
  - Predominantly associated with HPV 16, 18, and 33
  - Found in younger women

Presentation

- Early stage—vulvar mass/pruritis
- Advanced stage—pruritis, bleeding, pain, drainage, palpable groin nodes

Diagnosis and Workup

- H&P with EUA
  - Extent/depth/size/fixation of primary
- Colposcopic biopsy of cervix, vagina, and vulva bc of multifocal nature
  - Excisional bx for <1 cm
  - Wedge biopsy with surrounding skin, dermis, and subcutaneous tissue for larger lesions
- FNA or excisional bx of inguinal nodes (may be unilateral if well lateralized)
- CXR, CBC, chemistry, UA
- Cystoscopy, proctosigmoidoscopy, barium enema (BE), IVP for larger lesions/node involvement
- CT A/P can help identify inguinofemoral, pelvic, PA LNs, and tumor extent

Staging

Stage I	≤2 cm, confined to vulva/perineum
Stage IA	≤1-mm stromal invasion
Stage IB	>1-mm stromal invasion
Stage II	>2 cm, confined to vulva/perineum
Stage III	Spread to lower urethra, vagina, or anus and/or unilateral regional LN
Stage IVA	Spread to upper urethra, bladder mucosa, rectal mucosa, or pelvic bone and/or bilateral regional LN
Stage IVB	DM including pelvic LN

Treatment Overview

- VIN
  - Laser therapy, wide local excision (WLE), skinning vulvectomy, topical 5-FU (least preferable)
- IA (vulva/perineum, <2 cm, <1-mm stromal invasion)
  - WLE
- IB (>1-mm stromal invasion)
  - WLE + unilateral superficial inguinal node dissection
- II (>2 cm, no contiguous invasion, neg nodes)
  - WLE with b/l sup inguinal node dissection (unless well lateralized)
  - If unfavorable primary (<8-mm margins, LVSI, >5-mm stromal inv), treat central region only RT to 50.4
- III (contiguous invasion to the vagina/anus/lower urethra, or ipsilateral ing/fem nodes)
  - If ipsilateral nodes: WLE with b/l superior inguinal dissection, RT to pelvis/groin and central region
  - If contiguous invasion: definitive chemoRT
  - May consider preop chemoRT for smaller surgery (Moore)
- IVA (upper urethra, rectal, bladder, pubic bone, or b/l ing nodes):
  - Pelvic exenteration, radical vulvectomy, and b/l inguinal node dissection
  - Preop chemoRT for smaller surgery
  - Radical chemoRT
- IVB (pelvic nodes or other distant mets):
  - If IVB by positive pelvic nodes, radical chemoRT
  - If IVB by distant mets, palliative intent RT
- For Stage III/IV—can add chemo per Moore (cis/5-FU) (also extrapolating from other SCC sites).
- For stage III/IVA disease, can try preop chemoRT to improve operability (Moore).
- For medically inoperable disease, give radical RT to 70 Gy; consider concurrent chemo.

Radiation Therapy Technique

- Simulate frog leg, supine, wire nodes, and vulva
- Contour LNs on CT

- *Fields:*
  - AP/PA with photons
  - Supplement inguinal nodes with electrons (energy based on depth of nodes on CT)
  - Inf border: flash vulva 3 cm (2 cm below lesser trochanter)
  - Sup border: L4/L5 for pelvic nodes; ASIS for groin only
  - If positive pelvic LNs, L3/4
  - Lateral:
    - AP (6 MV)—line from ASIS to pubic tubercle, 2 cm above, 8 cm below
    - PA (15 MV)—2 cm beyond pelvic brim, exclude femoral heads
- IMRT
  - Beriwal. *IJROBP.* 2006; doi:10.1016/j.ijrobp.2005.11.007
  - 15 pts with vulvar cancer tx with IMRT 7 pre-op, 8 post-op
  - Nodal CTV: included bilateral external iliac, internal iliac, inguinofemoral regions
    - 1-cm margin around iliac vessels
    - 2-cm margin around inguinofemoral vessels
  - Vulvar CTV = entire vulva +1 cm
  - Bolus over vulva
- Dose:
  - Primary: Neg margin: 5040, Pos margin: 5940, Gross Dz: 6480
  - Nodes: Pos groin: 5040 to both groins, extracapsular extension (ECE): 5940, gross or extensive ECE: 6480.

Outcomes

- 5-year OS by stage:
  - I: 90%
  - II: 77%
  - III: 51%
  - IV: 18%
- Known prognostic factors:
  - *Nodal recurrence*
    - Size
    - Histologic grade
    - LVI
    - Clinical nodes
    - Ulceration
  - *Primary recurrence*
    - Margin <8 mm (1-cm fresh)
    - Size >4 cm
    - Grade
    - Depth of invasion >5 to 9 mm
    - LVI
  - *OS*
    - Stage
    - Nodal status (Inguinal/pelvic, # nodes, unilateral/bilateral, ECE, ulceration)
- If inguinal LNs involved, risk of pelvic LN involvement = 30%
- GOG 101: Moore *IJROBP.* 1998;42(1):79-85.
  - Phase II trial of planned split course of concurrent 5-FU/cisplatin + RT followed by surgical excision + bilateral groin dissection
  - 50% CR

- GOG 37: Homesley *Obst & Gynecol* 1986;68(6):733-740
  - Post-op pelvic/inguinal RT (45–50 Gy) versus PLND for N+ after radical vulvectomy + inguinal node dissection
  - *No RT to primary*
  - OS 2-year RT: 68% versus LND 54%
  - OS advantage to RT if matted nodes or 2+LN
  - OS benefit did not hold with longer FU
- GOG 88: Stehman *IJROBP*. 1992; doi:10.1016/0360-3016(92)90699-I
  - Groin LND versus groin RT for N0-1 Vulvar SCC after radical vulvectomy
  - Groin recurrence RT: 18% versus 0% surgery
  - Worse outcome for RT b/c prescribed to 3-cm depth (no CT planning, no pelvic RT)
- Dusenberry
  - 48% recurrence if central block is used—don't block primary when treating nodes.

Toxicity

- Lymphedema
- Skin changes
- Vaginal stricture/stenosis
- Bowel/bladder injury
- Femoral neck fracture

Follow-Up

- Interval H&P (including pelvic exam and Pap smear) every 3 months for 1 year, then every 4 months for 2nd year, then every 6 months for 3rd and 4th year, then annually after 5 years
- CXR annually

3.5 Ovary/Fallopian Tube

Epidemiology

- It is the second most common gynecological cancer and leading cause of cancer death in most developed countries.
- Peak incidence occurs in the eighth decade.
- It is highly curable if detected early; no cost-effective screening test.
- Risk factors include: family history (first-degree relative is strongest risk factor), nulliparity, late first parity >35 years, ovulation inducing drugs, hormone replacement therapy (HRT), dietary factors including coffee intake, high fat and high lactose diet, genetic predisposition (~5% of tumors result from genetic disposition).
- Protective factors include: Oral contraceptive pills (OCP) use, high parity, tubal ligation, lactation.
- Genetic syndromes with increased risk:
  - BRCA1: 35% to 45% lifetime risk
  - BRCA2: 15% to 25% lifetime risk
  - Lynch syndrome (HNPCC) or history of other gyn/GU tract cancers

Pathology

- 90% epithelial
  - Graded from borderline to undifferentiated
  - Histological subtypes: 50% serous, 20% endometrioid, 15% undifferentiated, 10% mucinous, 4% clear cell

- 4% to 8% stromal
- 24% germ cell

Presentation

- Tends to have indolent course
- Abdominal pain
- Nausea
- Early satiety
- Change in bowel habits
- Bloating/increased abdominal girth
- Pleural effusion
- Sister Mary Joseph nodule
- Blummer's shelf
- Stage at presentation
  - I: 25%
  - II:15%
  - III: 45%
  - IV: 15%

Diagnosis and Workup

- H+P including gynecological speculum exam with bimanual palpation
- Pap smear
- Endometrial biopsy if bleeding
- Labs—CBC, CMP including LFTs
- Tumor markers:
  - CA-125—elevated in 85% epithelial tumors
    - False positives can be due to pregnancy, endometriosis, adenomyosis, menstruation, pelvic inflammatory disease (PID), cirrhosis, other cancers.
  - CEA
  - CA19-9
  - Alpha feto protein (AFP) and β-human chorionic gonadotropin (β-HCG)—to rule out germ cell tumors
- Genetic counseling for family history
- Transvaginal ultrasound
- (Optional): CT/MRI abdomen, pelvis preoperatively to rule out advanced disease
- Cystoscopy, sigmoidoscopy, barium enema if indicated
- If patient is anemic, consider endoscopy to rule out Krukenburg tumor (metastasis to ovary from GI primary).
- Do not perform pre-op percutaneous assessment of mass or ascites; this may lead to tumor seeding.
- Staging is surgical—requires excision of intact mass for frozen section; if malignant, proceed to surgery.

Staging

Stage I	Limited to ovaries (one or both)
Stage IA	Tumor limited to one ovary, capsule intact, no tumor on ovarian surface, no malignant cells in ascites or peritoneal washings
Stage IB	Tumor limited to both ovaries, capsules intact, no tumor on ovarian surface, no malignant cells in ascites or peritoneal washings

(continued)

(continued)

Stage IC	Tumor limited to one or both ovaries with any of the following: capsule ruptured, tumor on ovarian surface, or malignant cells in ascites or peritoneal washings
Stage II	Tumor involves one or both ovaries with pelvic extension
Stage IIA	Extension and/or implants on uterus and/or tube(s). No malignant cells in ascites or peritoneal washings
Stage IIB	Extension to and/or implants on other pelvis tissues. No malignant cells in ascites or peritoneal washings
Stage IIC	Pelvic extension and/or implants with malignant cells in ascites or peritoneal washings
Stage III	Tumor involves one or both ovaries with microscopically confirmed peritoneal metastasis outside the pelvis
Stage IIIA	Microscopic peritoneal metastases beyond the pelvis (no macroscopic tumor)
Stage IIIC	Peritoneal metastasis beyond the pelvis >2 cm greatest dimension and/or regional lymph node metastasis
Stage IV	Distant metastasis (excluded peritoneal metastases)

Treatment Overview

- Surgical staging
  - TAH/BSO (except known stage IA, can preserve fertility with USO)
  - Sample ascites and peritoneal washings
  - Complete abdominal exploration
  - Omentectomy
  - Peritoneal biopsies
  - Pelvic/aortic LN sampling
  - Optimal debulking (affects overall survival)
- Adjuvant chemo (i.e., taxane/carboplatin) recommended for all but IA/B grade 1
- RT has limited role; whole abdominal RT (WART) reserved for nonchemo candidates
- Tumor-directed RT for palliation of symptomatic tumor deposits

Radiation Therapy Technique

- For WART, must cover entire peritoneal cavity
- Open field preferable to moving strip
- AP/PA borders:
  - Superior: above dome of diaphragm
  - Inferior: below obturator foramen
  - Lateral: cover peritoneal reflection based on CT
- 30 Gy at 1.2- to 1.5-Gy fractions
- Block kidneys at 15 Gy
- Block liver at 25 Gy (controversial)
- PA field boosted to 45 Gy
- Pelvis boosted to 45 to 55 Gy

Outcomes

- 5-year overall survival by stage:
  - I: ~80% (>90% IA/B)
  - II: ~60%
  - III: ~25% overall
    - ~30% to 50% minimal residual
    - ~10% bulky residual
  - IV: ~5% to 15%

Toxicity

- Acute:
  - Nausea/vomiting
  - Diarrhea
  - Leukopenia
  - Thrombocytopenia

- Chronic:
  - Chronic diarrhea
  - Pneumonitis
  - Small bowel obstruction
  - Transient elevation of LFTs

Follow-Up

- Interval H&P (including pelvic exam) every 2 to 4 months for 2 years, then 3 to 6 months for 3 years, then annually after 5 years
- CA-125 + other tumor markers at each visit if initially elevated
- Genetic referral if not already done
- CBC and CMP if clinically indicated
- Imaging only as clinically indicated: CXR, CT A/P, MRI, PET/CT

3.6   Palliation of Gynecological Cancer

Epidemiology

- Multiple reasons for palliative intent:
  - Systemic disease
  - Advanced age
  - Poor condition
  - Refusal of radical treatments

Presentation

- Pelvic pain
- Vaginal bleeding
- Malodorous discharge
- Lower extremity swelling
- Failure to thrive

Diagnosis and Workup

- Biopsy and staging workup as clinically indicated to identify primary and determine treatment options
- CBC to determine need for transfusion
- Imaging as clinically indicated (x-ray, CT, MR, PET/CT)

Treatment Overview

- Symptom-directed therapy
- Tumor-directed palliative RT

Radiation Therapy Technique

- Field designed to cover symptomatic mass
- Common fractionation schemes:
  - 30 Gy in 10 fractions
  - 20 to 25 Gy in 5 fractions
  - 10 Gy in 1 fraction
  - 3.7-Gy BID × 2 days = "Quad shot"
- Fraction size determined by life expectancy and proximity to organs at risk (OAR)
  - For life expectancy <3 months, monthly high-dose regimen (10 Gy × 1) more appropriate
  - For life expectancy >3 months, smaller fractionation regimen reasonable

Outcomes

- Onsrud et al. *Gynecol Oncol.* 2001;82:167-171
  - 10 Gy × 1, repeated monthly up to three courses if exam showed no progression
  - Bleeding cessation in 90%
  - Discharge cessation in 39%
  - No effect on pelvic pain
  - Bleeding control correlated with # fractions delivered
  - Risk of grade 3+ acute and chronic toxicities correlated with # fractions
  - Time to late toxicities = 9 to 10 months
- RTOG 8502
  - 3.7 Gy twice daily × 2 days, repeated monthly up to three courses
  - Response rate correlated with # fractions
    - 14% CR, 31% PR, 40% SD, 7% PD
  - Bleeding cessation in 90% to 98%
  - Pain response 50% to 75% (better if 2-week break given instead of 4 weeks)
  - 6% developed late grade 3+ toxicity
  - All were GI toxicities
  - All were patient treated with three courses
  - Median time to toxicity-related complications = 9 months

Toxicity

- Loose stools/diarrhea
- Frequent urination
- Dysuria

- Skin irritation
- Fatigue
- Late toxicity higher with large fractionation size

Follow-Up

- As clinically indicated
- If pain/bleeding persists or recurs, consider retreatment

Chapter 3: Practice Questions

1. Expected 5-year survival for stage II endometrial cancer is approximately

   A. 90%
   B. 80%
   C. 70%
   D. 60%

2. Keratinizing vulvar cancer is NOT

   A. Related to HPV 16
   B. Generally found in older women
   C. Associated with vulvar dystrophy
   D. More common than classic or Bowenoid type of vulvar cancer

3. In terms of vulvar cancer, the risk of nodal recurrence is increased by the following EXCEPT

   A. Tumor size
   B. Age
   C. Grade
   D. Tumor ulceration

4. The most frequent vaginal tumor of the following is

   A. Melanoma
   B. Sarcoma
   C. Small cell
   D. Lymphoma

5. In terms of epithelial ovarian cancer, the most frequent histology seen is

   A. Serous
   B. Endometroid
   C. Undifferentiated
   D. Clear cell

6. Risk factors for the development of endometrium cancer include the following EXCEPT

   A. Multiparity
   B. Obesity
   C. Tamoxifen use
   D. Age

7. Ovarian cancer with positive washings is staged as

   A. IB
   B. IC
   C. IIA
   D. IIB

8. Stage III vaginal cancer is associated with the following nodal risk:

   A. 5%
   B. 25%
   C. 75%
   D. 85%

9. Parametrial involvement of a vaginal tumor is staged as

   A. I
   B. II
   C. III
   D. IV

10. Stage III ovarian cancer is associated with what 5-year survival?

    A. 10%
    B. 25%
    C. 50%
    D. 60%

11. The definition of point B for the prescription of cervix cancer treatment is defined at the following point:

    A. 3-cm superior to point A
    B. 3-cm inferior to point A
    C. 3-cm medial to point A
    D. 3-cm lateral to point A

12. The expected 5-year survival outcome with a stage III cervix cancer is

    A. 70%
    B. 60%
    C. 50%
    D. 40%

13. Prognostic factors of vaginal cancer include the following EXCEPT

    A. Age
    B. Stage
    C. Histology
    D. Lymphovascular invasion

14. Risk factors for the development of vulvar cancer include the following EXCEPT

    A. Smoking
    B. Paget's disease
    C. HPV infection
    D. Alcohol intake

15. Appropriate microscopic and macroscopic doses for treatment of endometrial cancer include the following, respectively:

    A. 45 and 60 Gy
    B. 40 and 70 Gy
    C. 45 and 70 Gy
    D. 60 and 70 Gy

16. All of the following are prognostic features for endometrial cancer EXCEPT

    A. Stage
    B. Grade
    C. Histology
    D. Age

17. The definition of point A for the prescription of cervix cancer treatment is defined at the following point:

    A. 2-cm cephalad and 2-cm lateral from external os
    B. 2-cm inferior and 2-cm lateral from external os
    C. 2-cm cephalad from external os
    D. 2-cm inferior from external os

18. Risk factors for the development of ovarian cancer include the following EXCEPT

    A. Family history
    B. Tubal ligation
    C. Genetic predisposition
    D. Dietary factors

19. In terms of endometrial adenocarcinoma, cervical stromal invasion is staged as the following:

    A. IA
    B. IB
    C. II
    D. IIIA

20. Adenocarcinoma of the cervix occurs in what percentage of all cervix cancer cases?

    A. 1% to 2%
    B. 10% to 20%
    C. 50% to 60%
    D. 80% to 90%

Chapter 3: Answers

1. B
The 5-year survival expected from a stage II endometrial cancer is 80%.

2. A
The Keratinizing, differentiated, or simplex type is
    More common
    Occurs in older women
    Not related to HPV infection
    Associated with vulvar dystrophies

3. B
Known prognostic factors for nodal recurrence:
    Size
    Histologic grade
    LVI
    Clinical nodes
    Ulceration

4. A
Pathology of vaginal tumors:
    80% to 90% squamous cell CA
    5% to 15% clear cell adenoCA or other adenoCAs
    5% melanoma, most frequent in the lower 1/3rd
    1% to 2% adult sarcomas, small cell, papillary serous, lymphoma

5. A
Pathology of ovarian tumors:
    90% epithelial
    Histological subtypes: 50% serous, 20% endometrioid, 15% undifferentiated, 10% mucinous, 4% clear cell

6. A
Risk factors for the development of endometrial cancer include: obesity, unopposed estrogen exposure, nulliparity, tamoxifen use, advanced age, LVSI, lower uterine segment involvement, genetic factors including Lynch syndrome.

7. B
Stage IC ovarian cancer is defined as tumor limited to one or both ovaries with any of the following: capsule ruptured, tumor on ovarian surface, or malignant cells in ascites or peritoneal washings.

8. C
Risk of LN involvement by stage:
    Stage I: 5%
    Stage II: 25%
    Stage III: 75%
    Stage IV: 85%

9. B
Staging of vaginal tumors:
    Stage I: Confined to vagina
    Stage II: Paravaginal/parametrial extension
    Stage III: Pelvic sidewall extension or pelvic/inguinal LN mets
    Stage IVA: Invasion into bladder/rectal mucosa
    Stage IVB: Distant mets

10. B
5-year overall survival by stage for ovarian cancer:
    I: ~80% (>90% IA/B)
    II: ~60%

III: ~25% overall
  ~30% to 50% minimal residual
  ~10% bulky residual
IV: ~5% to 15%

11. D

Point B is defined as 3-cm lateral to Pt A, fixed Pt even if Pt A is off-center (obturator nodes), measured from midline, gets dose of approximately 55 Gy.

12. D

The expected results associated with stage III cervix cancer include the following:
  Pelvic LN: 50%
  PA LN: 30%
  5-year LC: 70%
  5-year OS: 40% to 45%

13. D

Prognostic factors related to vaginal cancer:
  Stage
  Age
  Tumor size (>1/3 length)
  Location (upper 1/3 better)
  Histology (adenoCA)
  Grade
  Use of brachytherapy, RT dose >75 Gy
  Shorter treatment time

14. D

Risk factors for the development of vulvar cancer include:
  HPV 16, 18, 33
  VIN (2%–5% progress to CA)
  Bowen's disease (Cis)
  Paget's disease
  Erythroplasia
  Chronic irritant vaginitis
  Leukoplakia
  Prior GU cancer
  Employment in laundry and cleaning industry
  Smoking

15. A

Tumor-directed EBRT 45 to 50.4 Gy ± Intracavitary brachytherapy boost 6 Gy × 3 fractions is considered reasonable. Consider boost to involved LNs to 60 Gy using IMRT.

16. D

Prognostic features related to endometrium cancer include: stage, grade, histology (clear cell/serous worse), depth of myometrial invasion, cervical involvement, and LVSI.

17. A

Point A is defined as 2-cm cephalad and 2-cm lat from external os (parametria)—measured from the phlange and receives ~85-Gy total dose.

18. B

Risk factors for ovarian cancer development: family history (first-degree relative is strongest risk factor), nulliparity, late first parity >35 years, ovulation-inducing drugs, HRT, dietary factors including coffee intake, high fat and high lactose diet, genetic predisposition (~5% of tumors result from genetic disposition).

19. C

In terms of endometrial cancer, the following staging system applies:

IA: <50% myometrial invasion

IB: ≥50% myometrial invasion

II: cervical stromal involvement

IIIA: extension to serosa or adnexa (direct involvement or mets)

20. B

Pathology of cervix cancer:

80% to 90% of invasive tumors are SCC

10% to 20% are adenocarcinomas

1% to 2% are clear cell carcinomas

Recommended Reading

Aalders J, Abeler V, Kolstad P, Onsrud M. Postoperative external irradiation and prognostic parameters in stage I endometrial carcinoma: clinical and histopathologic study of 540 patients. Obstet Gynecol. 1980;56(4):419-427.

Beriwal S, Heron DE, Kim H, et al. Intensity-modulated radiotherapy for the treatment of vulvar carcinoma: a comparative dosimetric study with early clinical outcome. *Int J Radiat Oncol Biol Phys.* 2006;64(5):1395-1400.

Creutzberg CL, Nout RA, Lybeert ML, et al. Fifteen-year radiotherapy outcomes of the randomized PORTEC-1 trial for endometrial carcinoma. *Int J Radiat Oncol Biol Phys.* 2011;81(4):e631-e638.

Dimopoulos JC, Petrow P, Tanderup K, et al. Recommendations from Gynaecological (GYN) GEC-ESTRO Working Group (IV): basic principles and parameters for MR imaging within the frame of image based adaptive cervix cancer brachytherapy. *Radiother Oncol.* 2012;103(1):113-122.

Dusenbery KE, Carlson JW, LaPorte RM, et al. Radical vulvectomy with postoperative irradiation for vulvar cancer: therapeutic implications of a central block. *Int J Radiat Oncol Biol Phys.* 1994;29(5):989-998.

Eifel PJ, Winter K, Morris M, et al. Pelvic irradiation with concurrent chemotherapy versus pelvic and para-aortic irradiation for high-risk cervical cancer: an update of radiation therapy oncology group trial (RTOG) 90-01. J Clin Oncol. 2004;22(5):872-880.

Frank SJ, Jhingran A, Levenback C, Eifel PJ. Definitive radiation therapy for squamous cell carcinoma of the vagina. *Int J Radiat Oncol Biol Phys.* 2005;62(1):138-147.

Homesley HD, Bundy BN, Sedlis A, Adcock L. Radiation therapy versus pelvic node resection for carcinoma of the vulva with positive groin nodes. Obstet Gynecol. 1986;68(6):733-740.

Keys HM, Roberts JA, Brunetto VL, et al. A phase III trial of surgery with or without adjunctive external pelvic radiation therapy in intermediate risk endometrial adenocarcinoma: a Gynecologic Oncology Group study. Gynecol Oncol. 2004;92(3):744-751.

Klopp A, Smith BD, Alektiar K, et al. The role of postoperative radiation therapy for endometrial cancer: executive summary of an American Society for Radiation Oncology evidence-based guideline. *Pract Radiat Oncol.* 2014;4(3):137-144.

Landoni F, Maneo A, Colombo A, et al. Randomised study of radical surgery versus radiotherapy for stage Ib-IIa cervical cancer. Lancet. 1997;350(9077):535-540.

Moore DH, Thomas GM, Montana GS, Saxer A, Gallup DG, Olt G. Preoperative chemoradiation for advanced vulvar cancer: a phase II study of the Gynecologic Oncology Group. Int J Radiat Oncol Biol Phys. 1998;42(1):79-85.

Nout RA, Putter H, Jürgenliemk-Schulz IM, et al. Five-year quality of life of endometrial cancer patients treated in the randomised Post Operative Radiation Therapy in Endometrial Cancer (PORTEC-2) trial and comparison with norm data. Eur J Cancer. 2012;48(11):1638-1648.

Onsrud M, Hagen B, Strickert T. 10-Gy single-fraction pelvic irradiation for palliation and life prolongation in patients with cancer of the cervix and corpus uteri. *Gynecol Oncol.* 2001;82(1):167-171.

Rotman M, Sedlis A, Piedmonte MR, et al. A phase III randomized trial of postoperative pelvic irradiation in Stage IB cervical carcinoma with poor prognostic features: follow-up of a gynecologic oncology group study. *Int J Radiat Oncol Biol Phys.* 2006;65(1):169-176.

Spanos WJ, Jr, Clery M, Perez CA, et al. Late effect of multiple daily fraction palliation schedule for advanced pelvic malignancies (RTOG 8502). *Int J Radiat Oncol Biol Phys.* 1994;29(5):961-967.

Stehman FB, Ali S, Keys HM, et al. Radiation therapy with or without weekly cisplatin for bulky stage 1B cervical carcinoma: follow-up of a Gynecologic Oncology Group trial. Am J Obstet Gynecol. 2007;197(5):503.e1-503.e6.

Stehman FB, Bundy BN, Thomas G, et al. Groin dissection versus groin radiation in carcinoma of the vulva: a Gynecologic Oncology Group study. *Int J Radiat Oncol Biol Phys*. 1992;24(2):389-396.

Viswanathan AN, Erickson B, Gaffney DK, et al. Comparison and consensus guidelines for delineation of clinical target volume for CT- and MR-based brachytherapy in locally advanced cervical cancer. *Int J Radiat Oncol Biol Phys*. 2014;90(2):320-328.

Genitourinary Malignancies

Timothy N. Showalter and Daniel M. Trifiletti

4.1 Kidney

Epidemiology and Risk Factors

- Several genetic conditions can predispose to the development of renal cell carcinoma (RCC).
  - o Von Hippel–Lindau disease (VHL); autosomal dominant mutation of the VHL gene (3p25.3); commonly associated with RCC, hemangioblastoma, pheochromocytoma, and pancreatic cysts
  - o Dirt–Hogg–Dubé syndrome; associated with RCC, renal and pulmonary cysts, and fibrofolliculoma of the skin
  - o Tuberous sclerosis; mutation of TSC1 or TSC2, tumor suppressor genes; predisposes to various tumors including RCC as well as developmental delay
- Sporadic RCC; point mutations in the VHL tumor suppressor gene on 3p25.

Anatomy and Patterns of Spread

- Tumors can spread by direct extension into the renal capsule or through the renal vein. They can also spread to regional lymph nodes or to distant sites (primarily lung, liver, bone, and brain).

Presentation

- Classic triad of RCC: hematuria, flank pain, mass
- Paraneoplastic syndromes occur in about 20% of patients and usually consist of elevated calcium, hypertension, and transaminitis.

Diagnosis and Workup

- Pathologic subtypes: clear cell (70% of cases), chromophilic, chromophobic, collecting duct
  - o History and physical exam
  - o Basic laboratory studies
- Renal ultrasound
- CT chest/abd/pelv with contrast
- ± Renal MRI
- Bone scan or brain MRI if indicated

Staging (AJCC 7th Edition)

- **T1**— ≤7 cm, kidney only
  - ○ T1a— ≤4 cm
  - ○ T1b—4 to 7 cm
- **T2**— >7 cm, kidney only
  - ○ T2a—7 to 10 cm
  - ○ T2b—>10 cm
- **T3**—into major veins or perinephric tissues
  - ○ T3a—into renal vein or perirenal fat
  - ○ T3b—into vena cava below diaphragm
  - ○ T3c—into vena cava above the diaphragm or wall of vena cava
- **T4**—invades Gerota's fascia (including adrenal gland)

- **N1**—renal hilum, caval (para/pre/retrocaval), interaortocaval, aortic (para/pre/retroaortic)

- **M1**—distant metastasis

AJCC 7th Edition Group Staging				
	T1	T2	T3	T4
N0	I	II	III	IV
N1	III			
M1	IV			

Treatment Overview

- Locoregional disease is usually treated with surgery alone.
  - ○ Partial or radical nephrectomy
  - ○ Active surveillance in select cT1aN0 patients
  - ○ Data that adjuvant radiation therapy (RT) improves locoregional control in patients with pT3 tumors; not commonly performed
- Metastatic disease
  - ○ Consider upfront palliative cytoreductive nephrectomy.
  - ○ Several targeted agents have demonstrated antitumoral activity in renal cell carcinoma:
    - ■ Sunitinib, sorafenib (multi-TKIs)
    - ■ Temsirolimus (mTOR inhibitor)
    - ■ Bevacizumab (anti-VEGF receptor)
    - ■ Interferons (cytokines)
    - ■ Nivolumab (anti-PD1)
  - ○ RT for palliation of metastases; technique and dose dependent on intent
    - ■ 30-39 Gy in 10 to 13 fractions for palliation
    - ■ Consider SRS or SBRT for low-volume metastatic disease

4.2   Bladder

Epidemiology and Risk Factors

- Risk factors: smoking, dyes, and chronic irritation (foley catheter)
- 93% TCC (5% SCC, 2% adenocarcinoma)
- 75% Ta, Tis, T1 at presentation
- Cystectomy: en block removal of bladder, perivesicular tissue, urethra, prostate (or uterus)

Anatomy and Patterns of Spread

- Tumors can spread by direct extension into the perivesicular fat, prostate, vagina, and rectum. They can also spread to regional lymph nodes or to distant sites.

Presentation

Most common presenting symptom is painless hematuria.

Diagnosis and Workup

- History and physical exam
- Basic laboratory studies
- Urinalysis, urine cytology, alkaline phosphatase
  - Cystoscopy, biopsy, bladder mapping; can consider exam under anesthesia
  - If superficial, CT pelvis with contrast and intravenous pyelogram
  - If muscle invasive, CT chest/abd/pelv, ± pelvic MRI, ± bone scan

Staging (AJCC 7th Edition)

- **Tis, Ta**—CIS, non-invasive, papillary
- **T1**—subepithelial invasion
- **T2**—muscularis propria invasion
  - T2a—inner half
  - T2b—outer half
- **T3**—perivesical tissue invasion
  - T3a—microscopic
  - T3b—macroscopic
- **T4**—adjacent organs
  - T4a—prostatic stroma, uterus, vagina
  - T4b—pelvic wall, abd wall

- **N1**—single LN below common iliac
- **N2**—multiple LNs below common iliac
- **N3**—common iliac LN involvement

- **M1**—distant metastasis

AJCC 7th Edition Group Staging						
	Ta, Tis	T1	T2	T3	T4a	T4b
N0	0a, 0is	I	II	III	III	IV
N+	IV					

Treatment Overview

- Tis, Ta tumors are usually treated with maximal TURBT, then single dose intravesicular chemotherapy (i.e., BCG) or observation in select patients. Tumor grade should guide the decision for adjuvant therapy.
- T1N0 tumors are usually treated with TURBT + BCG. An upfront cystectomy for T1N0 high-grade tumors may be appropriate.

- Stages II to III disease patients have several options:
  - o Neoadjuvant chemotherapy + radical cystectomy
    - consider adjuvant chemotherapy for pT3-4 or N+
    - consider post-op RT for positive margin or pT3-4 or N+
  - o Bladder preservation approach
    - Relative contraindications include multifocal disease, clinical extravesicular disease, component of Tis, hydronephrosis, subtotal TURBT
- cT4b or N+ can be treated with induction chemotherapy or CRT, followed by surgery, if appropriate.
- M1: palliative chemotherapy
- Recent preliminary evidence identifies high rate of regional nodal recurrence after cystectomy, and ongoing NRG/RTOG study aims to evaluate potential new role of adjuvant pelvic nodal irradiation.

Bladder Preservation Technique

- There are several common approaches.
- Overall survival at 5 years is 50% to 60% depending on stage.
- In general 2/3 of patients survive, and 2/3 of survivors avoid cystectomy.
- Usually consists of:
  - o Maximal TURBT (to negative margin)
  - o Concurrent chemoradiotherapy
    - 45 Gy to whole bladder + regional nodes
    - concurrent cisplatin or 5 FU/mitomycinC
  - o Cystoscopy w/ biopsies and cytology 3 weeks after 45 Gy:
    - ~70% of patients will have a clinical CR at this time (cT0 and negative cytology).
    - Radical cystectomy is indicated if residual disease is found on cystoscopy after 45 Gy.
    - Consider skipping mid-treatment cystoscopy for medically inoperable patients or those who refuse potential salvage cystectomy.
  - o Boost to 60to 65 Gy if clinical CR:
    - Shrinking field techniques can include partial bladder boost or treatment to whole bladder.

Follow-Up and Late Effects

- After a bladder-preserving approach, cystoscopy and urine cytology should be performed at 3-month intervals for 2 years.

4.3   Low-Risk Prostate Cancer

Epidemiology and Risk Factors

- There are 230,000 cases annually accounting for 27,000 deaths.
- Common risk factors include age, African American race, obesity, and high-fat diets.

Anatomy and Patterns of Spread

- The prostate is divided into four zones: peripheral, transitional (BPH), central, and anterior fibromuscular stroma.
  - o Two-thirds of cancers develop in the peripheral zone (posterior zone).
- Tumors can spread by direct extension into the periprostatatic tissues. They can also spread to regional lymph nodes (obtruators and internal iliacs) or to distant sites (primarily bone).
- Prostate-specific antigen (PSA):
  - o Normal levels vary by age and prostate volume, but generally less than 4 ng/mL can serve as a guide.
  - o Half-life is 2 to 3 days.

o   PSA velocity has been shown to increase the likelihood of Gleason 7+ disease (≥ 2 ng/mL/yr).
o   PSA density (PSA/gland volume) has been shown to predict for prostate cancer (over 7%).
o   Low free PSA (unbound PSA) is associated with an increased likelihood of prostate cancer (less than 25% can serve as a threshold).
o   Screening with PSA is debated, but the American Cancer Society recommends PSA screening every 1 to 2 years for men over 50 years old, or for younger men at high risk.

Presentation

- Most prostate cancers in the United States are diagnosed through screening PSA.
- Advanced disease can present with urinary obstruction, hematuria, or bone pain.

Diagnosis and Workup

- History and physical exam with digital rectal exam
- Transrectal ultrasound guided sextant biopsy
  o   Patients with low-risk prostate cancer should not undergo routine staging imaging unless there is a reason to suspect more advanced disease (bone pain, etc.).

Staging (AJCC 7th Edition)

- **T1**—clinically unapparent
  o   T1a—incidental less than 5% of tissue resected
  o   T1b—incidental greater than 5% of tissue resected
  o   T1c—needle biopsy ($\uparrow$PSA)
- **T2**—confined within prostate
  o   T2a—$\leq\frac{1}{2}$ of one lobe
  o   T2b—greater than ½ of one lobe
  o   T2c—both lobes
- **T3**—through capsule
  o   T3a—EPE or microscopic invasion of bladder neck
  o   T3b—seminal vesicles
- **T4**—invades adjacent structures: bladder neck, external sphincter, rectum, levator muscles, and/or pelvic wall

- **N1** —pelvic, hypogastric, obturator, iliac (internal, external), sacral

- **M1a**—non-regional lymph nodes
- **M1b**—bone metastasis
- **M1c**—other sites

AJCC 7th Edition Group Staging

T	1–2a	2b	2c	3	4
GS	<7	7	>7	–	–
PSA	<10	10–20	≥20	–	–
N, M	–	–	–	–	N1, M1
Group	I	IIA	IIB	III	IV
10 yr bPFS	90%	85%	60%	30–50%	<20%

Treatment Overview

- Active surveillance is the preferred approach for men with low-risk prostate cancer, regardless of life expectancy.
- For men who opt for definitive therapy, there are several options:
  o Radical prostatectomy (RP)
  o External beam radiation therapy (EBRT)
  o Brachytherapy, either low-dose rate (LDR) or high-dose rate (HDR)
- Watchful waiting (observation) is appropriate for men with a limited life expectancy (<10 years) as they are likely to die from another disease before clinically significant progression of their prostate cancer occurs.

Active Surveillance Approach

- Active Surveillance usually consists of:
  o PSA every 6 months
  o DRE every 12 months
  o Repeat biopsy every 12 months (25% will end up getting treated)
- Generally, 25% of patients under active surveillance will be definitively treated for their prostate cancer.
- While generally recommended for all low-risk patients, active surveillance is particularly appropriate for the NCCN "very low risk" group, as defined by Epstein's Criteria:
  o cT1c, Gleason less than 7, PSA, 10 ng/mL, fewer than three cores positive, less than 50% cancer in any core, PSA density less than 0.15 ng/mL/g.

Prostatectomy Techniques

- Approach can be retropubic (most common) or perineal.
- If the risk of N+ disease is greater than 2%, an extended pelvic lymph node dissection is preferred to provide more complete staging.
- It can be performed via an open, laparoscopic or robotic-assisted technique.
- Nerve-sparing techniques can reduce impotence.

External Beam Radiation Therapy Techniques

- Several trials have demonstrated a ~10% improved bPFS with EBRT doses of at least 74 Gy although these failed to demonstrate an overall survival benefit.
- There is no role for elective nodal irradiation (whole pelvis RT) in patients with low-risk prostate cancer.
- NCCN guidelines recommend EBRT doses from 75.6 to 79.2 Gy when delivered with conventional fractionation.
- There are several methods of modest and extreme hypofractionation in prostate cancer which could exploit its low alpha/beta ratio. These methods are considered cautionary and should be restricted to centers with expertise in this area.

Common EBRT Dose Constraints at 2 Gy/fx

Rectum		Bladder	
V75	15%	V80	15%
V70	20%	V75	25%
V65	30%	V70	35%
V50	50%	V65	50%
Bowel		Femoral head	
V45 <195 mL		V50 <5%	

Brachytherapy Techniques

- 5 mm TRUS slices, 5 mm PTV expansion (3 mm ant, 0 mm post)
- Postimplant dosimetry (usually at day 1 or 30)
- Relative contraindications:
  - Previous RT or TURP
  - Intermediate or high risk (consider combination therapy with supplemental EBRT)
  - Seminal vesicle invasion
  - Pubic arch interference
  - Median lobe
  - Large gland (greater than 60 mL)
  - AUA greater than 15 (increases risk of postbrachytherapy urinary toxicity)
  - Diabetes mellitus
- In intermediate risk prostate cancer, can consider LDR monotherapy if: Gleason 3 + 4, PSA less than 10, ≤4/12 cores, ≤T2a, ≤50% each core, between 20 and 65 mL gland
- Common isotopes:
  - ^{103}Pd: 17 day half-life, 21 keV energy, 125 Gy monotherapy, 100 Gy combo
  - ^{125}I: 60 day half-life, 28 keV energy, 145 Gy monotherapy, 110 combo
  - ^{192}Ir: 74 day half-life, 3.8 MeV energy, several reported dose/fx

Common LDR Dose Constraints

PTV		Urethra	
D90	>105%		
V100	>95%	V125	<50%
V150	<70%	V150	0%
V200	<40%	V200	0%
Rectum V100% <1 mL			

4.4   Intermediate-Risk Prostate Cancer

Workup

- Same as for low-risk prostate cancer, but should consider bone scan and pelvic CT/MRI more advanced disease.
- Biopsy suspicious nodes
- Prostate cancer staging (see Section 4.3)

Treatment Overview

- If there is a limited life expectancy, observation may be appropriate.
- Active surveillance is generally not recommended for patients with intermediate-risk disease.
- Definitive options for therapy include:
  - RP (with extended pelvic lymph node dissection if risk >2%)
  - EBRT with short course androgen deprivation therapy (ADT, 4–6 months)
    - Can be combined with brachytherapy
  - Brachytherapy alone in select patients (Gleason 3 + 4, PSA <10, ≤4/12 cores, ≤T2a, ≤50% each core, between 20 and 65 mL gland)

Androgen Deprivation Therapy

- Several phase III randomized trials have demonstrated that short course ADT (4–6 months in intermediate risk disease) improves long-term overall survival in patients with intermediate-risk prostate cancer by 5% to 10%.
- Of note, these trials were performed in patients treated with EBRT doses now considered inferior (66–70 Gy).
- Ongoing trial (RTOG 08-15) aims to answer the question of whether short-term ADT improves overall survival for patients receiving dose-escalated radiation therapy (79.2 Gy in 44 fractions or combination therapy with brachytherapy boost).
- There are several methods of ADT:
  - Castration
  - GnRH agonists
    - Goserelin (Zoladex)
    - Leuprolide (Lupron)
    - Triptorelin (Trelstar)
  - Antiandrogens: bicalutamide (Casodex)
  - Nonsteroidal antiandrogen: Flutamide
  - Estrogens
  - Ketoconazole: blocks P450
  - Degarelix: GnRH antagonist, no initial flare
- One common ADT strategy is to prescribe bicalutamide starting a few days prior to the first dose of leuprolide. This serves to minimize the risk of a GnRH-induced testosterone flare.

Radiation Therapy Technique

- The role of elective pelvic nodal RT in patients with intermediate-/high-risk prostate cancer is controversial.
  - Many of the historic trials on patients with intermediate-/high-risk prostate cancer included elective pelvic nodal irradiation.
  - Randomized trials have generally failed to identify a subset of patients with a clear benefit.
- NCCN guidelines recommend EBRT doses from 75.6 to 81.0 Gy when delivered with conventional fractionation.

4.5 High-Risk Prostate Cancer

Workup

- Similar to intermediate risk
- Bone scan if PSA greater than 20 ng/mL, Gleason score ≥ 8, T3/T4, symptomatic, or T2 plus PSA 10 ng/mL
- Pelvic MRI or CT if T3/T4 or T1–T2 and nomogram-based prediction of lymph node involvement greater than 10%
- Prostate cancer staging (see 4.3)

Treatment Overview

- In the setting of high-risk disease, evidence exists supporting the role for RT (in addition to ADT) through a ~10% improvement in long-term OS.
- There also exists evidence demonstrating a similar improvement in long-term OS in patients treated with long-term ADT (in addition to RT).
- Combination therapy with EBRT, brachytherapy, and ADT also can be considered, and recent ASCENDE-RT study support bPFS improvement at cost of higher rates of grade 3+ late GU toxicity.

- Consolidative docetaxel may be considered for very high-risk patients after EBRT and long-term ADT.
- Ongoing trial (RTOG 0924) aims to evaluate whether pelvic nodal irradiation improves survival for selected patients when added to ADT and dose-escalated RT.

4.6   Adjuvant/Salvage and Metastatic Prostate Cancer

PSA Failure Definitions

- After RP: ≥0.2 ng/mL
- 1996 ASTRO definition: three consecutive rises, then back-dated
- 2005 Phoenix definition: rise of 2 ng/mL over nadir

Adjuvant Radiation Therapy

- Three randomized trials have reported informed on the role of adjuvant RT in patients with adverse pathologic feature (pT3 and/or positive margin).
- All three demonstrated improved disease-specific control, and one demonstrated improved long-term overall survival (~10%).
- RT technique:
  - Common doses range from 64 to 70 Gy conventionally fractionated.
  - Target includes the postprostatectomy bed, vesicourethral anastomosis, and seminal vesicles. Target volumes can be adjusted based on pathologic factors.

Salvage Radiation Therapy

- While adjuvant RT improves outcomes, it risks over-treating patients.
- This leads some patients to a potential increase in treatment-related toxicity without an improvement in disease-specific outcome.
- Salvage RT can be used for patients with biochemical evidence of disease progression following surgery.
- While this strategy reduces the risk of over-treatment, it risks delaying some patients' potentially curative therapy.
- The optimum patient selection and timing of postoperative RT is the subject of several current phase III trials.

Node Positive Prostate Cancer

- Long-term ADT improves overall survival for patients with involved lymph nodes.
- In pN1 patients following RP, median survival is improved by 2 years with ADT.
- In cN1 patients treated with RT, long-term OS was improved by ~20% with ADT.

Metastatic Prostate Cancer

- First line therapy: generally ADT alone
- Second line therapy (castrate resistant prostate cancer): Docetaxel/Prednisone
- ^{223}Ra (Alpharadin):
  - FDA approved for bone-only metastases from castrate resistant prostate cancer
  - 11.4 day half life, alpha emitter, 5.8 MeV avg
  - Prescription typically 50 kBq/kg Q4weeks × 6 treatments
  - Requires:
    - Absolute neutrophil count ≥1.5 × 10^9/L
    - Platelet count ≥100 × 10^9/L
    - Hemoglobin ≥10 g/dL

Follow-Up and Late Effects

- After definitive therapy:
  - PSA every 6 to 12 months for 5 years, then every year
  - DRE every year
- PSA bounce: about 15% of patients treated with EBRT develop a transient rise in PSA of about 15% above nadir. This usually occurs 18 to 24 months following therapy.
- RP toxicity:
  - Erectile dysfunction, incontinence, stricture (~50% potent, ~75% continent)
- RT toxicity:
  - Erectile dysfunction, urinary frequency, proctitis (~50% potent, ~1% late GI/GU toxicity)
- ADT toxicity:
  - Hot flashes, decreased libido, fatigue, gynecomastia, metabolic syndrome (obesity, hyperlipidemia, diabetes, coronary artery disease)

4.7   Testis

Epidemiology and Risk Factors

- Several risk factors exist including cryptorchidism, polyvinyl chloride, Down syndrome, Klinefelter's syndrome, HIV.
- It most commonly occurs in young adult men.
- Histopathology:
  - Most testicular cancers are germ cell tumors (either seminoma or non-seminomatous germ cell tumors; NSGCT).
    - In elderly men, lymphoma is the most common testicular cancer.
  - Seminoma: bHcG can be ↑ (15%) but NEVER AFP
  - NSGCTs consist of a group of histologies:
    - Embryonal carcinoma (most common)
    - Yolk sac (↑AFP, Schiller Duval bodies)
    - Choriocarcinoma (↑bHcG)
    - Teratoma
    - Mixed (60%)
  - Others:
    - Sertoli cell: commonly increased estrogen
    - Leydig cell: commonly increased androgens
    - Lymphomas (elderly), sarcomas
- Tumor markers are commonly used to aid in diagnosis and staging.
  - bHcG
    - Can be elevated in some seminomas and NSGCTs
    - Half-life 24 hours
  - AFP:
    - Very uncommonly elevated in seminomas
    - Can be elevated in NSGCTs
    - Half life 5 days

Anatomy and Patterns of Spread

- Tumors can spread by direct extension through the tunica vaginalis and into the scutum. They can also spread to regional lymph nodes (paraaortic and pelvic) or to distant sites (primarily lungs, bone).

- Based on embryologic origin, the first echelon nodal drainage of the testes is to the paraaortic lymph nodes.
  - The first echelon lymph node from the left testicle is the left renal vein.
- Workup: H&P, sperm banking, bHcG, AFP, LDH, labs, CT abd/pelv ± chest, ± PET. Do not biopsy.

Presentation

Most common presenting symptom is painless testicular mass.

Diagnosis and Workup

- History and physical exam including transillumination
- Basic laboratory studies
- AFP, bHcG, LDH
- Testicular ultrasound
- Chest x-ray
- CT abd/chest typically done postoperatively
- ± brain MRI, bone scan
- Discuss sperm banking

Staging (AJCC 7th Edition)

- **T1**—testis, epididymis, no LVSI, no vaginalis
- **T2**—T1 + LVSI or vaginalis
- **T3**—spermatic cord
- **T4**—scrotum

- **N1**—N+, all ≤2 cm (path ≤5 nodes)
- **N2**—N+, all 2 to 5 cm (path >5 nodes or ECE)
- **N3**—N+, >5 cm

- **M1a**—nonregional nodes or lung mets
- **M1b**—distant

- **S0**—normal serum markers (all postorchiectomy)
- **S1**—LDH <1.5 ULN   AND hCG <5,000   AND   AFP <1,000
- **S2**—LDH 1.5 to 10 ULN   OR hCG 5,000 to 50,000   OR   AFP 1,000 to 10,000
- **S3**—LDH >10 ULN   OR hCG >50,000   OR   AFP >10,000

AJCC 7th Edition Staging					
	T1	T2	T3	T4	10 yr RFS
N0	IA (S0)	IB (S0)			98%
N1	IIA (S0–1)				92%
N2	IIB (S0–1)				86%
N3	IIC (S0–1)				70%
M1a	IIIA (S0-1, any N)				90% OS
S2	IIIB				

(continued)

AJCC 7th Edition Staging (*continued*)					
	T1	T2	T3	T4	10 yr RFS
S3	IIIC				80% OS
M1b					
IS—Any T N0 M0 S1-3					

Treatment Overview

Pure Seminoma

- The primary initial therapy for testicular cancer is orchiectomy.
  - Radical transinguinal orchiectomy with high ligation of the spermatic cord
  - Repeat tumor markers post-op to complete staging
- Transcrotal biopsy should not be performed.
- For stage I disease, postoperative surveillance is the preferred approach, although historically single agent carboplatin and RT to 20 Gy have been used.
  - 16% of patients will fail locoregionally during observation for stage I disease.
- For stage IIA disease, postoperative RT to 30 Gy is preferred. Alternatively chemotherapy (BEP) may be appropriate.
- For stage IIB disease, postoperative chemotherapy (BEP) is preferred. Alternatively RT to 36 Gy may be appropriate.
- For stage III/IV disease, the primary therapy is chemotherapy with RT used typically for salvage, and/or palliation.

Non-Seminomatous Germ Cell Tumors

- The primary initial therapy for testicular cancer is orchiectomy.
- Transcrotal biopsy should not be performed.
- For early stage disease, a paraaortic lymph node dissection is usually performed.
- Most patients (beside stage IA) receive primary chemotherapy (BEP).
- Radiation in NSGCT is typically limited to palliative of symptoms.

Radiation Technique for Seminoma

- A scrotal shield should be employed.
- All doses should be delivered using 3D-CRT delivered AP/PA.
- In stage I disease, multiple trials have informed the standard of care:
  - There is evidence that a dogleg field and a PA only field have identical relapse-free and overall survival.
  - In stage I disease, there is evidence that 20 Gy in 10 fractions is equivalent to 30 Gy in 15 fractions.
  - PA field to 20 Gy in 10 fractions:
    - Superior border: bottom of T11
    - Inferior border: bottom of L5
    - Lateral borders: tips of transverse processes
    - Consider partial renal block based on individual anatomy
- In stage IIA disease:
  - Dog leg field to 20 Gy in 10 fractions with a 10 Gy boost to GTV + 2 cm to block edge

- Superior border: bottom of T11
- Inferior border: top of acetabulum
- Lateral borders: tips of transverse processes superiorly; inferiorly, connect the lateral and medial borders to the lateral acetabulum and the medial obturator foramen, respectively (goal is at least 2.5 cm from vessels to beam edge)
  - Consider partial renal block based on individual anatomy
- In stage IIB disease:
  - Dog leg field to 20 Gy in 10 fractions with a 16 Gy boost to GTV + 2 cm to block edge

Treatment fields: Similar to stage IIA disease

Follow-Up and Late Effects

- Follow-up depends on tx, but generally labs/CT Q3 m for 2 years, then Q6 m for 2 years, then annually for 5 years.
- Based on therapy tolerance and the risk of secondary malignancy, at many centers adjuvant chemotherapy is preferred compared to adjuvant RT.
- In this population with a generally excellent prognosis, late RT-induced toxicity including renal and gastrointestinal toxicity should be carefully considered against the toxicity of chemotherapy and the risks associated with observation.

4.8 Penis

Epidemiology and Risk Factors

- Risk factors include uncircumcised, phimosis, poor hygiene, HPV (16 and 18), trauma, and smoking.
- 5 cm penile length is needed for sexual intercourse.
- 3 cm penile length is needed to urinate standing.

Anatomy and Patterns of Spread

- Tumors can spread by direct extension into the corpora, urethra and bladder. They can also spread to regional lymph nodes (inguinal and pelvic) or to distant sites (primarily paraortic lymph nodes, lungs, liver).
- The clinically significant layers of the penis:
  - Skin
  - Fascia (Buck's)
  - Corpus cavernosa (there is no cavernosa at the glans penis)
  - Corpus spongiosum
  - Urethra
- Anatomic inguinal node borders:
  - Superior: inguinal ligament
  - Interior: fossa ovalis
  - Lateral: sartorius muscle
  - Medially: adductor longus muscle
- Significant discrepancy can exist between clinical and pathologic inguinal nodal findings:
  - 20 % of patients with cN0 inguinal lymph nodes will be pN+
  - 30%–50% of patients with cN+ inguinal lymph nodes will be pN0

Presentation

- Usually presents as an ulcerative mass or an exophytic mass.
- Secondary infection can cause foul smell.
- Urethral obstruction is quite uncommon.

Diagnosis and Workup

- H&P exam
- Basic laboratory studies
  - Biopsy
  - EUA if advanced
  - ultrasound or MRI of primary
  - CXR

Staging (AJCC 7th Edition)

- Tis, Ta: CIS, noninvasive verrucous
- **T1**
  - T1a—subepithelial, no LVSI, no G3-4
  - T1b—subepithelial, +LVSI or G3-4
- **T2**—spongiosum or cavernosum
- **T3**—urethra
- **T4**—adj structures (inc prostate)

- **N1**—unilateral inguinal
- **N2**—multiple or bilateral inguinal
- **N3**—fixed or pelvic (ECE)

AJCC 7th Edition Staging

	Tis, Ta	T1a	T1b	T2	T3	T4
N0	0	I			II	
N1	–			IIIA		IV
N2	–			IIIB		
N3				IV		
M1						

Early Stage EBRT

- Grabstald & Kelly (1980): 10 pts, stages I to II: 90 % LC
- McLean 1993: 26 pts, stages I to II: mostly 50/20: 5 year DFS 50%

Early Stage Brachy

- Crook 2005: 49 pts, T1 to T3, Ir-192 to 55 and 65 Gy. 5 year LC 85%, OS 78%, penile preservation 86%
- Mazeron 1984: T1 to T3 Ir-192 to ~65 Gy, LC 78%, penile preservation 74%

Locally Advanced

- Krieg 1981: 17 pts stages I to IV, surgery ± LND ± RT, but 88% of pts without nodal treatment failed in nodes
- Sarin 1997: 101 pts stages I to IV, mixed treatments, 10-year OS 39%, LC 55%, validated use of RT with surgical salvage. Two patients attempted suicide after penectomy.

Treatment Overview

- The historic management of early stage penile cancer is surgery (partial vs. total penectomy).
  - Inguinal lymph node dissection is indicated if T1b or greater.
  - Pelvic lymph node dissection is indicated if at least two inguinal nodes are positive.
- Organ preservation options exist for early stage disease including laser therapy and RT (with or without chemotherapy).
- Locally advanced disease (N2+ or T4) is typically treated with neoadjuvant chemotherapy followed by evaluation for surgery, or with chemoradiotherapy upfront.

Radiation Therapy Technique

- Pre-RT circumcision is critical in minimizing risk of late phimosis.
- Simulation is usually supine (frog leg) with foley, bolus.
- Consider sperm banking and scrotal shielding as appropriate.
- If treating pelvic nodes, taping the penis up can improve coverage.
- Brachytherapy is preferred if <4 0 cm, either by mold or interstitial technique.
- Dose limits:
  - Urethra 60 Gy
  - Testes 3 Gy
- Typical EBRT dose is 45 to 50 Gy with a cone down to 60 to 70 Gy

Follow-Up and Late Effects

- Typically followed with clinical exam every 3 months for 2 years, then every 6 and 12 months for 5 to 10 years.
- CT imaging is appropriate for advanced nodal stages.
- Late effects include penile phimosis, urethral stenosis, infertility, testosterone deficiency.

Chapter 4: Practice Questions

1. The majority of prostate cancers develop within the

   A. Peripheral zone
   B. Transitional zone
   C. Central prostate zone
   D. Anterior fibromuscular stroma

2. Prostatic invasion of a bladder tumor is staged as

   A. T3a
   B. T3b
   C. T4a
   D. T4b

3. A kidney cancer that invades into the perirenal fat is staged as

   A. T3c
   B. T3a
   C. T3b
   D. T4

4. The current post-RT primary disease PSA failure definition is

A. ≥0.2 ng/mL
B. ≥0.4 ng/mL
C. 3 consecutive rises
D. Rise of 2 ng/mL over nadir

5. Temsirolimus is an example of a

A. mTOR inhibitor
B. Anti-PD1 inhibitor
C. Tyrosine kinase inhibitor
D. Anti-VEGF receptor inhibitor

6. Leydig cell carcinomas are usually associated with elevated

A. AFP
B. bHCG
C. Estrogen
D. Androgens

7. A T4aN0M0 bladder cancer is stage grouped as

A. II
B. III
C. IV
D. IVA

8. The half-life of alpha feto protein (AFP) is

A. 1 day
B. 5 days
C. 14 days
D. 28 days

9. The following is a contraindication for low-dose rate prostate brachytherapy:

A. PSA < 10 ng/mL
B. Gleason 4 + 4 disease
C. T2a disease
D. 50 mL gland size

10. Scrotal involvement of a testicular cancer is T staged as

A. T1
B. T2
C. T3
D. T4

11. All of the following are potentially useful in the diagnosis of prostate cancer EXCEPT

A. High PSA level
B. High PSA velocity
C. Low levels of bound PSA level
D. High PSA density

12. What is the most common presentation of bladder cancer?

A. Abdominal mass
B. Painless hematuria
C. Microscopic hematuria
D. Anemia

13. The first echelon nodal drainage for testicular tumors is

    A. Pelvic nodes
    B. Inguinal nodes
    C. Paraaortic nodes
    D. Femoral nodes

14. All of the following are GnRH/LHRH agonists EXCEPT

    A. Goserelin
    B. Leuprolide
    C. Bicalutamide
    D. Triptorelin

15. The Epstein criteria for very low-risk prostate cancer has all the following factors EXCEPT

    A. Gleason 2–6
    B. PSA < 6 ng/mL
    C. <3 cores positive
    D. cT1c disease

16. Using dose-escalated external beam radiation therapy (EBRT) for low to intermediate risk prostate cancer has been shown to have the following benefit:

    A. Benefit to biochemical control and survival
    B. Benefit to survival only
    C. Benefit to biochemical control only
    D. No benefit to biochemical control or survival

17. The zones of the prostate include the following EXCEPT

    A. Peripheral
    B. Posterior fibromuscular stroma
    C. Transitional
    D. Central

18. The most frequent histological subtype of bladder cancer is

    A. Squamous cell carcinoma
    B. Adenocarcinoma
    C. Transitional cell carcinoma
    D. Small cell carcinoma

19. Common iliac nodes in the context of a bladder cancer is staged as

    A. N1
    B. N2a
    C. N2b
    D. N3

20. All of the following dose fractionation schedules are considered usual standard of care for bladder cancer EXCEPT

    A. 60 Gy in 30 fractions
    B. 66 Gy in 33 fractions
    C. 55 Gy in 20 fractions
    D. 45 Gy in 30 fractions BID

Chapter 4: Answers

1. A
Two thirds of cancers develop in the peripheral zone.

2. C
The staging of locally advanced bladder cancers is as following:
T3—perivesical tissue invasion
  T3a—microscopic
  T3b—macroscopic
T4—adjacent organs
  T4a—prostatic stroma, uterus, vagina
  T4b—pelvic wall, abdominal wall

3. B
T staging of locally advance kidney cancer involves the following:
T3—into major veins or perinephric tissues
  T3a—into renal vein or perirenal fat
  T3b—into vena cava below diaphragm
  T3c—into vena cava above the diaphragm or wall of vena cava
T4—invades Gerota's fascia (including adrenal gland)

4. D
PSA Failure Definitions:
After RP: ≥0.2 ng/mL
1996 ASTRO definition: three consecutive rises, then back-dated
2005 Phoenix definition: rise of 2 ng/mL over nadir

5. A
Several targeted agents have demonstrated antitumoral activity in renal cell carcinoma:
Sunitinib, sorafenib (multi-TKIs)
Temsirolimus (mTOR inhibitor)
Bevacizumab (anti-VEGF receptor)
Interferons (cytokines)
Nivolumab (anti-PD1)

6. D
Yolk sac (AFP)
Choriocarcinoma (bHcG)
Sertoli cell: commonly increased estrogen
Leydig cell: commonly increased androgens

7. B
Both T3 and T4a N0M0 bladder cancers are staged as stage III.

8. B
AFP is very uncommonly elevated in seminomas but can be elevated in NSGCTs with a half life of 5 days.

9. B
In intermediate risk prostate cancer, can consider LDR monotherapy if: Gleason 3 + 4, PSA <10, ≤4/12 cores, ≤T2a, ≤50% each core, between 20 and 65 mL gland.

10. D
The T staging of testicular cancer is:
T1—testis, epididymis, no LVSI, no vaginalis
T2—T1 + LVSI or vaginalis
T3—spermatic cord
T4—scrotum

11. C

Prostate-specific antigen (PSA):

Normal levels vary by age and prostate volume, but generally less than 4 ng/mL can serve as a guide

PSA velocity has been shown to increase the likelihood of Gleason 7+ disease (≥2 ng/mL/yr)

PSA density (PSA/gland volume) has been shown to predict for prostate cancer (over 7%)

Low free PSA (unbound PSA) is associated with an increased likelihood of prostate cancer (less than 25% can serve as a threshold)

12. B

The most common presenting symptom of bladder cancer is painless hematuria.

13. C

Based on embryologic origin, the first echelon nodal drainage of the testes is to the paraaortic lymph nodes. The first echelon lymph node from the left testicle is the left renal vein.

14. C

Bicalutamide is an antiandrogen.

15. B

The Epstein criteria include the following: cT1c, Gleason less than seven, PSA, 10 ng/mL, fewer than three cores positive, less than 50% cancer in any core, PSA density less than 0.15 ng/mL/g.

16. C

Several trials have demonstrated a ~10% improved bPFS with EBRT doses of at least 74 Gy although these failed to demonstrate an overall survival benefit.

17. B

The prostate is divided into four zones: peripheral, transitional (BPH), central, and anterior fibromuscular stroma.

18. C

Ninety-three percent of bladder cancers are transitional cell in origin.

19. D

The nodal staging of locally advanced bladder cancers is as following:

N1—single LN below common iliac

N2—multiple LNs below common iliac

N3—common iliac LN involvement

20. D

Usual total dose to bladder cancer given in 1.8 to 2.0 Gy/day is in the range of 60 to 66 Gy. The MRC trial used 55 Gy in 20 fractions.

Recommended Reading

Chung P, Warde P. Contemporary management of stage I and II seminoma. *Curr Urol Rep.* 2013;14(5):525-533.

Crook JM, Haie-Meder C, Demanes DJ, et al. American Brachytherapy Society–Groupe Europeen de Curietherapie–European Society of Therapeutic Radiation Oncology (ABS–GEC–ESTRO) consensus statement for penile brachytherapy. *Brachytherapy.* 2013;12(3):191-198.

Davis BJ, Horwitz EM, Lee WR, et al. American Brachytherapy Society consensus guidelines for transrectal ultrasound-guided permanent prostate brachytherapy. *Brachytherapy.* 2012;11(1):6-19.

Harris VA, Staffurth J, Naismith O, et al. Consensus guidelines and contouring atlas for pelvic node delineation in prostate and pelvic node intensity modulated radiation therapy. *Int J Radiat Oncol Biol Phys.* 2015;92(4): 874-883.

Hasan S, Francis A, Hagenauer A, et al. The role of brachytherapy in organ preservation for penile cancer: a meta-analysis and review of the literature. *Brachytherapy.* 2015;14(4):517-524.

Hsu IC, Yamada Y, Assimos DG, et al. ACR appropriateness criteria high-dose-rate brachytherapy for prostate cancer. *Brachytherapy*. 2014;13(1):27-31.

Jani AB, Efstathiou JA, Shipley WU. Bladder preservation strategies. *HematolOncol Clin North Am*. 2015;29(2):289-300, ix.

Kothari G, Foroudi F, Gill S, et al. Outcomes of stereotactic radiotherapy for cranial and extracranial metastatic renal cell carcinoma: a systematic review. *Acta Oncol*. 2015;54(2):148-157.

Nguyen PL, Aizer A, Assimos DG, et al. ACR appropriateness criteria definitive external-beam irradiation in stage T1 and T2 prostate cancer. *Am J Clin Oncol*. 2014;37(3):278-288.

Lymphoma/Myeloma

Jeffrey Q. Cao

5.1 Hodgkin's Lymphoma

Epidemiology

- Hodgkin's lymphoma (HL) was referred to formerly as Hodgkin's disease.
- It accounts for about 10% of all lymphoma diagnoses and about 0.6% of all cancer diagnoses globally annually.
- There was an estimate of 9,190 new cases and 1,180 deaths from HL in the United States in 2014.
- Bimodal age distribution (~20 and ~65 years) may differ with geography, level of industrialization, and race.
- There is a slight male predominance.
- Risk factors:
  - Socioeconomic status (SES) varies by subtype (increased risk of nodular sclerosis [NS] with higher SES but increased risk of mixed cellularity [MC] with lower SES).
  - Environmental or infectious agents such as mononucleosis due to Epstein–Barr virus (EBV) are also a risk factor.
  - Smoking
  - Immunosuppression associated with transplantation or due to immunosuppressive drugs or HIV infection
  - Autoimmune disorders such as rheumatoid arthritis (RA), systemic lupus erythematosus (SLE), sarcoidosis, ulcerative colitis
  - Family history due either to genetics or common environmental exposure are other risk factors.
- Possible protective effect from:
  - Childhood infectious illnesses (e.g., chickenpox, measles-mumps-rubella [MMR], pertussis)
  - Breastfeeding
  - Aspirin use
- Prognostic factors:
  - Presence or absence of systemic symptoms
  - Stage of disease
  - Presence of large masses
  - Quality and suitability of treatment administered
  - Age
  - Sex
  - Erythrocyte sedimentation rate (ESR)
  - Extent of abdominal involvement
  - Hematocrit
  - Absolute number of nodal sites of involvement

- For advanced stage HL, the International Prognostic Score (IPS) is based on seven adverse risk factors:
  - Albumin less than 4.0 g/dL
  - Hemoglobin less than 10.5 g/dL
  - Male sex
  - Age ≥45 years
  - Stage IV disease
  - White blood cell (WBC) count ≥15,000/mm^3
  - Absolute lymphocytic count less than 600/mm^3 or a lymphocyte count less than 8% of total WBC count

Pathology

- Pathologists currently use the World Health Organization (WHO) modification of the Revised European-American Lymphoma (REAL) classification for the histologic classification.
- Two major subgroups, based on cell appearance and immunophenotype:
  - Classical HL (divided into four subtypes in order of incidence and prevalence)
    - NS ~70%
    - MC ~20% to 25%
    - Lymphocyte rich (LR) ~5 to 10
    - Lymphocyte depleted (LD) ~less than 1%
  - Nodular lymphocyte predominant HL (NLPHL)
- Typical immunophenotype for classical HL: CD15+, CD30+, PAX-5+ (weak), CD3−, CD20− (majority), CD45−, CD79a−
- Typical immunophenotype for NLPHL: CD20+, CD45+, CD79a+, BCL6+, PAX-5+, CD3−, CD15−, CD30−
- Diagnostic hallmark for classical HL is presence of Reed–Sternberg cells in inflammatory background.
- NLPHL usually presents as asymptomatic cervical or inguinal nodal involvement among young males but without mediastinal involvement.
- NLPHL have earlier-stage disease, longer survival, and fewer treatment failures compared to classical HL.
- NLPHL has tendency for histologic transformation to diffuse large B-cell lymphoma in ~10% of patients by ~10 years.

Diagnosis and Workup

- History: B symptoms, alcohol intolerance, pruritus, fatigue, performance status
- Physical examination: lymphoid regions, spleen, liver
- Bloodwork: complete blood count (CBC), differential, erythrocyte sedimentation rate (ESR), lactate dehydrogenase (LDH), liver function tests (LFTs), albumin, blood urea nitrogen (BUN), creatinine
- HIV test (in selected cases)
- Pregnancy test for women of childbearing age
- Imaging: Chest x-ray (CXR), contrast-enhanced CT neck, thorax, abdomen, pelvis, whole body PET-CT
- Excisional biopsies preferred with immunohistochemistry evaluation (large core needle biopsies may be adequate if diagnostic but fine needle aspiration alone is to be avoided)
- Bone marrow (BM) biopsy if B symptoms, myelosuppression, or advanced stage (involvement ~5% of patients)
- Multigated acquisition (MUGA) scan to test ejection fraction (EF) prior to doxorubicin-containing chemotherapy regimens
- Pulmonary function tests (PFTs) to test DLCO prior to bleomycin-containing chemotherapy regimens
- Counseling: fertility, smoking cessation, psychosocial

Staging

- American Joint Committee on Cancer (AJCC) has designated staging using the Ann Arbor classification system.

Stage I	Involvement of a single lymphatic site (i.e., nodal region, Waldeyer's ring, thymus, or spleen) (I).
	Localized involvement of a single extralymphatic organ or site in the absence of any lymph node involvement (IE) (rare in HL).
Stage II	Involvement of ≥two lymph node regions on the same side of the diaphragm (II).
	Localized involvement of a single extralymphatic organ or site in association with regional lymph node involvement with or without involvement of other lymph node regions on the same side of the diaphragm (IIE).
	The number of regions involved may be indicated by a subscript numeral, as in, for example, II_3.
Stage III	Involvement of lymph node regions on both sides of the diaphragm (III), which also may be accompanied by extralymphatic extension in association with adjacent lymph node involvement (IIIE) or by involvement of the spleen (IIIS), or both (IIIE, S).
	Splenic involvement is designated by the letter S.
Stage IV	Diffuse or disseminated involvement of one or more extralymphatic organs, with or without associated lymph node involvement.
	Isolated extralymphatic organ involvement in the absence of adjacent regional lymph node involvement, but in conjunction with disease in distant site(s).
	Stage IV includes any involvement of the liver or BM, lungs (other than by direct extension from another site), or cerebrospinal fluid.
A	Asymptomatic.
B	B symptoms: Unexplained loss of more than 10% of body weight in the 6 months before diagnosis, unexplained fever with temperatures above 38°C, drenching night sweats.

BM, bone marrow; HL, Hodgkin's lymphoma.

- Lugano classification recommends modification of the Ann Arbor classification for anatomic description of disease extent for primary nodal lymphomas.

Stage	Involvement	Extranodal (E) Status
Limited		
I	One node or a group of adjacent nodes	Single extranodal lesions without nodal involvement
II	Two or more nodal groups on the same side of the diaphragm	Stage I or II by nodal extent with limited contiguous extranodal involvement
II bulky*	II as above with "bulky" disease	Not applicable
Advanced		
III	Nodes on both sides of the diaphragm; nodes above the diaphragm with spleen involvement	Not applicable

(continued)

(continued)

Stage	Involvement	Extranodal (E) Status
IV	Additional noncontiguous extralymphatic involvement	Not applicable

Note: Extent of disease is determined by PET-CT for avid lymphomas and CT for nonavid histologies. Tonsils, Waldeyer's ring, and spleen are considered nodal tissue.

*Whether stage II bulky disease is treated as limited or advanced disease may be determined by histology and a number of prognostic factors.

- Ann Arbor Anatomical regions for the staging of HL
- Lymph nodes above the diaphragm
  - Waldeyer ring
  - Tonsils, adenoids (nasopharynx), lingual tonsils
  - Cervical[neck] (occipital, submental, preauricular, submandibular, internal jugular)
  - Infraclavicular
  - Supraclavicular (scalene)
  - Axillary, pectoral
  - Mediastinal (peritracheal, thymic region)
  - Hilar
  - Epitrochlear, brachial
  - Upper abdomen (splenic hilar, celiac, porta hepatis)
  - Lower abdomen (iliac, paraaortic, retroperitoneal, mesenteric, abdominal, NOS)
  - Iliac
  - Inguinal
  - Femoral
  - Popliteal
  - Spleen

Treatment Overview

- Regardless of stage, general practice is to treat patients based on limited (stages I and II, nonbulky) or advanced (stage III or IV) disease, with stage II bulky disease considered as limited or advanced disease based on a number of prognostic factors.
- Primary treatment for classical HL is based on clinical staging system and risk factors.
- Unfavorable risk factors vary by different organizations such as German Hodgkin Study Group (GHSG), European Organization for the Research and Treatment of Cancer (EORTC), National Cancer Institute of Canada (NCIC), and National Comprehensive Cancer Network (NCCN).

Risk Factor	GHSG	EORTC	NCCN	NCIC
Large mediastinal mass	Mediastinal mass ratio >0.33	Mediastinal thoracic ratio ≥0.35	Mediastinal mass ratio >0.33	Mediastinal mass ratio >0.33 or >10 cm
Elevated ESR or B symptoms	>50 mm/h if A or >30 mm/h if B symptoms	>50 mm/h if A or >30 mm/h if B symptoms	>50 mm/h or any B symptoms	>50 mm/h or any B symptoms

(continued)

(*continued*)

Risk Factor	GHSG	EORTC	NCCN	NCIC
Number of nodal sites involved	≥3 nodal areas (out of 11 GHSG areas)	≥4 nodal areas (out of five supra-diaphragmatic EORTC areas)	≥4 nodal regions (out of 16 Ann Arbor regions)	≥4 nodal regions (out of 16 Ann Arbor regions)
Extranodal involvement	Any extranodal disease			
"Bulky" disease			>10 cm	
Age		≥50		≥40
Histology				MC or LD

EORTC, European Organization for the Research and Treatment of Cancer; ESR, erythrocyte sedimentation rate; GHSG, German Hodgkin Study Group; LD, lymphocyte depleted; MC, mixed cellularity; NCCN, National Comprehensive Cancer Network; NCIC, National Cancer Institute of Canada.

- Note that the EORTC includes the infraclavicular/subpectoral nodal area with the axilla while the GHSG includes it with the cervical.
- Both EORTC and GHSG combine the mediastinum and both hila as a single region.

	Stage	Treatment
Early stage classical HL	Stage I–II favorable	• Combined modality therapy • ABVD × 2 cycles, then ISRT (20 Gy) • Alternative to ABVD is Stanford V × 8 weeks for combined modality therapy • Alternative for patients avoiding RT is ABVD × 2 cycles, then restaging PET-CT, if negative, then further ABVD × 2 cycles, if positive, then ISRT
	Stage I–II unfavorable, bulky (unfavorable RF include any of ESR >50, ESR >30 with B symptoms, ≥3 sites, or extranodal disease)	• ABVD × 4–6 cycles, then ISRT (30–36 Gy) • Alternative to ABVD is Stanford V × 12 weeks or Escalated BEACOPP × 2 + ABVD × 2 cycles for combined modality therapy
	Stage I–II unfavorable, nonbulky (unfavorable RF include any of ESR >50, ESR >30 with B symptoms, ≥3 sites, or extranodal disease)	• ABVD × 4–6 cycles, then ISRT (30 Gy) • Alternative to ABVD is Stanford V × 12 weeks or Escalated BEACOPP × 2 + ABVD × 2 cycles for combined modality therapy
Advanced stage classical HL	Stage III–IV, nonbulky	• ABVD × 6–8 cycles • Alternative dose-escalated BEACOPP × 6 cycles • Alternative is Stanford V × 12 weeks for selected cases if IPS <3
	Stage III–IV, bulky	• ABVD × 6–8 cycles, then ISRT to site of prior bulk • Alternative dose-escalated BEACOPP × 6 cycles, then ISRT to site of prior bulk

(*continued*)

(continued)

	Stage	Treatment
NLPHL	Stage IA, IIA, nonbulky	• ISRT
	Stage IA, IIA, bulky or Stage IB, IIB	• Chemotherapy + ISRT ± Rituximab • Chemotherapy options include ABVD or CHOP or CVP
	Stage IIIA, IVA	• Chemotherapy ± Rituximab ± ISRT
	Stage IIIB, IVB	• Chemotherapy ± Rituximab ± ISRT

ABVD, adriamycin, bleomycin, vinblastine, decarbazine; CHOP, cyclophosphamide, adriamycin, vincristine, prednisone; IPS, international prognostic score; ISRT, involved site radiation therapy; RT, radiation therapy.

Radiation Therapy Technique

Involved Site Radiation Therapy

- The recommended modern RT concept of involved site radiation therapy (ISRT) was developed by the international lymphoma radiation oncology group (ILROG) consensus on basis of involved node radiation therapy (INRT).
- The prechemotherapy gross target volume (GTV) determines clinical target volume (CTV).
- The irradiated volume is significantly smaller than with involved field radiation therapy (IFRT).
- ISRT accommodates cases in which optimal prechemotherapy imaging is not available.
- Clinical judgment and best available imaging are used to contour larger CTV compared to INRT to accommodate uncertainties in defining prechemotherapy GTV due to differences in positioning.
- CTV encompasses original lymphoma volume, modified for normal tissue boundaries and expanded to accommodate uncertainties in determining the prechemotherapy volume.
- In situations where RT is primary treatment, larger margins to encompass subclinical disease need to be applied.
- Internal target volume (ITV) should be added to the CTV where internal organ movement is of concern.
- Planning target volume (PTV) is based on institutional measures of patient setup error.

Involved Field Radiation Therapy

- For historical perspective, traditional IFRT concept involves treating a region, not an individual lymph node.
- Main involved field regions are neck (unilateral), mediastinum (including bilateral hilar regions), axilla (including supra- and infraclavicular nodes), spleen, para-aortic lymph nodes, and inguinal (including femoral and iliac nodes).
- The target initially involves prechemotherapy sites and volume, with exception of transverse diameter of mediastinal and para-aortic lymph nodes where usually reduced postchemotherapy volume is used.

General Dose Guidelines

Combine Modality Therapy

- Stages IA to IIA, nonbulky disease: 20 Gy (favorable) to 30 Gy (unfavorable) if treated with adriamycin, bleomycin, vinblastine, decarbazine (ABVD), 30 Gy if treated with Stanford V
- Stages IB to IIB, nonbulky disease: 30 Gy
- Stages I to IV, bulky disease: 30 to 36 Gy

RT Alone (for NLPHL)

- Involved regions: 30 to 36 Gy
- Uninvolved regions: 25 to 30 Gy

IFRT	Borders
Unilateral cervical/ supraclavicular region	Superior: 1–2 cm above the lower tip of mastoid process and midpoint through chin
	Inferior: 2 cm below bottom of clavicle
	Lateral: To include medial 2/3 of clavicle
	Medial: (a) Ipsilateral transverse process (if supraclavicular nodes not involved), or (b) to include entire vertebral body (if medial nodes seen), or (c) to contralateral transverse process (if supraclavicular nodes involved)
Bilateral cervical/ supraclavicular region	Treat both cervical and supraclavicular regions as described above
Mediastinum	Superior: C5–C6 interspace
	Inferior: The lower of (a) 5 cm below carina or (b) 2 cm below prechemotherapy inferior border
	Lateral: Postchemotherapy volume with 1.5-cm margin
	Hilar area: To be included with 1-cm margin, or 1.5-cm margin if initially involved
Mediastinum with cervical node involvement	Mantle field without axilla as described above
	If paracardiac nodes involved, treat whole heart with 14.4 Gy and initially involved nodes with 30.6 Gy
Axillary region	Superior: C5–C6 innerspace
	Inferior: The lower of (a) tip of scapula or (b) 2 cm below lowest axillary node
	Medial: Ipsilateral cervical transverse process (include vertebral bodies only if supraclavicular node involved)
	Lateral: Flash axilla
Spleen	Postchemotherapy volume with 1.5-cm margin
Abdomen (para-aortic nodes)	Superior: Top of T11 and at least 2 cm above prechemotherapy volume
	Inferior: Bottom of L4 and at least 2 cm below prechemotherapy volume
	Lateral: Edge of transverse processes and at least 2 cm from postchemotherapy volume
	Porta-hepatis region should be included if originally involved
Inguinal/femoral/ external iliac region	Superior: Middle of sacro-iliac joint
	Inferior: 5 cm below lesser trochanter
	Lateral: Greater trochanter and 2 cm lateral to initially involved nodes
	Medial: Medial border of obturator foramen with at least 2 cm medial to involved nodes
	Field should extend to L4–L5 interspace if common iliac nodes involved and at least 2 cm above the initially involved nodal border

Toxicity

- Dependent on radiation site or field
- Acute: generalized fatigue, radiation dermatitis, esophagitis, gastritis, nausea, vomiting, diarrhea, myelosupression

- Subacute: radiation pneumonitis, L'Hermitte's sign
- Late: hypothyroidism, pulmonary fibrosis, immunosuppression particularly with splenic irradiation, gastric ulceration, infertility, coronary artery disease, secondary malignancy

Follow-Up

- Follow-up after completion of treatment up to 5 years
- Interim H&P every 3 to 6 months for first 1 to 2 years, then every 6 to 12 months for years 3 to 5
- Laboratory studies (CBC, differential, ESR [if elevated at initial diagnosis], chemistry profile) with each clinic visit
- Thyroid-stimulating hormone (TSH) at least annually if RT is to neck
- Annual influenza vaccine
- PET-CT to confirm Deauville one to three but subsequent imaging only if there are clinical symptoms
- Annual mammogram for women less than 30 years beginning 8 to 10 years after RT

5.2 Non-Hodgkin's Lymphoma

Epidemiology

- Non-Hodgkin's lymphoma (NHL) is a diverse group of malignant neoplasms derived from B cell progenitors, T cell progenitors, mature B cells, mature T cells, or natural killer (NK) cells.
- NHL is divided into three broad classifications: (a) indolent, (b) aggressive, (c) very aggressive.
- Indolent lymphoma can present with slow-growing lymphadenopathy, hepatomegaly, splenomegaly, or cytopenias.
- Aggressive lymphoma usually have subacute or acute presentation with rapidly growing mass, constitutional symptoms or elevated LDH or uric acid.
- ~10% to 35% patients have primary extranodal disease at diagnosis.
- ~50% patients develop secondary extranodal disease during course of disease.
- Most common extranodal site is GI tract, followed by skin. Other sites include testis, bone, CNS, kidney, and rarely, prostate, bladder, ovary, orbit, heart, breast, salivary glands, and adrenals.
- Example of initial extranodal presentation: primary GI tract lymphoma, primary CNS lymphoma
- Lymphomas can present as oncological emergencies: spinal cord compression, pericardial tamponade, hypercalcemia, superior vena cava compression (SVCO), hyperleukocytosis, acute airway/intestinal/ureteral obstruction, hyperuricemia or tumor lysis syndrome, hyperviscosity syndrome, venous thromboembolic disease, or severe hepatic dysfunction or autoimmune hemolytic anemia/thrombocytopenia.
- Lymphomas can present with abnormal laboratory results: cytopenia, hypercalcemia, hyperuricemia, elevated serum LDH, monoclonal immunoglobulin peak.
- Up to 40% of patients present with constitutional (B) symptoms.
- More than two-thirds of patients present with painless peripheral lymphadenopathy.
- Prognosis is heterogeneous and dependent on histology and patient, disease, and treatment-related factors.
- International Prognostic Index (IPI) identified five pretreatment characteristics independently to design a model to predict an individual patient's risk of death:
  - Age greater than 60 years
  - Tumor stage III or IV [advanced disease]
  - Number of extranodal sites greater than one
  - Performance status ≥2
  - Serum LDH level greater than one times normal
- Four risk groups were identified: low risk (0–1 factors, 5-year OS 73%), low intermediate (2 factors, 5-year OS 51%), high intermediate (3 factors, 5-year OS 43%), and high risk (4–5 factors, 5-year OS 26%).

- Age-adjusted IPI model for patients 60 years or younger, based on tumor stage, lactate dehydrogenase level, and performance status, identified four risk groups based on zero to three factors with predicted five-year survival rates of 83%, 69%, 46%, and 32%.
- Follicular Lymphoma International Prognostic Index (FLIPI) identified five adverse prognostic factors:
  - Age greater than 60 years
  - Ann Arbor stages III to IV
  - Hemoglobin level less than 120 g/L
  - Number of nodal areas greater than four
  - Serum LDH level above normal
- Three FLIPI risk groups were defined: low risk (0–1 adverse factor, HR 1.0, 5-year OS 90.6%), intermediate risk (2 factors, HR 2.3, 5-year OS 77.6%), and poor risk (>3 adverse factors, HR 4.3, 5-year OS 52.5%).

Pathology

NHL is divided into three broad classifications: (a) indolent, (b) aggressive, (c) very aggressive.

	B-cell	T-cell
Indolent	Follicular, grades 1, 2, 3a	MF/SS
	Small lymphocytic (CLL)	Primary cutaneous, CD30+
	Marginal zone, extranodal (MALT)	Primary cutaneous PTCL, CD30–
	Splenic marginal zone	T-cell large granular lymphocytic leukemia
	Marginal zone, nodal (monocytoid B-cell)	
	Lymphoplasmacytic (Waldenström's macroglobulinemia)	
	Primary cutaneous, follicle center	
	Hairy cell leukemia	
Aggressive	Diffuse large B-cell	Peripheral T-cell, unspecified
	• T-cell/histocyte-rich DLBCL	Angioimmunoblastic (AILD)
	• Primary DLBCL of the CNS	Enteropathy associated T-cell
	• Primary cutaneous DLBCL, leg	Hepatosplenic T-cell
	• EBV-positive DLBCL of the elderly	Subcutaneous panniculitis-like
	DLBCL associated with chronic inflammation	Anaplastic large cell (CD30+) ALK+
	Lymphomatoid granulomatosis	Anaplastic large cell (CD30+) ALK-
	Primary mediastinal large B-cell	Extranodal NK/T-cell, nasal type
	Intravascular large B-cell	
	ALK positive large B-cell	
	Plasmablastic lymphoma	
	LBCL in HHV8-associated Castleman disease	
	Primary effusion lymphoma	
	Follicular grade 3b (large cell)	

(continued)

(*continued*)

	B-cell	T-cell
Special	Burkitt lymphoma	T lymphoblastic leukemia/lymphoma
	Intermediate between DLBCL and BL	
	Intermediate between DLBCL and HL	ATL/L-HTLV-1+ (adult T-cell leukemia/lymphoma)
	High-grade Burkitt-like	T prolymphocytic leukemia
	B lymphoblastic leukemia/lymphoma	
	B prolymphocytic leukemia	
	Mantle cell	
	Lymphomas associated with HIV infection	
	Lymphomas associated with primary immune disorders	
	Posttransplant lymphoproliferative disorders (PTLD)	
	• Plasmacytic hyperplasia and infectious mononucleosis-like PTLD • Polymorphic PTLD • Monomorphic PTLD • Classical Hodgkin-type PTLD	
	Other iatrogenic immunodeficiency-associated lymphomas	

BF, Burkitt lymphoma; DLBCL, diffuse large B-cell lymphoma; HL, Hodgkin's lymphoma; LBCL, large B-cell lymphoma; MF, mycosis fungoides; PTCL, peripheral T-cell lymphoma; SS, Sézary syndrome.

Diagnosis and Workup

- History: B symptoms, alcohol intolerance, pruritus, fatigue, performance status
- Physical examination: lymphoid regions, spleen, liver
- Bloodwork: CBC, differential, ESR, LDH, LFTs, albumin, BUN, creatinine
- HIV test (in selected cases)
- Pregnancy test for women of childbearing age
- Imaging: CXR, contrast-enhanced CT neck, thorax, abdomen, pelvis, whole body PET-CT
- Excisional biopsies preferred with immunohistochemistry evaluation (large core needle biopsies may be adequate if diagnostic but fine needle aspiration alone is to be avoided)
- BM biopsy if B symptoms, myelosupression, or advanced stage (involvement ~5% of patients)
- MUGA scan to test EF prior to doxorubicin-containing chemotherapy regimens
- PFTs to test DLCO prior to bleomycin-containing chemotherapy regimens
- Counseling: fertility, smoking cessation, psychosocial

Staging

- AJCC has designated staging using the Ann Arbor classification system.
- Lugano classification recommends modification of the Ann Arbor classification for anatomic description of disease extent for primary nodal lymphomas.

Treatment Overview

- Regardless of stage, general practice is to treat patients based on limited (stages I and II, nonbulky) or advanced (stage III or IV) disease, with stage II bulky disease considered as limited or advanced disease based on histology and a number of prognostic factors.

Stage I   Involvement of a single lymphatic site (i.e., nodal region, Waldeyer's ring, thymus, or spleen) (I).

Localized involvement of a single extralymphatic organ or site in the absence of any lymph node involvement (IE) (rare in Hodgkin's lymphoma).

Stage II   Involvement of ≥2 lymph node regions on the same side of the diaphragm (II).

Localized involvement of a single extralymphatic organ or site in association with regional lymph node involvement with or without involvement of other lymph node regions on the same side of the diaphragm (IIE).

The number of regions involved may be indicated by a subscript numeral, as in, for example, II_3.

Stage III   Involvement of lymph node regions on both sides of the diaphragm (III), which also may be accompanied by extralymphatic extension in association with adjacent lymph node involvement (IIIE) or by involvement of the spleen (IIIS) or both (IIIE, S).

Splenic involvement is designated by the letter S.

Stage IV   Diffuse or disseminated involvement of one or more extralymphatic organs, with or without associated lymph node involvement.

Isolated extralymphatic organ involvement in the absence of adjacent regional lymph node involvement, but in conjunction with disease in distant site(s).

Stage IV includes any involvement of the liver or BM, lungs (other than by direct extension from another site), or cerebrospinal fluid.

A   Asymptomatic.

B   B Symptoms: Unexplained loss of more than 10% of body weight in the 6 months before diagnosis, unexplained fever with temperatures above 38°C, drenching night sweats.

Stage	Involvement	Extranodal (E) Status
Limited		
I	One node or a group of adjacent nodes	Single extranodal lesions without nodal involvement
II	Two or more nodal groups on the same side of the diaphragm	Stage I or II by nodal extent with limited contiguous extranodal involvement
II bulky*	II as above with "bulky" disease	Not applicable
Advanced		
III	Nodes on both sides of the diaphragm; nodes above the diaphragm with spleen involvement	Not applicable
IV	Additional noncontiguous extralymphatic involvement	Not applicable

Note: Extent of disease is determined by PET-CT for avid lymphomas and CT for nonavid histologies. Tonsils, Waldeyer's ring, and spleen are considered nodal tissue.

*Whether stage II bulky disease is treated as limited or advanced disease may be determined by histology and a number of prognostic factors.

Follicular lymphoma	Stage I–II		• ISRT • Immunotherapy ± chemotherapy • Immunotherapy ± chemotherapy + ISRT • Observation
	Stage II Bulky, Stage III–IV		• Observation • Consider treatment with chemotherapy if symptomatic, threatened end-organ function, cytopenia secondary to lymphoma, bulky disease, steady progression, or candidate for clinical trial
Marginal zone lymphoma	Gastric MALT Lymphoma	Stage IE–IIE, H. pylori positive	Antibiotic therapy for H. pylori ISRT or Rituximab if ISRT contraindicated
		Stage IE–IIE, H. pylori negative	Observe or treat symptomatic
		Stage IIIE–IV	
	Nongastric MALT Lymphoma	Stage I–II	• ISRT • Surgery • Rituximab • Observation
		Extranodal (multiple sites)	• RT • Observation
		Stage III–IV	Observe or treat symptomatic
		Stage I–IV, MALT coexist with large cell lymphoma	Manage as DLBCL
	Nodal Marginal Zone Lymphoma	Stage I–II	• ISRT • Immunotherapy ± chemotherapy • Immunotherapy ± chemotherapy + ISRT • Observation
		Stage II Bulky, Stage III–IV	• Observation • Consider treatment with chemotherapy if symptomatic, threatened end-organ function, cytopenia secondary to lymphoma, bulky disease, steady progression, or candidate for clinical trial
	Splenic Marginal Zone Lymphoma		• Observation • Splenectomy • Rituximab
Mantle cell lymphoma	Stage I–II		• Chemotherapy ± RT • RT
	Stage II bulky, III–IV		• Observation • Chemotherapy

DLBCL

Stage I–II	Nonbulky (<10 cm)	• RCHOP × 3 cycles + ISRT • RCHOP × 6 cycles ± ISRT
	Bulky (≥10 cm)	• RCHOP × 6 cycles ± ISRT
Stage III–IV		• RCHOP × 6 cycles ± ISRT
Relapsed/refractory disease		• Second-line chemotherapy • High-dose therapy with autologous stem cell rescue ± RT pre- or posttransplant • IFRT/ISRT

DLBCL, diffuse large B-cell lymphoma; IFRT, involved field radiation therapy; ISRT, involved site radiation therapy.

Radiation Therapy Technique

Involved Site Radiation Therapy

- The recommended modern RT concept of ISRT was developed by ILROG consensus on basis of INRT.
- The prechemotherapy GTV determines CTV.
- The irradiated volume is significantly smaller than with IFRT.
- ISRT accommodates cases in which optimal prechemotherapy imaging is not available.
- Clinical judgment and best available imaging is used to contour larger CTV compared to INRT to accommodate uncertainties in defining prechemotherapy GTV due to differences in positioning.
- CTV encompasses original lymphoma volume, modified for normal tissue boundaries and expanded to accommodate uncertainties in determining the prechemotherapy volume.
- In situations where RT is primary treatment, larger margins to encompass subclinical disease need to be applied.
- ITV should be added to the CTV where internal organ movement is of concern.
- PTV is based on institutional measures of patient setup error.

General Dose Guidelines

- Localized CLL/SLL: 24 to 30 Gy
- FL: 24 to 30 Gy
- MZL:
  o Gastric: 30 Gy
  o Other extranodal sites: 24 to 30 Gy
  o Nodal MZL: 24 to 30 Gy
- Early-stage MCL: 30 to 36 Gy
- Mini-dose RT (2 Gy × 2) for palliation/local control of CLL/SLL, FL, MZL, MCL
- Diffuse large B-cell lymphoma (DLBCL) or peripheral T-cell lymphoma (PTCL):
  o Consolidation RT after chemotherapy CR: 30 to 36 Gy
  o Complimentary RT after PR: 40 to 50 Gy
  o Primary RT for refractory or noncandidates for chemotherapy: 45 to 55 Gy
- Primary cutaneous anaplastic large cell lymphoma: 30 to 36 Gy

Toxicity

- Dependent on radiation site or field
- Acute: generalized fatigue, radiation dermatitis, esophagitis, gastritis, nausea, vomiting, diarrhea, myelosupression

- Subacute: radiation pneumonitis, L'hermitte's sign
- Late: hypothyroidism, pulmonary fibrosis, immunosuppression particularly with splenic irradiation, gastric ulceration, infertility, coronary artery disease, secondary malignancy

Follow-Up

- Follow-up after completion of treatment up to 5 years
- Interim H&P every 3 to 6 months for first 1 to 2 years, then every 6 to 12 months for years 3 to 5
- Laboratory studies (CBC, differential, ESR [if elevated at initial diagnosis], chemistry profile) with each clinic visit
- TSH at least annually if RT to neck
- Annual influenza vaccine
- PET-CT to confirm Deauville one to three but subsequent imaging only if clinical symptoms
- Annual mammogram for women less than 30 years beginning 8 to 10 years after RT

5.3   Cutaneous Lymphoma

Epidemiology

- Primary cutaneous lymphomas (PCLs) are a heterogeneous group of T- and B-cell lymphomas with considerable variation in histology, phenotype, and prognosis.
- PCL must be distinguished from nodal or systemic lymphomas, for which cutaneous involvement is secondary.
- WHO-EORTC classification is based on clinical, histologic, and immunophenotypic criteria.
- ~75% to 80% of PCLs are T-cell origin in Western world, with mycosis fungoides (MF) the most common type, and cutaneous B-cell lymphomas ~20% to 25%.
- In Asia, cutaneous T-cell lymphomas other than MF, in particular cutaneous NK/T-cell lymphomas, are much more common, whereas cutaneous B-cell lymphomas are much more uncommon.
- Mycosis Fungoides (MF) and Sézary syndrome (SS) are most common subtypes of cutaneous T-cell lymphoma (CTCL).
- Primary cutaneous CD30+ lymphoproliferative disorders are second most common group of CTCL.
- Primary cutaneous B cell lymphoma (PCBCL) has three main subtypes:
  - Primary cutaneous follicle center lymphoma (PCFCL)—most common PCBCL, presentation on head or trunk, indolent course, excellent prognosis
  - Primary cutaneous large B-cell lymphoma (PCLBCL), leg-type presentation on legs, older age at diagnosis, most commonly elderly women, aggressive lymphoma, intermediate prognosis
  - Primary cutaneous marginal zone lymphoma (PCMZL)—indolent PCBCL

Pathology

- CTCL: MF, primary cutaneous anaplastic large-cell lymphoma (PCALCL), subcutaneous panniculitis-like T-cell lymphoma, primary cutaneous gamma-delta T-cell lymphoma, and primary cutaneous NK/T-cell lymphoma, nasal type
- Cutaneous B-cell lymphomas: PCFCL, PCMZL, and primary cutaneous diffuse large B-cell lymphoma, leg type
- MF represents most common form of CTCL
- Malignant cell is derived from post-thymic T-cell typically with CD4+ helper/memory antigen
- Characterized by erythematous patches in sun-protected areas progressing to plaques or tumors
- SS is aggressive leukemic and erythrodermic form of CTCL
- Characterized by circulating atypical, malignant T lymphocytes with cerebriform nuclei (Serezy cells)
- Sezary cells have mature memory T-cell phenotype (CD3+, CD4+) with loss of CD7 and CD26

Diagnosis and Workup

- Delineation of skin involvement with photographs
- Skin biopsy (histopathology, immunophenotyping, and T-cell receptor (TCR) gene analysis)
- CBC differential
- Peripheral blood Sezary cell count
- Chemistry panel with LDH
- Consider peripheral blood flow cytometry (CD4/CD8 ratio), TCR gene analysis
- Lymph node and BM biopsy (histopathology, immunophenotyping, TCR gene analysis)
- Consider diagnostic imaging with CT or PET-CT
- Consider serologic testing (HTLV-1 and HIV)

Staging

- MF and SS have formal staging system by International Society for Cutaneous Lymphoma (ISCL) and EORTC.
- Other cutaneous non-HLs are staged using same system as HL and NHL.

ISCL/EORTC Revision to Classification of MF and SS

Skin (T)	
T1	Limited patches*, papules, and/or plaques† covering <10% of the skin surface; may further stratify into T1a (patch only) versus T1b (plaque ± patch)
T2	Patches, papules, or plaques covering ≥10% of the skin surface; may further stratify into T2a (patch only) versus T2b (plaque ± patch)
T3	One or more tumors‡ (≥1-cm diameter)
T4	Confluence of erythema covering ≥80% body surface area
Node (N)	
N0	No clinically abnormal lymph nodes§; biopsy not required
N1	Clinically abnormal lymph nodes; histopathology Dutch grade 1 or NCI LN0-2
N1a	Clone negative‖
N1b	Clone positive‖
N2	Clinically abnormal lymph nodes; histopathology Dutch grade 2 or NCI LN3
N2a	Clone negative‖
N2b	Clone positive‖
N3	Clinically abnormal lymph nodes; histopathology Dutch grades 3–4 or NCI LN4; clone positive or negative
NX	Clinically abnormal lymph nodes; no histologic confirmation
Visceral (M)	
M0	No visceral organ involvement
M1	Visceral involvement (must have pathology confirmation¶ and organ involved should be specified)

(continued)

ISCL/EORTC Revision to Classification of MF and SS (*continued*)

Skin (T)

Blood (B)	
B0	No significant blood involvement: ≤5% of Sézary cells. For clinical trials, B0 may also be defined as <250/microL Sézary cells; CD4+CD26− or CD4+CD7− cells or CD4+CD26− and CD4+CD7− cells <15% by flow cytometry
B0a	Clone negative
B0b	Clone positive
B1	Low blood tumor burden: Does not meet the criteria of B0 or B2
B1a	Clone negative
B1b	Clone positive
B2	High blood tumor burden: Positive clone[#] plus one of the following: ≥1,000/microL Sézary cells; CD4/CD8 ≥10; CD4+CD7− cells ≥40%; or CD4+CD26− cells ≥30%. For clinical trials, B2 may also be defined as >1,000/microL CD4+CD26− or CD4+CD7− cells.

[*]For skin, patch indicates any size lesion without significant elevation or induration. Presence/absence of hypo- or hyperpigmentation, scale, crusting, and/or poikiloderma should be noted.

[†]For skin, plaque indicates any size skin lesion that is elevated or indurated. Presence or absence of scale, crusting, and/or poikiloderma should be noted. Histologic features such as folliculotropism or large-cell transformation (>25% large cells), CD30+ or CD30−, and clinical features such as ulceration are important to document.

[‡]For skin, tumor indicates at least 1-cm diameter solid or nodular lesion with evidence of depth and/or vertical growth. Note total number of lesions, total volume of lesions, largest size lesion, and region of body involved. Also note if histologic evidence of large-cell transformation has occurred. Phenotyping for CD30 is encouraged.

[§]For node, abnormal lymph node(s) indicates any lymph node that on physical examination is firm, irregular, clustered, fixed, or 1.5 cm or larger in diameter or on imaging is >1.5 cm in the long axis or >1 cm in the short axis. Node groups examined on physical examination include cervical, supraclavicular, epitrochlear, axillary, and inguinal.

[||]A T cell clone is defined by PCR or Southern blot analysis of the TCR gene.

[¶]For viscera, spleen and liver may be diagnosed by imaging criteria alone.

[#]The clone in the blood should match that of the skin. The relevance of an isolated clone in the blood or a clone in the blood that does not match the clone in the skin remains to be determined.

This research was originally published in *Blood*, Olsen E, Vonderheid E, Pimpinelli N, et al. Revisions to the staging and classification of mycosis fungoides and Sezary syndrome: a proposal of the International Society for Cutaneous Lymphomas (ISCL) and the cutaneous lymphoma task force of the European Organization of Research and Treatment of Cancer (EORTC). *Blood*. 2007;110:1713. Copyright © the American Society of Hematology.

Additional data from: Olsen EA, Whittaker S, Kim YH, et al. Clinical end points and response criteria in mycosis fungoides and Sézary syndrome: a consensus statement of the International Society for Cutaneous Lymphomas, the United States Cutaneous Lymphoma Consortium, and the Cutaneous Lymphoma Task Force of the European Organisation for Research and Treatment of Cancer. *J Clin Oncol*. 2011;29:2598.

Clinical Staging for MF/SS

Clinical Stage	T	N	M	Peripheral Blood Involvement
IA	1	0	0	0,1
IB	2	0	0	0,1

Clinical Stage	T	N	M	Peripheral Blood Involvement
IIA	1,2	1,2	0	0,1
IIB	3	0–2	0	0,1
IIIA	4	0–2	0	0
IIIB	4	0–2	0	1
IVA1	1–4	0–2	0	2
IVA2	1–4	3	0	0–2
IVB	1–4	0-3	1	0–2

TNM Classification of Cutaneous Lymphoma Other Than MF/SS

T1	Solitary skin involvement
T1a	A solitary lesion <5-cm diameter
T1b	A solitary lesion >5-cm diameter
T2	Regional skin involvement: multiple lesions limited to one body region or two contiguous body regions
T2a	All disease encompassing in a <15-cm diameter circular area
T2b	All disease encompassing in a >15-cm and <30-cm diameter circular area
T2c	All disease encompassing in a >30-cm diameter circular area
T3	Generalized skin involvement
T3a	Multiple lesions involving two noncontiguous body regions
T3b	Multiple lesions involving ≥3 body regions
N0	No clinical or pathologic lymph node involvement
N1	Involvement of one peripheral lymph node region that drains an area of current or prior skin involvement
N2	Involvement of two or more peripheral lymph node regions or involvement of any lymph node region that does not drain an area of current or prior skin involvement
N3	Involvement of central lymph nodes
M0	No evidence of extracutaneous nonlymph node disease
M1	Extracutaneous nonlymph node disease present

Treatment Overview

PCBCL	Stage	Treatment
PCFCL/PCMZL/PCALCL	Solitary/regional T1-2	• Local RT • Excision • Observation • Topicals • Intralesional steroids
	Generalized disease (skin only) T3	• Observation • Rituximab • Topicals • Palliative RT • Intralesional steroids • Palliative chemotherapy
	Extracutaneous	• Manage as FL
PC-DLBCL, Leg type	Solitary regional T1–2	• CHOP-R + local RT • Local RT • Clinical trial
	Generalized disease (skin only) T3	• CHOP-R ± local RT • Clinical trial
	Extracutaneous disease	Manage as DLCBL

PCALCL, primary cutaneous anaplastic large-cell lymphoma; PCFCL, primary cutaneous follicle center lymphoma; PCMZL, primary cutaneous marginal zone lymphoma; RT, radiation therapy.

CTCL	Stage	Treatment
MF/SS	Limited/localized skin involvement	Skin-directed therapies • Topical corticosteroids • Topical chemotherapy • Local RT (8–36 Gy) • Topical retinoids • Phototherapy (UVB, narrow-band UVB, PUVA) • Topical imiquimod
	Generalized skin involvement	Skin-directed therapies • Topical corticosteroids • Topical chemotherapy • Local RT (8–36 Gy) • Topical retinoids • Phototherapy (UVB, narrow-band UVB, PUVA) • TSEBT (total skin electron beam therapy) (12–36 Gy)
	Histologic evidence of folliculotropic or large-cell transformation	Systemic therapy
	Stage IV Non-Sézary or visceral disease	Systemic therapy
	Sézary syndrome	Systemic therapy

Radiation Therapy Technique

- PCFCL, PCMZL, PCALCL are managed similarly.
- Margins beyond area of clinically evident erythema/induration will vary depending on lesion size and body site and must take into account beam dosimetry.
- EORTC/ISCL/ILROG recommends a margin of 1 to 1.5 cm.
- Thickness of lesions must be determined to ensure adequate coverage also in depth.
- Intact bone and/or fascia are not expected to harbor microscopic disease and may reduce the need for depth coverage.
- Most lesions can be treated effectively with electrons, usually 6 to 9 MeV.
- Alternatively, low energy x-rays (~100 kV) may be used.
- Bolus required to avoid skin sparing.
- For deep and bulky tumors or for circumferential lesions, higher energy photon fields and opposed field treatment (with bolus) may be required to provide adequate coverage.
- EORTC/ISCL recommends dose range of 20 to 36 Gy for PCMZL and 30 Gy for PCFCL.
- NCCN recommends dose of 24 to 30 Gy for PCMZL.
- ILROG recommends 24 to 30 Gy for PCFCL and PCMZL as well as PCALCL.
- PC-DLBCL, leg type, has a more aggressive behavior and is dealt with differently.
- CTV includes prechemotherapy GTV with margins of 1 to 2 cm.
- Most lesions can be treated effectively with electrons, usually 6 to 9 MeV.
- Bolus is required to avoid skin sparing.
- For certain body surfaces, higher energy photon fields and opposed-field treatment (with bolus) may be required to provide adequate coverage.
- 36 to 40 Gy is recommended but if no systemic treatment is given, dose of 40 Gy is recommended.

Mycosis Fungoides

- Local RT is effective for eradication of unilesional disease or palliation of multisite disease.
- Unilesional MF: ILROG encourages doses of 20 to 24 Gy and given "curative" nature of this treatment, margins greater than 2 cm are generally used.
- Otherwise local palliation treatment includes the lesion of interest plus 1 to 2 cm margins.
- Patches and plaques may be treated with 6- to 9-MeV electrons (plus bolus), but exophytic tumors may require even higher energy electrons, depending on their thickness.
- Alternatively, low energy x-rays may be used (~100 kV).
- Occasional localizations of disease on extremities or very complex contoured surfaces may require treatment with higher energy photons (~6 MV) and multiple field arrangements to ensure homogeneity of dose distribution.

Total Skin Electron Beam Therapy (TSEBT)

- Comprehensive programs of TSEBT may be used for effective palliation.
- It is technically challenging and requires careful attention to dosimetric technique.
- Variety of techniques may be used to ensure total skin coverage, including large electron field techniques, rotational techniques, and techniques involving patient or beam movement during RT.
- This generally requires treating patients in standing position on a rotating platform or else assuming multiple different positions to expose as much as possible of all body surfaces.
- Techniques for degrading electron beams to make them suitable for total skin treatment vary.
- Goal is to achieve dose homogeneity in the coronal plane, a Dmax at the skin surface (where the dose is prescribed), and an 80% dose at 0.7- to 1-cm depth.
- "Shadowed" areas such as top of the scalp, soles, and perineum, as well as areas under the breasts, beneath a pannus, etc., especially if involved, require supplemental treatment.
- Supplemental boost treatment may be delivered to tumors early during the course of TSEBT, to decrease their thickness and enhance penetration by the TSEBT.
- As appropriate for individuals, shielding of the eyes may be with either internal or external shields and the scalp may be shielded selectively.

Toxicity

- Dependent on radiation site or field
- Acute: generalized fatigue, radiation dermatitis, or alopecia
- Late: hyperpigmentation, skin fibrosis, secondary malignancy
- TSEBT
- Acute: onychoptosis or onycholysis, anhydrosis, epistaxis, parotiditis
- Late: nail dystrophy, xerosis, telangiectasias, alopecia, infertility, secondary malignancy

Follow-Up

- Follow-up after completion of treatment up to 5 years
- Interim H&P every 3 to 6 months for first 1 to 2 years, then every 6 to 12 months for years 3 to 5
- Laboratory studies (CBC, differential, LDH [if elevated at initial diagnosis], chemistry profile) with each clinic visit

5.4   Multiple Myeloma/Plasmacytoma

Epidemiology

- Multiple myeloma (MM) is a malignant neoplasm of plasma cells that accumulate in BM resulting in bone destruction and marrow failure.
- There is an estimate of 22,350 new cases and 10,710 deaths in United States in 2013.
- Mean age is 62 years in men and 61 years in women.
- 5-year survival rates ~34% according to SEER database.
- It is not considered curable unless solitary plasmacytoma (SP).
- SP is further classified as osseous or extraosseous.
- Osseous plasmacytoma is defined as emanating from bone without other evidence of disease.
- SP derived from soft tissue are termed solitary extraosseous plasmacytoma (SEP).

Pathology

- MM consists of a spectrum of diseases ranging from monoclonal gammopathy of unknown significance (MGUS) to plasma cell leukemia.
- Malignant plasma cells produce monoclonal paraprotein (M-protein).
- M-protein is IgG in ~55% of cases and IgA in ~20%.
- ~55% to 60% patients also have Bence Jones proteinuria.
- IgD myeloma accounts for about 1% of cases.
- Variant expressions of MM include:
  o Extramedullary plasmacytoma
  o SP of bone
  o Osteosclerotic myeloma (POEMS syndrome): polyneuropathy (chronic inflammatory), organomegaly (hepatomegaly, splenomegaly, or lymphadenopathy), endocrinopathy (e.g., gynecomastia, testicular atrophy), M-protein, and skin changes (e.g., hyperpigmentation, excess hair)
  o Nonsecretory myeloma (absence of M-protein in serum and urine, presence of M-protein in plasma cells)

Diagnosis and Workup

- H&P
- Labs: CBC, differential, BUN/creatinine (assess kidney function), electrolytes, LDH (assess tumor cell burden), calcium, albumin, beta-2 microglobulin (reflects tumor mass and now considered standard measure of tumor burden)
- Serum and urine analyses for monoclonal protein: serum quantitative immunoglobulins (IgG, IgA, and IgM), serum protein electrophoresis (SPEP), serum immunofixation electrophoresis (IFE), serum free light chain (FLC) assay (quantitative monitoring with prognostic value), 24-hour urine for total protein, urine protein electrophoresis (UPEP), urine IFE

- Skeletal survey to evaluate lytic bone lesions
- BM aspirate & biopsy, including BM immunohistochemistry and/or BM flow cytometry
- Chromosome analysis by conventional karyotyping (cytogenetics) and FISH [del 13, del 17p13, t(4;14), t(11;14), t(14;16), 1q21 amplification]
- Consider other imaging depending on circumstance: CT (avoid contrast), MRI, PET/CT
- Consider tissue biopsy to diagnose solitary osseous or SEP
- Consider baseline bone densitometry if treating bisphosphonate therapy
- Consider plasma cell labeling index (identify fraction of myeloma cell population that is proliferating)
- Consider staining of BM and fat pad for amyloid as well as serum viscosity if hyperviscosity is suspected
- Consider HLA typing in selected patients for allogeneic stem cell transplantation

Staging

MM is classified as either smoldering (asymptomatic) disease or active (symptomatic) disease.

Definition of MM (Smoldering and Active)	International Myeloma Working Group (IMWG) Criteria

Smoldering (Asymptomatic) Myeloma	• M-protein in serum
	  o IgG value ≥3 g/dL
	  o IgA value <1 g/dL
	  o Bence Jones protein >1 g/24h
	  AND/OR
	• BM clonal plasma cells ≥10%
	• No related organ or tissue impairment (no end organ damage, including bone lesions) or symptoms

Active (Symptomatic) Myeloma	Requires any of the criteria for smoldering (asymptomatic) myeloma be present AND one or more of the following: • Calcium elevation (>11.5 mg/dL) [>2.65 mmol/L] • Renal insufficiency (creatinine >2 mg/dL) [177 micromol/L or more] • Anemia (hemoglobin <10 or 2 g/dL less than normal) [<12.5 or 1.25 mmol/L less than normal] • Bone disease (lytic or osteopenic)

Active disease is further categorized according to Durie-Salmon staging system or International Staging System (ISS) criteria.

Stage	Durie-Salmon Criteria	ISS Criteria

I	All of the following:
	
	• Hemoglobin >10 g/dL
	• Serum calcium value normal or ≤12 mg/dL
	• Bone x-ray, normal bone structure or solitary bone plasmacytoma only
	• Low M-component production rate
	  o IgG value <5 g/dL
	  o IgA value <3 g/dL
	  o Bence Jones protein <4 g/24 h
		Serum beta-2 microglobulin <3.5 mg/L
		Serum albumin ≥3.5 g/dL

II	Neither fitting stage I nor stage III	Neither fitting stage I nor stage III

(continued)

Active disease is further categorized according to Durie-Salmon staging system or International Staging System (ISS) criteria. (*continued*)

Stage	Durie-Salmon Criteria	ISS Criteria
III	One or more of the following:	Serum beta-2 microglobulin ≥5.5 mg/L
	• Hemoglobin value <8.5 g/dL	
	• Serum calcium value >12 mg/dL	
	• Advanced lytic bone lesions	
	• Low M-component production rate	
	o IgG value >7 g/dL	
	o IgA value >3 g/dL	
	o Bence Jones protein >12 g/24 h	

Subclassification Criteria

A: Normal renal function (serum creatinine level <2.0 mg/dL)

B: Abnormal renal function (serum creatinine level ≥2.0 mg/dL)

ISS, International Staging System.

Treatment Overview

Solitary osseous plasmacytoma	Involved field radiation therapy (≥45 Gy)
SEP	Involved field radiation therapy (≥45 Gy) initially and surgery if necessary

SEP, solitary extraosseous plasmacytoma.

Radiation Therapy Technique

For SP: Involved Field Radiation Therapy

- Include involved bone with 2- to 3-cm margin
- Consider including primary lymphatic drainage for SEP
- Dose 45 to 50 Gy in 1.8 to 2.0 Gy per fraction

For MM: Palliative RT for Uncontrolled Pain, Impending Pathologic Fracture, or Impending Spinal Cord Compression

- Dose 10 to 30 Gy in 1.5 to 2.0 Gy per fraction

Toxicity

- Dependent on radiation site or field
- Acute: generalized fatigue, radiation dermatitis, tumor pain flare, esophagitis, gastritis, nausea, vomiting, diarrhea, myelosupression
- Late: myelosuppression, infertility, secondary malignancy

Follow-Up

- SPs have a 50% chance of developing into systemic MM in 10 years
- Follow-up after completion of treatment up to 5 years
- Interim H&P every 3 to 6 months for first 1 to 2 years, then every 6 to 12 months for years 3 to 5

- Laboratory studies (CBC, differential, serum chemistry for creatinine, albumin, corrected calcium, LDH as clinically indicated, beta-2 microglobulin as clinically indicated) with each clinic visit
- Serum FLC assay
- 24 hours urine for total protein, UPEP, urine IFE
- Serum quantitative immunoglobulins, SPEP, serum IFE
- BM aspirate and biopsy as clinically indicated
- Bone survey as clinically indicated or annually
- MRI and/or CT and/or PET/CT as clinically indicated

Chapter 5: Practice Questions

1. All of the following are important factors for the classification of active myeloma EXCEPT

    A. Hypocalcemia
    B. Renal insufficiency
    C. Anemia
    D. Bone disease

2. Mycosis fungoides is an

    A. Indolent B cell lymphoma
    B. Aggressive B cell lymphoma
    C. Indolent T cell lymphoma
    D. Aggressive T cell lymphoma

3. Anaplastic large cell lymphoma is an

    A. Indolent B cell lymphoma
    B. Aggressive B cell lymphoma
    C. Indolent T cell lymphoma
    D. Aggressive T cell lymphoma

4. Non-Hodgkin's lymphoma consists of malignancies involving the following immune cells EXCEPT

    A. B cells
    B. T cells
    C. NK cells
    D. Plasma cells

5. The most common site of extranodal Non-Hodgkin's lymphoma is in the

    A. GI tract
    B. GU tract
    C. CNS space
    D. MSK system

6. The International Prognostic Score for advanced stage Hodgkin's lymphoma consists of how many total factors?

    A. 6
    B. 7
    C. 8
    D. 9

7. Stages I to IIA favorable Hodgkin's disease is usually treated with the following radiation dose:

    A. 20 Gy
    B. 30 Gy
    C. 36 Gy
    D. 40 Gy

8. What proportion of non-Hodgkin's lymphoma patients will present with extranodal disease at some point in their disease course?

    A. 25%
    B. 50%
    C. 75%
    D. 100%

9. What proportion of non-Hodgkin's lymphoma patients present with B symptoms?

    A. <5%
    B. 20%
    C. 40%
    D. 60%

10. Risk factors related to Hodgkin's lymphoma include the following EXCEPT

    A. Immunosuppression
    B. Alcohol intake
    C. Autoimmune disorders
    D. Socioeconomic status

11. The risk of bone marrow positivity with Hodgkin's lymphoma with high-risk features (e.g., advanced stage or B symptoms) is

    A. 1%
    B. 5%
    C. 10%
    D. 15%

12. Plasmablastic lymphoma is an

    A. Indolent B cell lymphoma
    B. Aggressive B cell lymphoma
    C. Indolent T cell lymphoma
    D. Aggressive T cell lymphoma

13. Stages I to IV bulky Hodgkin's disease are usually treated with the following radiation dose:

    A. 20 Gy
    B. 25 Gy
    C. 36 Gy
    D. 40 Gy

14. Stages I to IIA unfavorable Hodgkin's disease are usually treated with the following radiation dose:

    A. 20 Gy
    B. 30 Gy
    C. 36 Gy
    D. 40 Gy

15. In terms of lymphoma, anatomical staging regions of all of the following are considered upper abdominal nodes EXCEPT

    A. Splenic hilar
    B. Celiac
    C. Porta hepatis
    D. Para-aortic

16. Prognostic factors associated with Hodgkin's lymphoma outcomes include the following EXCEPT

    A. Sex
    B. Age
    C. Systemic symptoms
    D. Platelet count

17. Sezary cells have the following phenotypes EXCEPT

    A. CD3+
    B. CD4+
    C. CD7+
    D. CD26-

18. A cutaneous lymphoma with 100 Sezary cells per microliter is B classified as

    A. B0
    B. B1a
    C. B1b
    D. B2

19. The least frequently observed form of classical Hodgkin's lymphoma is

    A. Nodular sclerosis
    B. Mixed cellularity
    C. Lymphocyte rich
    D. Lymphocyte depleted

20. A grade 3 node associated with a cutaneous lymphoma is N staged as

    A. N1
    B. N2a
    C. N2b
    D. N3

Chapter 5: Answers

1. A
Active myeloma requires any of the criteria for smoldering (asymptomatic) myeloma be present and one or more of the following:
   Calcium elevation (>11.5 mg/dL) [>2.65 mmol/L]
   Renal insufficiency (creatinine >2 mg/dL) [177 micromol/L or more]
   Anemia (hemoglobin <10 or 2 g/dL less than normal) [<12.5 or 1.25 mmol/L less than normal]
   Bone disease (lytic or osteopenic)

2. C
Indolent T cell lymphomas include:
   Mycosis fungoides/Sezary syndrome
   Primary cutaneous, CD30+
   Primary cutaneous PTCL, CD30–
   T-cell large granular lymphocytic leukemia

3. D
Aggressive T-cell lymphomas include:
   Peripheral T-cell, unspecified
   Angioimmunoblastic (AILD)
   Enteropathy associated T-cell
   Hepatosplenic T-cell
   Subcutaneous panniculitis-like
   Anaplastic large cell (CD30+) ALK+
   Anaplastic large cell (CD30+) ALK–
   Extranodal NK/T-cell, nasal type

4. D
Non-Hodgkin's lymphoma (NHL) is a diverse group of malignant neoplasms derived from B cell progenitors, T cell progenitors, mature B cells, mature T cells, or NK cells.

5. A
Most common extranodal site is GI tract, followed by skin. Other sites include testis, bone, CNS, kidney, and rarely, prostate, bladder, ovary, orbit, heart, breast, salivary glands, and adrenals.

6. B
There are seven total factors for the International Prognostic Score for Hodgkin's lymphoma:
   Albumin <4.0 g/dL
   Hemoglobin <10.5 g/dL
   Male sex
   Age ≥45 years
   Stage IV disease
   WBC count ≥15,000/mm^3
   Absolute lymphocytic count <600/mm^3 or a lymphocyte count <8% of total WBC count

7. A
Treatment of early stage favorable disease is combined modality therapy, ABVD × 2 cycles, then 20 Gy.

8. B
~50% patients develop secondary extranodal disease during course of disease. Most common extranodal site is GI tract, followed by skin. Other sites include testis, bone, CNS, kidney, and rarely, prostate, bladder, ovary, orbit, heart, breast, salivary glands, and adrenals.

9. C
Up to 40% of patients with non-Hodgkin's lymphoma present with constitutional (B) symptoms.

10. B

The following are risk factors for the development of Hodgkin's lymphoma:

    Socioeconomic status (SES)

    Environmental or infectious agents

    Smoking

    Immunosuppression autoimmune disorders such as RA, SLE, sarcoidosis, ulcerative colitis

    Family history

11. B

Bone marrow biopsy if B symptoms, myelosupression, or advanced stage (involvement ~5% of patients).

12. B

Aggressive B-cell lymphomas include:

    Diffuse large B-cell

    Diffuse large B-cell lymphoma (DLBCL) associated with chronic inflammation

    Lymphomatoid granulomatosis

    Primary mediastinal large B-cell

    Intravascular large B-cell

    ALK positive large B-cell

    Plasmablastic lymphoma

    Large B-cell lymphoma (LBCL) in HHV8-associated Castleman disease

    Primary effusion lymphoma

    Follicular grade 3b (large cell)

13. A

Treatment of early stage favorable disease is combined modality therapy with 30 to 36 Gy.

14. A

Treatment of early stage unfavorable disease is which 30 Gy combined modality therapy.

15. D

Upper abdomen (splenic hilar, celiac, porta hepatis)

Lower abdomen (iliac, paraaortic, retroperitoneal, mesenteric, abdominal, NOS)

16. D

Prognostic factors for Hodgkin's lymphoma:

    Presence or absence of systemic symptoms

    Stage of disease

    Presence of large masses

    Quality and suitability of treatment administered

    Age

    Sex

    Erythrocyte sedimentation rate (ESR)

    Extent of abdominal involvement

    Hematocrit

    Absolute number of nodal sites of involvement

17. C

Sezary cells have mature memory T-cell phenotype (CD3+, CD4+) with loss of CD7 and CD26.

18. A

A cutaneous lymphoma with 100 Sezary cells per microliter is B classified as B0.

19. D

Classical HL (divided into four subtypes in order of incidence and prevalence):

    Nodular sclerosis (NS) ~70%

    Mixed cellularity (MC) ~20% to 25%

Lymphocyte rich (LR) ~5 to 10

Lymphocyte depleted (LD) ~<1%

20. D

N staging of cutaneous lymphoma:

N1 Clinically abnormal lymph nodes; histopathology Dutch grade 1 or NCI LN0-2

N2 Clinically abnormal lymph nodes; histopathology Dutch grade 2 or NCI LN3 (a vs. b for clone positivity)

N3 Clinically abnormal lymph nodes; histopathology Dutch grades 3 to 4 or NCI LN4; clone positive or negative

Recommended Reading

Aleman BM, Raemaekers JM, Tirelli U, et al. Involved-field radiotherapy for advanced Hodgkin's lymphoma. *N Engl J Med.* 2003;348(24):2396-2406.

Aleman BM, Raemaekers JM, Tomišič R, et al. Involved-field radiotherapy for patients in partial remission after chemotherapy for advanced Hodgkin's lymphoma. *Int J Radiat Oncol Biol Phys.* 2007;67(1):19-30.

Behringer K, Goergen H, Hitz F, et al. Omission of dacarbazine or bleomycin, or both, from the ABVD regimen in treatment of early-stage favourable Hodgkin's lymphoma (GHSG HD13): an open-label, randomised, non-inferiority trial. *Lancet.* 2015;385(9976):1418-1427.

Boivin JF, Hutchison GB, Zauber AG, et al. Incidence of second cancers in patients treated for Hodgkin's disease. *J Natl Cancer Inst.* 1995;87:732-741.

Bonnet C, Fillet G, Mounier N, et al. CHOP alone compared with CHOP plus radiotherapy for localized aggressive lymphoma in elderly patients: a study by the Groupe d'Etude des Lymphomes de l'Adulte. *J Clin Oncol.* 2007;25(7):787-792.

Borchmann P, Haverkamp H, Diehl V, et al. Eight cycles of escalated-dose BEACOPP compared with four cycles of escalated-dose BEACOPP followed by four cycles of baseline-dose BEACOPP with or without radiotherapy in patients with advanced-stage Hodgkin's lymphoma: final analysis of the HD12 trial of the German Hodgkin Study Group. *J Clin Oncol.* 2011;29(32):4234-4242.

Chan EK, Fung S, Gospodarowicz M, et al. Palliation by low-dose local radiation therapy for indolent non-Hodgkin lymphoma. *Int J Radiat Oncol Biol Phys.* 2011;81(5):e781-e786.

Cheson BD, Fisher RI, Barrington SF, et al. Recommendations for initial evaluation, staging, and response assessment of Hodgkin and non-Hodgkin lymphoma: the Lugano classification. *J Clin Oncol.* 2014;32:3059-3068.

Cheson BD, Horning SJ, Coiffier B, et al. Report of an International Workshop to standardize response criteria for non-Hodgkin's lymphomas: NCI Sponsored International Working Group. *J Clin Oncol.* 1999;17:1244-1253.

Cheson BD, Pfistner B, Juweid ME, et al. Revised response criteria for malignant lymphoma. *J Clin Oncol.* 2007;25:579-586.

Chinn DM, Chow S, Kim YH, Hoppe RT. Total skin electron beam therapy with or without adjuvant topical nitrogen mustard or nitrogen mustard alone as initial treatment of T2 and T3 mycosis fungoides. *Int J Radiat Oncol Biol Phys.* 1999;43(5):951-958.

Creach KM, Foote RL, Neben-Wittich MA, Kyle R. Radiotherapy for extramedullary plasmacytoma of the head and neck. *Int J Radiat Oncol Biol Phys.* 2009;73(3):789-794.

Diehl V, Franklin J, Pfreundschuh M, et al. Standard and increased-dose BEACOPP chemotherapy compared with COPP-ABVD for advanced Hodgkin's disease. *N Engl J Med.* 2003;348(24):2386-2395.

Dimopoulos MA, Goldstein J, Fuller L, Delasalle K, Alexanian R. Curability of solitary bone plasmacytoma. *J Clin Oncol.* 1992;10(4):587-590.

Dores GM, Landgren O, McGlynn KA, Curtis RE, Linet MS, Devesa SS. Plasmacytoma of bone, extramedullary plasmacytoma, and multiple myeloma: incidence and survival in the United States, 1992-2004. *Br J Haematol.* 2009;144(1):86-94.

Eich HT, Diehl V, Görgen H, et al. Intensified chemotherapy and dose-reduced involved-field radiotherapy in patients with early unfavorable Hodgkin's lymphoma: final analysis of the German Hodgkin Study Group HD11 trial. *J Clin Oncol.* 2010;28(27):4199-4206.

Eich HT, Müller RP, Engenhart-Cabillic R, et al. Involved-node radiotherapy in early-stage Hodgkin's lymphoma: definition and guidelines of the German Hodgkin Study Group (GHSG). *Strahlenther Onkol.* 2008;184(8):406-410.

Engert A, Haverkamp H, Kobe C, et al. Reduced-intensity chemotherapy and PET-guided radiotherapy in patients with advanced stage Hodgkin's lymphoma (HD15 trial): a randomised, open-label, phase 3 non-inferiority trial. *Lancet.* 2012;379(9828):1791-1799.

Engert A, Plütschow A, Eich HT, et al. Reduced treatment intensity in patients with early-stage Hodgkin's lymphoma. *N Engl J Med.* 2010;363(7):640-652.

Fabian CJ, Mansfield CM, Dahlberg S, et al. Low-dose involved field radiation after chemotherapy in advanced Hodgkin disease: a Southwest Oncology Group randomized study. *Ann Intern Med.* 1994;120(11):903-912.

Federico M, Bellei M, Marcheselli L, et al. Follicular lymphoma international prognostic index 2: a new prognostic index for follicular lymphoma developed by the international follicular lymphoma prognostic factor project. *J Clin Oncol.* 2009;27(27):4555-4562.

Franklin J, Pluetschow A, Paus M, et al. Second malignancy risk associated with treatment of Hodgkin's lymphoma: meta-analysis of the randomized trials. *Ann Oncol.* 2006;17:1749-1760.

Friedberg JW, Byrtek M, Link BK, et al. Effectiveness of first-line management strategies for stage I follicular lymphoma: analysis of the National LymphoCare Study. *J Clin Oncol.* 2012;30(27):3368-3375.

Gerry D, Lentsch EJ. Epidemiologic evidence of superior outcomes for extramedullary plasmacytoma of the head and neck. *Otolaryngol Head Neck Surg.* 2013;148(6):974-981.

Grange F, Bekkenk MW, Wechsler J, et al. Prognostic factors in primary cutaneous large B-cell lymphomas: a European multicenter study. *J Clin Oncol.* 2001;19:3602-3610.

Harrison C, Young J, Navi D, et al. Revisiting low-dose total skin electron beam therapy in mycosis fungoides. *Int J Radiat Oncol Biol Phys.* 2011;81(4):e651-e657.

Hasenclever D, Diehl V. A prognostic score for advanced Hodgkin's disease: international prognostic factors project on advanced Hodgkin's disease. *N Engl J Med.* 1998;339:1506-1514.

Heinzerling LM, Urbanek M, Funk JO, et al. Reduction of tumor burden and stabilization of disease by systemic therapy with anti-CD20 antibody (rituximab) in patients with primary cutaneous B-cell lymphoma. *Cancer.* 2000;89:1835-1844.

Held G, Murawski N, Ziepert M, et al. Role of radiotherapy to bulky disease in elderly patients with aggressive B-cell lymphoma. *J Clin Oncol.* 2014;32(11):1112-1118.

Held G, Zeynalova S, Murawski N, et al. Impact of rituximab and radiotherapy on outcome of patients with aggressive B-cell lymphoma and skeletal involvement. *J Clin Oncol.* 2013;31(32):4115-4122.

Hoppe RT. Mycosis fungoides: radiation therapy. *Dermatol Ther.* 2003;16:347-354.

Horning SJ, Weller E, Kim K, et al. Chemotherapy with or without radiotherapy in limited-stage diffuse aggressive non-Hodgkin's lymphoma: Eastern Cooperative Oncology Group study 1484. *J Clin Oncol.* 2004;22(15):3032-3038.

Hoskin SJ, Weller E, Kim K, et al. 4 Gy versus 24 Gy radiotherapy for patients with indolent lymphoma (FORT): a randomised phase 3 non-inferiority trial. *Lancet Oncol.* 2014;15(4):457-463.

Hu K, Yahalom J. Radiotherapy in the management of plasma cell tumors. *Oncology (Williston Park).* 2000;14(1):101-108, 111; discussion 111-112, 115.

Illidge T, Specht L, Yahalom J, et al. Modern radiation therapy for nodal non-Hodgkin lymphoma-target definition and dose guidelines from the International Lymphoma Radiation Oncology Group. *Int J Radiat Oncol Biol Phys.* 2014;89(1):49-58.

Johnson PW, Sydes MR, Hancock BW, et al. Consolidation radiotherapy in patients with advanced Hodgkin's lymphoma: survival data from the UKLG LY09 randomized controlled trial (ISRCTN97144519). *J Clin Oncol.* 2010;28(20):3352-3359.

Jones GW, Kacinski BM, Wilson LD, et al. Total skin electron radiation in the management of mycosis fungoides: consensus of the European Organization for Research and Treatment of Cancer (EORTC) Cutaneous Lymphoma Project Group. *J Am Acad Dermatol.* 2002;47:364-370.

Kelsey SM, Newland AC, Hudson GV, Jelliffe AM. A British National Lymphoma Investigation randomised trial of single agent chlorambucil plus radiotherapy versus radiotherapy alone in low grade, localised non-Hodgkin's lymphoma. *Med Oncol.* 1994;11(1):19-25.

Kempf W, Pfaltz K, Vermeer MH, et al. EORTC, ISCL, and USCLC consensus recommendations for the treatment of primary cutaneous CD30-positive lymphoproliferative disorders: lymphomatoid papulosis and primary cutaneous anaplastic large-cell lymphoma. *Blood.* 2011;118:4024-4035.

Kim YH, Willemze R, Pimpinelli N, et al. TNM classification system for primary cutaneous lymphomas other than mycosis fungoides and Sezary syndrome: a proposal of the International Society for Cutaneous Lymphomas (ISCL) and the Cutaneous Lymphoma Task Force of the European Organization of Research and Treatment of Cancer (EORTC). *Blood.* 2007;110:479-484.

Klimm B, Franklin J, Stein H, et al. Lymphocyte-depleted classical Hodgkin's lymphoma: a comprehensive analysis from the German Hodgkin study group. *J Clin Oncol.* 2011;29(29):3914-3920.

Knowling MA, Harwood AR, Bergsagel DE, et al. Comparison of extramedullary plasmacytomas with solitary and multiple plasma cell tumors of bone. *J Clin Oncol.* 1983;1(4):255-262.

Lister TA, Crowther D, Sutcliffe SB, et al. Report of a committee convened to discuss the evaluation and staging of patients with Hodgkin's disease: Cotswolds Meeting. *J Clin Oncol.* 1989;7:1630-1636.

Lowry L, Smith P, Qian W, et al. Reduced dose radiotherapy for local control in non-Hodgkin lymphoma: a randomised phase III trial. *Radiother Oncol.* 2011;100(1):86-92.

Meyer RM, Gospodarowicz MK, Connors JM, et al. ABVD alone versus radiation-based therapy in limited-stage Hodgkin's lymphoma. *N Engl J Med*. 2012;366(5):399-408.

Micaily B, Miyamoto C, Kantor G, et al. Radiotherapy for unilesional mycosis fungoides. *Int J Radiat Oncol Biol Phys*. 1998;42:361-364.

Miller TP, Dahlberg S, Cassady JR, et al. Chemotherapy alone compared with chemotherapy plus radiotherapy for localized intermediate- and high-grade non-Hodgkin's lymphoma. *N Engl J Med*. 1998;339(1):21-26.

Neelis KJ, Schimmel EC, Vermeer MH, et al. Low-dose palliative radiotherapy for cutaneous B- and T-cell lymphomas. *Int J Radiat Oncol Biol Phys*. 2009;74:154-158.

Ng AK, Bernardo MP, Weller E, et al. Long-term survival and competing causes of death in patients with early-stage Hodgkin's disease treated at age 50 or younger. *J Clin Oncol*. 2002;20:2101-2108.

Olsen E, Vonderheid E, Pimpinelli N, et al. Revisions to the staging and classification of mycosis fungoides and Sezary syndrome: a proposal of the International Society for Cutaneous Lymphomas (ISCL) and the cutaneous lymphoma task force of the European Organization of Research and Treatment of Cancer (EORTC). *Blood*. 2007;110:1713-1722.

Persky DO, Unger JM, Spier CM, et al. Phase II study of rituximab plus three cycles of CHOP and involved-field radiotherapy for patients with limited-stage aggressive B-cell lymphoma: Southwest Oncology Group study 0014. *J Clin Oncol*. 2008;26(14):2258-2263.

Pfreundschuh M, Ho AD, Cavallin-Stahl E, et al. Prognostic significance of maximum tumour (bulk) diameter in young patients with good-prognosis diffuse large B-cell lymphoma treated with CHOP-like chemotherapy with or without rituximab: an exploratory analysis of the MabThera International Trial Group (MInT) study. *Lancet Oncol*. 2008;9(5):435-444.

Pfreundschuh M, Schubert J, Ziepert M, et al. Six versus eight cycles of bi-weekly CHOP-14 with or without rituximab in elderly patients with aggressive CD20+ B-cell lymphomas: a randomised controlled trial (RICOVER-60). *Lancet Oncol*. 2008;9(2):105-116.

Phan J, Mazloom A, Medeiros LJ, et al. Benefit of consolidative radiation therapy in patients with diffuse large B-cell lymphoma treated with R-CHOP chemotherapy. *J Clin Oncol*. 2010;28(27):4170-4176.

Piotrowski T, Milecki P, Skorska M, et al. Total skin electron irradiation techniques: a review. *Postepy Dermatol Alergol*. 2013;30:50-55.

Pugh TJ, Ballonoff A, Newman F, Rabinovitch R. Improved survival in patients with early stage low-grade follicular lymphoma treated with radiation: a surveillance, epidemiology, and end results database analysis. *Cancer*. 2010;116(16):3843-3851.

Radford J, Illidge T, Counsell N, et al. Results of a trial of PET-directed therapy for early-stage Hodgkin's lymphoma. *N Engl J Med*. 2015;372(17):1598-1607.

Raemaekers JM, André MP, Federico M, et al. Omitting radiotherapy in early positron emission tomography-negative stage I/II Hodgkin lymphoma is associated with an increased risk of early relapse: clinical results of the preplanned interim analysis of the randomized EORTC/LYSA/FIL H10 trial. *J Clin Oncol*. 2014;32(12):1188-1194.

Reed V, Shah J, Medeiros LJ, et al. Solitary plasmacytomas: outcome and prognostic factors after definitive radiation therapy. *Cancer*. 2011;117(19):4468-4474.

Reyes F, Lepage E, Ganem G, et al. ACVBP versus CHOP plus radiotherapy for localized aggressive lymphoma. *N Engl J Med*. 2005;352(12):1197-1205.

Rosenberg SA. Validity of the Ann Arbor staging classification for the non-Hodgkin's lymphomas. *Cancer Treat Rep*. 1977;61:1023-1027.

Senff NJ, Noordijk EM, Kim YH, et al. European Organization for Research and Treatment of Cancer and International Society for Cutaneous Lymphoma consensus recommendations for the management of cutaneous B-cell lymphomas. *Blood*. 2008;112:1600-1609.

Solal-Céligny P, Roy P, Colombat P, et al. Follicular lymphoma international prognostic index. *Blood*. 2004;104(5):1258-1265.

Solal-Céligny P, Lepage E, Brousse N, et al. Doxorubicin-containing regimen with or without interferon alfa-2b for advanced follicular lymphomas: final analysis of survival and toxicity in the Groupe d'Etude des Lymphomes Folliculaires 86 Trial. *J Clin Oncol*. 1998;16(7):2332-2338.

Specht L. Very long-term follow-up of the Danish National Hodgkin Study Group's randomized trial of radiotherapy (RT) alone vs. combined modality treatment (CMT) for early stage Hodgkin lymphoma, with special reference to second tumors and overall survival. *Blood*. 2003;102(suppl 2351a. abstract).

Specht L, Dabaja B, Illidge T, et al. Modern radiation therapy for primary cutaneous lymphomas: field and dose guidelines from the International Lymphoma Radiation Oncology Group. *Int J Radiat Oncol Biol Phys*. 2015;92(1):32-39.

Specht L, Yahalom J, Illidge T, et al. Modern radiation therapy for Hodgkin lymphoma: field and dose guidelines from the International Lymphoma Radiation Oncology Group (ILROG). *Int J Radiat Oncol Biol Phys*. 2014;89(4):854-862.

Swerdlow SH, Campo E, Harris NL. *WHO Classification of Tumours of Haematopoietic and Lymphoid Tissues*. 4th ed. Lyon, France: IARC; 2008.

The International Non-Hodgkin's Lymphoma Prognostic Factors Project: a predictive model for aggressive non-hodgkin's lymphoma. *N Engl J Med.* 1993;329:987-994.

Thomas TO, Agrawal P, Guitart J, et al. Outcome of patients treated with a single-fraction dose of palliative radiation for cutaneous T-cell lymphoma. *Int J Radiat Oncol Biol Phys.* 2013;85:747-753.

Tournier-Rangeard L, Lapeyre M, Graff-Caillaud P, et al. Radiotherapy for solitary extramedullary plasmacytoma in the head-and-neck region: a dose greater than 45 Gy to the target volume improves the local control. *Int J Radiat Oncol Biol Phys.* 2006;64(4):1013-1017.

Trautinger F, Knobler R, Willemze R, et al. EORTC consensus recommendations for the treatment of mycosis fungoides/Sezary syndrome. *Eur J Cancer.* 2006;42:1014-1030.

van Leeuwen FE, Klokman WJ, Veer MB, et al. Long-term risk of second malignancy in survivors of Hodgkin's disease treated during adolescence or young adulthood. *J Clin Oncol.* 2000;18:487-497.

Viviani S, Zinzani PL, Rambaldi A, et al. ABVD versus BEACOPP for Hodgkin's lymphoma when high-dose salvage is planned. *N Engl J Med.* 2011;365(3):203-212.

von Tresckow B, Plütschow A, Fuchs M, et al. Dose-intensification in early unfavorable Hodgkin's lymphoma: final analysis of the German Hodgkin Study Group HD14 trial. *J Clin Oncol.* 2012;30(9):907-913.

Willemze R, Elaine SJ, Günter B, et al. WHO-EORTC classification for cutaneous lymphomas. *Blood.* 2005;105:3768-3785.

Wilson LD, Jones GW, Kim D, et al. Experience with total skin electron beam therapy in combination with extracorporeal photopheresis in the management of patients with erythrodermic (T4) mycosis fungoides. *J Am Acad Dermatol.* 2000;43(1 pt 1):54-60.

Wilson LD, Kacinski BM, Jones GW. Local superficial radiotherapy in the management of minimal stage IA cutaneous T-cell lymphoma (Mycosis Fungoides). *Int J Radiat Oncol Biol Phys.* 1998;40:109-115.

Wobser M, Kneitz H, Bröcker EB, Becker JC. Primary cutaneous diffuse large B-cell lymphoma, leg-type, treated with a modified R-CHOP immunochemotherapy: diagnostic and therapeutic challenges. *J Dtsch Dermatol Ges.* 2011;9:204-211.

Yahalom J, Illidge T, Specht L, et al. Modern radiation therapy for extranodal lymphomas: field and dose guidelines from the International Lymphoma Radiation Oncology Group. *Int J Radiat Oncol Biol Phys.* 2015;92(1):11-31.

Yahalom J, Mauch P. The involved field is back: issues in delineating the radiation field in Hodgkin's disease. *Ann Oncol.* 2002;13(suppl 1):79-83.

Ysebaert L, Truc G, Dalac S, et al. Ultimate results of radiation therapy for T1-T2 mycosis fungoides (including reirradiation). *Int J Radiat Oncol Biol Phys.* 2004;58(4):1128-1134.

Yu JB, McNiff JM, Lund MW, Wilson LD, et al. Treatment of primary cutaneous CD30+ anaplastic large-cell lymphoma with radiation therapy. *Int J Radiat Oncol Biol Phys.* 2008;70:1542-1545.

Zhou Z, Sehn LH, Rademaker AW, et al. An enhanced International Prognostic Index (NCCN-IPI) for patients with diffuse large B-cell lymphoma treated in the rituximab era. *Blood.* 2014;123:837-842.

Head and Neck Malignancies

Mehee Choi, Emma B. Holliday, Alec M. Block,
Clifton D. Fuller, and Aidnag Z. Diaz

6.1 Nasopharynx

Epidemiology and Risk Factors

- There are only 5,000–6,000 new cases annually in the United States.
- It is more common in Southeast Asia, East Asia, Polynesia, North Africa, and for native peoples of the Artic.
- Worldwide, there are 87,000 cases annually and 51,000 deaths from the disease.
- It is male-predominant.
- Median age at diagnosis is 55 years.
- Epstein Barr Virus (EBV) is the strongest risk factor for the nonkeratinizing, undifferentiated form (WHO type 2b).
  - EBV titer has also been shown to be prognostic.
- Alcohol and tobacco increase risk of developing the keratinizing squamous cell carcinoma form (WHO type I).

Anatomy and Patterns of Spread

- Boundaries of the nasopharynx: anterior—nasal cavity; posterior—clivus and C1–C2 vertebral body; superior—sphenoid sinus; inferior—soft palate.
- Most commonly arises in the pharyngeal recess just posterior to the torus tubarius (fossa of Rosenmüller).
- May also invade the sphenoid sinus and skull base → cavernous sinus.
- Named nerve palsies syndromes:
  - Jacod's: direct extension through foramen lacerum to cavernous Sinus (containing CN III, IV, V1, V2, VI) resulting in eye symptoms and upper face pain/anesthesia
  - St Villaret's: metastases to parapharyngeal space, or compression from nodes resulting in CN IX–XII AND sympathetic chain
  - Collet-Sicard: CN IX–XII involved
  - Vernet's (jugular foramen): CN IX–XI involved
  - Jackson's: CN X–XII involved.
- High propensity for lymphatic spread (70%–80%):
  - Nasopharynx cancer has highest risk of retropharyngeal and level V lymph node metastases

Presentation

- Most commonly presents with a neck mass from cervical nodal metastasis.
- Other presenting symptoms include otitis and hearing loss (Eustachian tube obstruction); nasal obstruction and epistaxis (anterior extension).

- Other common presenting symptoms are: headaches, trismus, and nerve palsies (see anatomy and patterns of spread).
- Differential diagnosis includes carcinoma, lymphoma, minor salivary gland tumor, plasmacytoma, melanoma, chordoma, rhabdomyosarcoma, and juvenile angiofibroma.

Histology

- World Health Organization classification
  - WHO type 1: keratinizing squamous cell carcinoma (20% of U.S. cases)
    - Keratinizing squamous cell carcinoma has highest risk for local failure and lowest risk for distant failure.
  - WHO type 2a: nonkeratinizing squamous cell carcinoma (uncommon)
  - WHO type 2b: undifferentiated carcinoma (99% of endemic cases)
    - Lymphoepithelioma: distinct entity with high lymphoid component. Easier to control locoregionally but equivalent survival due to higher rates of distant metastases.

Diagnosis and Workup

- History and physical exam including complete head and neck exam with fiberoptic nasopharyngolaryngoscopy and otoscopy
- Biopsy of suspicious lesions
- Routine laboratory studies. Consider EBV titer
- CT head/neck
- MRI skull base
- Chest X ray (CXR) for stage III/IV
- Consider PET/CT if stage III/IV (most will be)
- Dental evaluation, nutrition evaluation, speech and swallowing evaluation, and audiology testing
  - Consider prophylactic feeding tube placement in patients receiving chemoradiation

Staging (AJCC 7th Edition)

T-stage	
Tx	Primary tumor cannot be assessed
T0	No evidence of primary tumor
Tis	Carcinoma in situ
T1	Tumor confined to the nasopharynx, or extends to oropharynx and/or nasal cavity without parapharyngeal extension*
T2	Tumor with parapharyngeal extension*
T3	Tumor involves bony structures of skull base and/or paranasal sinuses
T4	Tumor with intracranial extension and/or involvement of cranial nerves, hypopharynx, orbit, or with extension to the infratemporal fossa/masticator space

N-stage	
N0	No regional lymph node metastasis
N1	Unilateral metastasis in lymph node(s), 6 cm or less in greatest dimension, above the supraclavicular fossa, and/or unilateral or bilateral, retropharyngeal lymph nodes, 6 cm or less, in greatest dimension†
N2	Bilateral metastasis in lymph node(s), 6 cm or less in greatest dimension, above the supraclavicular fossa†
N3	Metastasis in a lymph node(s)† greater than 6 cm and/or extension to supraclavicular fossa
N3a	Greater than 6 cm in dimension
N3b	Extension to the supraclavicular fossa

(continued)

(continued)

M-stage

M0	No distant metastases
M1	Distant metastases

* Parapharyngeal extension denotes posterolateral infiltration of tumor.
† Midline nodes are considered ipsilateral nodes.

Group Stage	T	N	M
0	Tis	N0	M0
I	T1	N0	M0
II	T1	N1	M0
	T2	N0–1	M0
III	T1–2	N2	M0
	T3	N0–2	M0
IVA	T4	N0–3	M0
IVB	Any T	N3	M0
IVC	Any T	Any N	M1

Treatment Overview

- Stage I: Radiation therapy (RT) alone.
- Stages II to IVB: concurrent chemoradiation → adjuvant chemotherapy.
  - Concurrent chemotherapy: cisplatin 100 mg/m^2 q21 days × 3 cycles.
  - Adjuvant chemotherapy: cisplatin 80 mg/m^2 + 5-FU 1,000 mg/m^2 × 4 days q21 days × 3 cycles.
- Stage IVC: platinum-based combination chemotherapy → chemoradiation if complete response (CR).
- Recurrent disease: RT options include intensity modulated radiation therapy (IMRT), HDR brachytherapy or radiosurgery (30–50 Gy in 3–5 fractions show reasonable efficacy and safety).
- Consider salvage surgery if primary has less than CR or residual neck mass by imaging or physical examination at 6 to 12 weeks posttreatment.
- Toxicities:
  - Acute: fatigue, mucositis, xerostomia, dermatitis, nausea, dysphagia, odynophagia, and dysgeusia.
  - Late: soft tissue fibrosis, trismus, hearing loss, dysphagia, xerostomia, hypothyroidism, temporal lobe necrosis, osteoradionecrosis of skull base, delayed bulbar palsy, hypopituitarism, and RT-associated malignancy.

Radiation Therapy Techniques

- Simulation: supine, shoulder pulls, head, and shoulder mask
  - Wire lymph nodes
  - Mouthguards
- MRI and PET/CT fused for treatment planning
- Full-field simultaneous-integrated boost IMRT will be used to three target volumes treated over 33 fractions.
  - Gross tumor volume (GTV) will be gross primary disease and all nodes greater than 1 cm, with a necrotic center, or active on PET.
  - CTV70 will include a 5 mm expansion on GTV trimmed around critical structures. Planning target volume (PTV) will be an additional 5 mm expansion. Margin may be reduced when abutting critical structures such as the brainstem.
  - CTV59.4 will include CTV70 with a minimum 1 cm margin except when against critical structures. CTV59.4 will also include the entire nasopharynx, anterior 2/3 of clivus (all if involved), skull base covering foramen rotundum and foramen ovale, pterygoid fossa, pterygopalatine fossa, parapharyngeal space (to hyoid), inferior sphenoid sinus (all in T3/4 disease), posterior 1/3 of maxillary sinus/nasal

cavity, cavernous sinus if T3/4 or bulky or involves roof of nasopharynx, bilateral retropharyngeal, and level IB-V lymph nodes.
- Bilateral IB lymph nodes can be spared if patient is node-negative.
  - o CTV54 will include CTV59.4 and uninvolved low neck nodal regions.
- 95% of PTV receives prescription dose.
- No more than 5% of tissue outside of targets can receive 70 Gy.
- No more than 1 mL of unspecified tissue can receive 77 Gy or more.
- Organs at risk
  - o Planning organ at risk volume (PRV)
    - Spinal cord + 5 mm
    - Brainstem + 1 mm
    - Optic apparatus + 1 mm
  - o Brachial plexus: max 66 Gy
  - o Mandible: max 70 Gy. If not possible, then V75 Gy less than 1 mL
  - o Optic nerves/chiasm: max 50 Gy. PRV: max 54 Gy
  - o Spinal cord: max 45 Gy. 1% PRV: max 50 Gy
  - o Brainstem: max 54 Gy. PRV: max 60 Gy
  - o Parotids: mean less than 26 Gy in at least one gland, or at least 50% of one gland less than 30 Gy
  - o Glottic/supraglottic larynx: mean less than 37 Gy
  - o Esophagus: mean less than 45 Gy
  - o Cochlea: V55 Gy less than 5%

6.2   Oral Cavity

Epidemiology and Risk Factors

- There are approximately 30,000 new cases annually in the United States.
- It accounts for 30% of head and neck cancers.
- Subsites of oral cavity include: lips, oral tongue, floor of mouth, alveolar ridge, buccal mucosa, hard palate, and retromolar trigone.
- Distribution by subsite:

Location	Percentage
Lips	45
Oral tongue	16
Floor of mouth	12
Alveolar ridge	12
Buccal mucosa	10
Hard palate	5

- Risk factors:
  - o Alcohol and tobacco
  - o Poor oral hygiene
  - o Betel and areca nut chewing
  - o UV radiation (lip)
  - o Genetic predisposition: Plummer–Vinson syndrome, Fanconi's anemia, Li Fraumeni syndrome
  - o History of premalignant lesions (leukoplakia, erythroplakia)
- Oral cavity cancer carries extraordinary risk of metachronous primary cancers.
- Oral tongue cancers carry the worst prognosis of all oral cavity cancers.

Anatomy and Patterns of Spread

- Boundaries of the oral cavity: superior—hard palate, superior alveolar ridge, maxillary teeth; lateral—cheeks; posterior—anterior tonsillar pillars, circumvallate papillae; inferior—mylohyoid muscle, inferior alveolar ridge, teeth.
- Lymph node involvement is common.
  - Incidence of skip metastases for oral tongue lesions is approximately 15%.
  - Increasing depth of invasion, T-stage, and grade are associated with greater risk of lymph node involvement.
- Lymphatic drainage:
  - Upper lip: facial and level IB
  - Lower lip: I to III
  - Floor of mouth: I to III
  - Buccal mucosa: I to III
  - Alveolar ridge: levels I to III
  - Oral tongue: I to IV

Presentation

- Signs and symptoms:
  - Early: asymptomatic, slightly elevated red lesions with ill-defined borders, ill-fitting dentures
  - Late: ulcerated mass, pain, bleeding, difficulty with speech or swallowing secondary to tongue fixation, trismus, otalgia
- Referred otalgia:

Cranial Nerve	Primary
CN X (auricular (Arnold) nerve → postauricular)	Larynx, hypopharynx
CN IX (nerve of Jacobson → tympanic cavity)	Base of tongue
CN V_3 (auriculotemporal nerve → preauricular)	Oral tongue

Histology

- 95% are squamous cell carcinomas.
- Other histologies include: minor salivary gland tumors greater than melanoma, ameloblastoma, lymphoma, sarcoma, and plasmacytoma.

Diagnosis and Workup

- History and physical exam including complete head and neck exam with careful inspection and palpation of oral cavity and anterior oropharynx, fiberoptic nasopharyngolaryngoscopy, and palpation of all neck levels
- Biopsy of lesion
- CT head/neck if greater than T1
- CXR for stages III/IV
- Consider PET/CT and MRI
- Routine laboratory studies
- Dental evaluation, nutrition evaluation, speech and swallowing evaluation, and audiology testing
  - Consider prophylactic feeding tube placement in patients receiving chemoradiation.

Staging (AJCC 7th Edition)

T-stage

Tx	Primary tumor cannot be assessed
T0	No evidence of primary tumor
Tis	Carcinoma in situ
T1	Tumor 2 cm or less in greatest dimension
T2	Tumor greater than 2 cm but not more than 4 cm in greatest dimension
T3	Tumor more than 4 cm in greatest dimension
T4a	Moderately advanced local disease
	(lip) Tumor invades through cortical bone, inferior alveolar nerve, floor of mouth, or skin of face, that is, chin or nose
	(oral cavity) Tumor invades adjacent structures only (e.g., through cortical bone, [mandible or maxilla] into deep [extrinsic] muscle of tongue [genioglossus, hyoglossus, palatoglossus, and styloglossus], maxillary sinus, skin of face)
T4b	Tumor invades masticator space, pterygoid plates, or skull base and/or encases internal carotid artery

Note: Superficial erosion alone of bone/tooth socket by gingival primary is not sufficient to classify a tumor as T4.

N-stage

N0	No regional lymph node metastasis
N1	Metastasis in a single ipsilateral lymph node, 3 cm or less in greatest dimension
N2a	Metastasis in single ipsilateral lymph node more than 3 cm but not more than 6 cm in greatest dimension
N2b	Metastasis in multiple ipsilateral lymph nodes, none more than 6 cm in greatest dimension
N2c	Metastasis in bilateral or contralateral lymph nodes, none more than 6 cm in greatest dimension
N3	Metastasis in a lymph node more than 6 cm in greatest dimension

M-stage

M0	No distant metastases
M1	Distant metastases

Group Stage	T	N	M
0	Tis	N0	M0
I	T1	N0	M0
II	T1	N1	M0
	T2	N0–1	M0
III	T1–2	N2	M0
	T3	N0–2	M0
IVA	T4	N0–3	M0
IVB	Any T	N3	M0
IVC	Any T	Any N	M1

Treatment Overview

- Lip
  - Stages I to II: Surgery or RT.
  - Stages III to IVB: Prefer surgery with neck dissection; alternative is chemoradiation.
    - Preferred concurrent chemotherapy: cisplatin 100 mg/m^2 q21 days × 3 cycles.
  - Notes
    - Re-excise if feasible for positive surgical margin.
    - Postoperative RT indicated for T3/T4, close margin, greater than 1 LN involved, perineural invasion (PNI), Lympho vascular space invasion (LVSI), or level IV to V lymph node involvement.
    - Postoperative chemoradiation indicated for positive margin or extracapsular extension.
    - Consider salvage surgery if primary has less than CR or residual neck mass by imaging or physical examination at 6 to 12 weeks posttreatment.
- Oral cavity
  - Stages I to II: Surgery or RT.
  - Stage III (T3N0): Surgery.
  - Stages III (T3N1)–IVB: Surgery.
  - Unresectable: Chemoradiation
    - Preferred concurrent chemotherapy: cisplatin 100 mg/m^2 q21 days × 3 cycles.
  - Notes:
    - Re-excise if feasible for positive surgical margin.
    - Neck dissection—supraomohyoid dissection, levels I to III.
    - Elective neck dissection based on depth of invasion: if greater than 4 mm elective dissection should be strongly considered if RT is not planned. If less than 2 mm, elective dissection is indicated only in highly selective situations. If 2 to 4 mm, clinical judgement should be utilized (as to reliability of follow-up, etc.).
    - Postoperative RT indicated for T3/T4, close margin, greater than 1 LN involved, PNI, LVSI, or level IV–V lymph node involvement.
    - Postoperative chemoradiation indicated for positive margin or extracapsular extension.
    - Consider salvage surgery if primary has less than CR or residual neck mass by imaging or physical examination at 6 to 12 weeks posttreatment.
- Toxicities
  - Acute: fatigue, mucositis, xerostomia, dermatitis, nausea, dysphagia, odynophagia, and dysgeusia.
  - Late: pharyngocutaneous fistula, soft tissue fibrosis, dysphagia, xerostomia, hypothyroidism, osteoradionecrosis, and RT-associated malignancy.

Radiation Therapy Techniques

- Simulation: supine, shoulder pulls, head and shoulder mask
  - Wire lymph nodes, surgical scars, oral commissure
  - Bite block
  - Mouthguards
- Preoperative diagnostic imaging fused for treatment planning
- Full field simultaneous-integrated-boost IMRT will be used to target volumes.
  - Alternative techniques include split-field IMRT (match line just above arytenoids), sequential boost, brachytherapy boost, and 3D-conformal planning.
- Postoperative RT:
  - 60 Gy to high-risk areas and postoperative bed.
  - 54 Gy to intermediate-risk areas outside of operative bed and elective neck.
  - Consider 66 Gy for areas at very high risk (extra capsular extension [ECE], positive margin).
- Definitive RT:
  - GTV (for unresectable disease) will be gross primary disease and all nodes greater than 1 cm or with a necrotic center or active on PET.

- o PTV70 will be a 3 to 5 mm expansion on GTV.
  - ■ 60 to 66 Gy sufficient for T1 tumors.
  - ■ 66 to 70 Gy sufficient for T2 tumors.
  - o CTV63 will include GTV with a minimum 1 cm margin except when against critical structures and high-risk neck.
  - o CTV56 will include intermediate-risk areas and elective neck.
  - o Other RT options include: brachytherapy alone (LDR or HDR) or EBRT (50 Gy) + brachytherapy (16 Gy).
- Lips
  - o Small lesions can be treated orthovoltage photons, electrons, or brachytherapy.
    - ■ Consider bolus for superficial lesions, lead cutout, and lead shield to protect oral cavity and mandible.
  - o Upper lesions: consider covering perifacial lymphatics for advanced tumors.
- Oral tongue, floor of mouth
  - o Small lesions can be treated with brachytherapy.
  - o Bite block and mouthguards
- Buccal mucosa
  - o Wire oral commissures
  - o Bite block and mouthguards
- Alveolar ridge, hard palate, and retromolar trigone
  - o EBRT preferred to brachytherapy due to risk of osteoradionecrosis.
  - o Bite block and mouthguards
- Organs at risk
  - o Spinal cord: max 45 Gy
  - o Brainstem: max 54 Gy
  - o Parotids: combined mean less than 26 Gy, or mean less than 20 Gy in at least one gland
  - o Glottic/supraglottic larynx: mean less than 37 Gy
  - o Mandible: max 70 Gy

6.3 Oropharynx

Epidemiology and Risk Factors

- There are approximately 8,500 new cases of oropharynx cancer annually in the United States.
- Rising incidence occurs in middle-aged White males without alcohol or tobacco history.
- Subsites of oropharynx include: base of tongue, soft palate, palatine tonsils, tonsillar pillars, and lateral and posterior pharyngeal walls between nasopharynx and pharyngoepiglottic fold.
- Risk factors:
  - o HPV 16, 18, 31 infection
  - o Alcohol and tobacco
  - o Betel and areca nut chewing
- Risk of second primary cancers is very high (25%), especially in patients who continue to smoke.
- Risk stratification groups from RTOG 0129:
  - o Low Risk: p16+, no smoking history less than 10 pack years
    - ■ 3yr OS 94%
  - o Intermediate Risk: p16+ with smoking history less than 10 pack years, or p16– and no smoking history (<10 pack years)
    - ■ 3yr OS 67%
  - o High Risk: p16- with smoking history greater than 10 pack years
    - ■ 3yr OS 42%

Anatomy and Patterns of Spread

- Oropharynx bounded by soft palate superiorly, pharyngeal walls laterally, pharyngeal wall posteriorly, and hyoid bone inferiorly.
- Lymphatic drainage generally extensive: upper jugulodigastric, bilateral cervical, and retropharyngeal lymph nodes.
- Clinical nodal involvement at diagnosis:
  - BOT: 75%
  - Tonsillar fossa: 75%
  - Tonsillar pillar: 45%
  - Soft palate: 45%
  - Oropharyngeal wall: 70%

Presentation

- Most common presenting symptom is a neck mass.
- Other symptoms on presentation include a mucosal lesion with pain and bleeding, sore throat, dysphagia, globus sensation, referred otalgia, hoarse voice, poor articulation from fixed tumor, foul breath from ulceration and necrosis, trismus, and temporal pain.
- Referred otalgia

Cranial Nerve	Primary
CN X (auricular (Arnold) nerve $\rightarrow$ postauricular)	Larynx, hypopharynx
CN IX (nerve of Jacobson $\rightarrow$ tympanic cavity)	Base of tongue
CN V_3 (auriculotemporal nerve $\rightarrow$ preauricular)	Oral tongue

Histology

- 95% are squamous cell carcinoma.
- Other histologies include: non-Hodgkin's lymphoma, lymphoepithelioma, adenoid cystic carcinoma, mucoepidermoid carcinoma, adenocarcinoma, verrucous carcinoma, plasmacytoma, melanoma, and small-cell carcinoma.

Diagnosis and Workup

- History and physical exam including complete head and neck exam with careful inspection and palpation of oral cavity and anterior oropharynx, fiberoptic nasopharyngolaryngoscopy, and palpation of all neck levels
- Panendoscopy
- Biopsy of lesion
  - Perform HPV testing
- CT head/neck if greater than T1
- CXR for stages III/IV
- Consider PET/CT and MRI
- Routine laboratory studies
- Dental evaluation, nutrition evaluation, speech and swallowing evaluation, and audiology testing
  - Consider prophylactic feeding tube placement in patients receiving chemoradiation

Staging (AJCC 7th Edition)

T-stage

Tx	Primary tumor cannot be assessed
T0	No evidence of primary tumor
Tis	Carcinoma in situ
T1	Tumor 2 cm or less in greatest dimension
T2	Tumor more than 2 cm but not more than 4 cm in greatest dimension
T3	Tumor more than 4 cm in greatest dimension or extension to lingual surface of epiglottis
T4a	Moderately advanced local disease. Tumor invades the larynx, extrinsic muscle of tongue, medial pterygoid, hard palate, or mandible*
T4b	Very advanced local disease. Tumor invades lateral pterygoid muscle, pterygoid plates, lateral nasopharynx, or skull base or encases carotid artery

* Mucosal extension to lingual surface of epiglottis from primary tumors of the base of the tongue and vallecula does not constitute invasion of larynx.

N-stage

N0	No regional lymph node metastasis
N1	Metastasis in a single ipsilateral lymph node, 3 cm or less in greatest dimension
N2a	Metastasis in single ipsilateral lymph node more than 3 cm but not more than 6 cm in greatest dimension
N2b	Metastasis in multiple ipsilateral lymph nodes, none more than 6 cm in greatest dimension
N2c	Metastasis in bilateral or contralateral lymph nodes, none more than 6 cm in greatest dimension
N3	Metastasis in a lymph node more than 6 cm in greatest dimension

M-stage

M0	No distant metastases
M1	Distant metastases

Group Stage	T	N	M
0	Tis	N0	M0
I	T1	N0	M0
II	T2	N0	M0
III	T3	N0	M0
	T1–3	N1	M0
IVA	T4a	N0–1	M0
	T1–4a	N2	M0
IVB	Any T	N3	M0
	T4b	Any N	M0
IVC	Any T	Any N	M1

Treatment Overview

- T1–2, N0–1: RT or surgery ± neck dissection
  - Consider chemoradiation for T2N1
- T3–4a, N0–1: Concurrent chemoradiation (preferred) or surgery
- Any T, N2–3: Concurrent chemoradiation (preferred) or surgery
- T4b, any N, or unresectable: Concurrent chemoradiation
- Notes:
  - Preferred concurrent chemotherapy: cisplatin 100 mg/m^2 q21 days × 3 cycles.
  - Postoperative RT indicated for T3/T4, close margin, N2 or N3 disease, PNI, LVSI, or level IV to V lymph node involvement.
  - Postoperative chemoradiation indicated for positive margin or extracapsular extension.
  - Consider salvage surgery if primary has less than CR or residual neck mass by imaging or physical examination at 6 to 12 weeks posttreatment.

Radiation Therapy Techniques

- Simulation: supine, shoulder pulls, head and shoulder mask
  - Wire lymph nodes, surgical scars
  - Bite block
  - Mouthguards
- Preoperative diagnostic imaging fused for treatment planning
- Full field simultaneous-integrated-boost IMRT used to target volumes
  - Alternative techniques include split-field IMRT (match line just above arytenoids), sequential boost, brachytherapy boost, and 3D-conformal planning.
    - Split-field IMRT technique matched to a supraclavicular AP field with a half-beam block ONLY when there is no gross disease at the level of the arytenoids.
- Postoperative RT:
  - 60 Gy to tumor bed + ~1 cm margin.
  - 57 Gy to entire primary operative bed and involved neck nodal levels.
  - 54 Gy to intermediate-risk areas outside of operative bed and elective neck.
  - Consider 66 Gy for areas at very high risk (ECE, positive margin).
- Definitive RT:
  - GTV (for unresectable disease) will be gross primary disease and all nodes greater than 1 cm or with a necrotic center or active on PET.
  - PTV70 will be a 3–5 mm expansion on GTV.
    - 60 to 66 Gy sufficient for T1 tumors.
    - 66 to 70 Gy sufficient for T2 tumors.
  - CTV63 will include GTV with a minimum 1 cm margin except when against critical structures and high-risk neck.
  - CTV56 will include intermediate-risk areas and elective neck.
- Notes:
  - In general, treat bilateral neck (retropharyngeals, levels II–IV).
  - If more anterior tumor, consider treating level IB lymph nodes.
  - If tonsil primary with greater than 1 cm extension invasion into soft palate or base of tongue and N1–2a, treat ipsilateral neck only.
  - Treat ipsilateral IB if level II involved.
  - Treat ipsilateral level V for T3+ or N+.
- Organs at risk:
  - Spinal cord: max 45 Gy
  - Brainstem: max 54 Gy
  - Oral cavity: no hot spots

- o Parotids: combined mean less than 26 Gy, or mean less than 20 Gy in at least one gland
- o Glottic/supraglottic larynx: mean less than 37 Gy
- o Mandible: max 70 Gy

6.4   Hypopharynx

Epidemiology and Risk Factors

- There are approximately 3,000 new cases of hypopharynx cancer annually in the United States.
- Subsites of hypopharynx include: pyriform sinuses (most common), posterior pharyngeal walls, and postcricoid area (least common).
- Risk factors:
  - o Alcohol and tobacco
  - o Betel and areca nut chewing
  - o Iron, vitamin C, vitamin B12, and vitamin C deficiencies

Anatomy and Patterns of Spread

- Hypopharynx is pharynx from hyoid bone to bottom of cricoid.
- Lymph node drainage: usually to levels II to V, retropharyngeals, paratracheal, paraesophageal
  - o Low neck (level IV) lymph node involvement has a worse prognosis.
- Risk of lymph node involvement is 60% for early-stage disease and 85% for advanced-stage disease.

Presentation

- Typical presentation includes sore throat, otalgia, hoarse voice, dysphagia, odynophagia, and trismus.
- Referred otalgia

Cranial Nerve	Primary
CN X (auricular (Arnold) nerve → postauricular)	Larynx, hypopharynx
CN IX (nerve of Jacobson Symbol tympanic cavity)	Base of tongue
CN V$_3$ (auriculotemporal nerve Symbol preauricular)	Oral tongue

Histology

- 95% are squamous cell carcinoma.

Diagnosis and Workup

- History and physical exam including complete head and neck exam with careful inspection and palpation of oral cavity and anterior oropharynx, fiberoptic nasopharyngolaryngoscopy, and palpation of all neck levels
- Panendoscopy
- Bronchoscopy if clinically indicated
- Biopsy of lesion
- CT head/neck
- CXR for stage III/IV
- Consider PET/CT and MRI
- Routine laboratory studies
- Dental evaluation, nutrition evaluation, speech and swallowing evaluation, and audiology testing
  - o Consider prophylactic feeding tube placement in patients receiving chemoradiation

Staging (AJCC 7th Edition)

T-stage

Tx	Primary tumor cannot be assessed
T0	No evidence of primary tumor
Tis	Carcinoma in situ
T1	Tumor limited to one subsite of hypopharynx and/or 2 cm or less in greatest dimension
T2	Tumor invades more than one subsite of hypopharynx or an adjacent site, or measures more than 2 cm but not more than 4 cm in greatest dimension without fixation of hemilarynx
T3	Tumor more than 4 cm in greatest dimension or with fixation of hemilarynx or extension to esophagus
T4a	Tumor invades thyroid/cricoid cartilage, hyoid bone, thyroid gland, or central compartment soft tissue[†]
T4b	Tumor invades prevertebral fascia, encases carotid artery, or involves mediastinal structures

[†] Central compartment soft tissue includes prelaryngeal strap muscles and subcutaneous fat.

N-stage

N0	No regional lymph node metastasis
N1	Metastasis in a single ipsilateral lymph node, 3 cm or less in greatest dimension
N2a	Metastasis in single ipsilateral lymph node more than 3 cm but not more than 6 cm in greatest dimension
N2b	Metastasis in multiple ipsilateral lymph nodes, none more than 6 cm in greatest dimension
N2c	Metastasis in bilateral or contralateral lymph nodes, none more than 6 cm in greatest dimension
N3	Metastasis in a lymph node more than 6 cm in greatest dimension

M-stage

M0	No distant metastases
M1	Distant metastases

Group Stage	T	N	M
0	Tis	N0	M0
I	T1	N0	M0
II	T2	N0	M0
III	T3	N0	M0
	T1–3	N1	M0

(continued)

(continued)

Group Stage	T	N	M
IVA	T4a	N0–1	M0
	T1–4a	N2	M0
IVB	Any T	N3	M0
	T4b	Any N	M0
IVC	Any T	Any N	M1

Treatment Overview

- Most T1, N0; selected T2, N0 (not requiring total laryngectomy): RT or surgery.
  - Surgery is partial laryngopharyngectomy with neck dissection.
- T1, N+; T2–3, any N (requiring total laryngectomy): Induction chemotherapy → RT or chemoradiation (if complete or partial response) or surgery (if less than partial response) OR concurrent chemoradiation OR surgery.
  - Surgery is laryngopharyngectomy with neck dissection.
- T4a, any N (requiring total laryngectomy): surgery (preferred) OR induction chemotherapy → RT or chemoradiation (if complete or partial response) or surgery (if less than partial response) OR concurrent chemoradiation.
- T4b, any N, or unresectable
  - Concurrent chemoradiation
- Notes:
  - Induction chemotherapy: docetaxel, cisplatin, 5-FU.
    - If complete response or partial response at primary site and stable or improved disease in neck: chemoradiation
    - If less than partial response at primary site or progression in neck: salvage surgery
  - Following induction, concurrent chemotherapy: weekly platinums, weekly taxanes, or cetuximab.
  - Preferred concurrent chemotherapy without induction chemotherapy: cisplatin 100 mg/m^2 q21 days × 3 cycles.
  - Postoperative RT indicated for T3/T4, close margin, N2 or N3 disease, PNI, LVSI, or level IV–V lymph node involvement.
  - Postoperative chemoradiation indicated for positive margin or extracapsular extension.
  - Consider salvage surgery if primary has less than CR or residual neck mass by imaging or physical examination at 6 to 12 weeks posttreatment.

Radiation Therapy Techniques

- Simulation: supine, shoulder pulls, head and shoulder mask
  - Wire lymph nodes, surgical scars
  - Mouthguards
- Preoperative diagnostic imaging fused for treatment planning
- Full field simultaneous-integrated-boost IMRT will be used to target volumes.
  - Alternative techniques include split-field IMRT (match line just above arytenoids), sequential boost, brachytherapy boost, and 3D-conformal planning.
- Postoperative RT:
  - 60 Gy to high-risk areas and postoperative bed.
  - 54 Gy to intermediate-risk areas outside of operative bed and elective neck.
  - Consider 66 Gy for areas at very high risk (ECE, positive margin).

- Definitive RT:
  - GTV (for unresectable disease) will be gross primary disease and all nodes greater than 1 cm or with a necrotic center or active on PET.
  - PTV70 will be a 3 to 5 mm expansion on GTV.
    - 60 to 66 Gy sufficient for T1 tumors.
    - 66 to 70 Gy sufficient for T2 tumors.
  - CTV63 will include GTV with a minimum 1 cm margin except when against critical structures and high-risk neck.
  - CTV56 will include intermediate-risk areas and elective neck.
- Notes:
  - Treat bilateral neck (retropharyngeals, levels II–V) in all cases.
  - Boost tracheal stoma to 60 to 66 Gy if: emergent tracheostomy, subglottic extension, soft tissue invasion, ECE in level VI, scar crosses stoma, or close/positive margin.
- Organs at risk:
  - Spinal cord: max 45 Gy
  - Brainstem: max 54 Gy
  - Brachial plexus: max 66 Gy
  - Oral cavity: no hot spots
  - Parotids: combined mean less than 26 Gy, or mean less than 20 Gy in at least one gland
  - Mandible: max 70 Gy

6.5   Larynx

Epidemiology and Risk Factors

- There are approximately 13,000 new cases of larynx cancer annually in the United States and 3.600 cancer-related deaths annually.
- 2/3 are glottic, 1/3 are supraglottic, 2% are subglottic.
- It is more common in men.
- Synchronous primaries in aerodigestive tract up to 5%.
- Risk factors:
  - Alcohol and tobacco
  - Occupation based on voice

Anatomy and Patterns of Spread

- Subsites:
  - Supraglottis:
    - Epiglottis
    - Aryepiglottic folds
    - False cords
    - Ventricles
    - Arytenoids
  - Glottis:
    - True vocal cords
    - Anterior commissure
  - Subglottis:
    - 5 mm below true vocal cords to bottom of cricoid
- Lymph node drainage:
  - Supraglottis:
    - 55% are node positive at diagnosis
    - Levels II to IV most commonly involved

- o Glottis:
  - ▪ Less than 1% of T1 tumors, 2% to 5% of T2, and 20% to 30% of T3 to 4 are node positive at diagnosis
  - ▪ Levels II to IV most commonly involved
- o Subglottis:
  - ▪ Pretracheal (Delphian), paratracheal, and inferior jugular most commonly involved

Presentation

- Presentation:
  - o Supraglottis: dysphagia, odynophagia, persistent sore throat, otalgia
  - o Glottis: hoarse voice, persistent sore throat
  - o Subglottis: stridor, dyspnea
- Referred otalgia:

Cranial Nerve	Primary
CN X (auricular (Arnold) nerve → postauricular)	Larynx, hypopharynx
CN IX (nerve of Jacobson Symbol tympanic cavity)	Base of tongue
CN V$_3$ (auriculotemporal nerve Symbol preauricular)	Oral tongue

Histology

- 95% are squamous cell carcinomas.
  - o Verrucous carcinoma (1%–2%) is a variant that is low grade, infrequently metastasizes, and may undergo anaplastic transformation after RT (controversial). Surgery preferred.
- Other histologies include: minor salivary gland carcinomas, lymphoma, plasmacytoma, carcinoid, sarcoma, melanoma.

Diagnosis and Workup

- History and physical exam including complete head and neck exam with fiberoptic nasopharyngolaryngoscopy
  - o Consider videostroboscopy for functional evaluation and documentation of baseline tumor characteristics and vocal cord function.
- Biopsy of suspicious lesions
- Panendoscopy
- CT head and neck
- Consider MRI
- Consider PET/CT for stage III/IV disease
- Chest x-ray
- Pulmonary function tests for surgery candidates
- Dental evaluation, nutrition evaluation, speech and swallowing evaluation, and audiology testing
  - o Consider prophylactic feeding tube placement in patients receiving chemoradiation.

Staging (AJCC 7th Edition)

T-stage	
Tx	Primary tumor cannot be assessed
T0	No evidence of primary tumor
Tis	Carcinoma in situ

(continued)

(continued)

T-stage

Supraglottis

T1	Tumor limited to one subsite of supraglottis with normal vocal cord mobility
T2	Tumor invades mucosa of more than one adjacent subsite of supraglottis or glottis or region outside the supraglottis (e.g., mucosa of base of tongue, vallecula, medial wall of pyriform sinus) without fixation of the larynx
T3	Tumor limited to larynx with vocal cord fixation and/or invades any of the following postcricoid area, preepiglottic space, paraglottic space, and/or inner cortex of thyroid cartilage
T4a	Tumor invades through the thyroid cartilage and /or invades tissues beyond the larynx (e.g., trachea, soft tissues of neck including deep extrinsic muscle of the tongue, strap muscles, thyroid, or esophagus)
T4b	Tumor invades prevertebral space, encases carotid artery, or invades mediastinal structures

Glottis

T1a	Tumor limited to one vocal cord
T1b	Tumor involves both vocal cords
T2	Tumor extends to supraglottis and/or subglottis, and/or with impaired vocal cord mobility
T3	Tumor limited to the larynx with vocal cord fixation and/or invasion of paraglottic space, and/or inner cortex of the thyroid cartilage
T4a	Tumor invades through the outer cortex of the thyroid cartilage and/or invades tissues beyond the larynx (e.g., trachea, soft tissues of neck including deep extrinsic muscle of the tongue, strap muscles, thyroid, or esophagus)
T4b	Tumor invades prevertebral space, encases carotid artery, or invades mediastinal structures

Subglottis

T1	Tumor limited to the subglottis
T2	Tumor extends to vocal cord(s) with normal or impaired mobility
T3	Tumor limited to larynx with vocal cord fixation
T4a	Tumor invades cricoid or thyroid cartilage and/or invades tissues beyond the larynx (e.g., trachea, soft tissues of neck including deep extrinsic muscles of the tongue, strap muscles, thyroid, or esophagus)
T4b	Tumor invades prevertebral space, encases carotid artery, or invades mediastinal structures

N-stage

N0	No regional lymph node metastasis
N1	Metastasis in a single ipsilateral lymph node, 3 cm or less in greatest dimension
N2a	Metastasis in single ipsilateral lymph node more than 3 cm but not more than 6 cm in greatest dimension
N2b	Metastasis in multiple ipsilateral lymph nodes, none more than 6 cm in greatest dimension

(continued)

(continued)

N-stage

N2c	Metastasis in bilateral or contralateral lymph nodes, none more than 6 cm in greatest dimension
N3	Metastasis in a lymph node more than 6 cm in greatest dimension

M-stage

M0	No distant metastases
M1	Distant metastases

Group Stage	T	N	M
0	Tis	N0	M0
I	T1	N0	M0
II	T2	N0	M0
III	T3	N0	M0
	T1–3	N1	M0
IVA	T4a	N0–1	M0
	T1–4a	N2	M0
IVB	Any T	N3	M0
	T4b	Any N	M0
IVC	Any T	Any N	M1

Treatment Overview

- Glottic:
  - Tis: Endoscopic resection (preferred) or RT
  - T1–2N0, select T3 N0 (amenable to larynx preservation): Primary RT or partial laryngectomy
  - T3, Any N (requiring total laryngectomy): Chemoradiation or total laryngectomy
  - T4a, Any N: Total laryngectomy (preferred) or chemoradiation
  - T4b, Any N: Chemoradiation
- Supraglottic:
  - Amenable to larynx preservation:
    - T1–2N0, selected T3: Endoscopic resection or partial supraglottic laryngectomy or definitive RT
    - T1–2N+, selected T3N1: Partial supraglottic laryngectomy or chemoradiation or radiation
  - Requiring total laryngectomy:
    - T3N0: laryngectomy or chemoradiation
    - T3N2–3: Laryngectomy or chemoradiation
  - T4a, Any N: laryngectomy + RT or chemoradiation
  - T4b, Any N or unresectable: chemoradiation
- Subglottic:
  - Total laryngectomy + postoperative RT preferred
  - Primary chemoradiation may be considered

- Notes:
  - Re-excise if feasible for positive surgical margin.
  - Postoperative RT indicated for T3/T4, close margin, greater than 1 LN involved, PNI, LVSI, soft tissue invasion, emergent trach.
  - Postoperative chemoradiation indicated for positive margin or extracapsular extension.
  - Consider salvage surgery if primary has less than CR or residual neck mass by imaging or physical examination at 6 to 12 weeks posttreatment.
  - Induction chemotherapy can be considered for T3 and node positive cases:
    - Complete response at primary site: definitive RT
    - Partial response at primary site: definitive RT or chemoradiation
    - Less than partial response at primary site: surgery

Radiation Therapy Techniques

- Early glottic (T1 to 2N0):
  - Simulation: supine, shoulder pulls, neck extension, head and shoulder mask
  - Opposed lateral fields (5 cm × 5 cm or 6 cm × 6 cm), 4 to 6 MV photons, wedges
    - Superior border: thyroid notch
    - Inferior border: bottom of cricoid (about C6)
    - Posterior: anterior aspect of vertebral bodies
    - Anterior: flash skin
  - Dose
    - Tis: 66 Gy in 33 fractions or 60.75 Gy n 27 fractions
    - T1: 66 Gy in 33 fractions or 63 Gy in 28 fractions
    - T2: 70 Gy in 35 fractions (6 fractions per week) or 65.25 Gy in 29 fractions
  - Note: Keep total treatment time to less than 6 weeks.
- Advanced larynx:
  - Simulation: supine, shoulder pulls, head and shoulder mask
  - Wire lymph nodes, surgical scars
  - Preoperative diagnostic imaging fused for treatment planning
  - Full field simultaneous-integrated-boost IMRT will be used to target volumes
  - Postoperative RT:
    - 60 Gy to high-risk areas and postoperative bed
    - 54 Gy to intermediate-risk areas outside of operative bed and elective neck
    - Consider 66 Gy for areas at very high risk (ECE, positive margin)
  - Definitive RT:
    - GTV (for unresectable disease) will be gross primary disease and all nodes greater than 1 cm or with a necrotic center or active on PET.
    - PTV70 will include GTV plus 3 to 5 mm margin.
    - CTV63 will include GTV with a minimum 1 cm margin except when against critical structures and high-risk neck.
    - CTV56 will include intermediate-risk areas and elective neck.
    - *Consider altered fractionation for radiation alone.
  - Notes:
    - Except for early stage glottis cancers, treat bilateral neck (levels II–IV).
    - Boost tracheal stoma to 60 to 66 Gy if: emergent tracheostomy, subglottic extension, soft tissue invasion, ECE in level VI, scar crosses stoma, or close/positive margin.
  - Organs at risk:
    - Brachial plexus max dose 66 Gy
    - Mandible 70 Gy; if not possible, then V75 Gy <1 mL
    - Spinal cord max 45 Gy; 1% PRV max 50 Gy
    - Brainstem max 54 Gy; PRV max 60 Gy

- Parotids mean dose less than 26 in at least one, or at least 50% of one gland less than 30 Gy
- Esophagus mean dose less than 45 Gy

6.6 Thyroid

Epidemiology and Risk Factors

- Thyroid tumors are the most common endocrine neoplasms.
- There are approximately 30,000 new cases annually in the United States.
- Papillary and follicular histologies are more than twice as common in women than in men.
- Risk factors:
  - Prior ionizing radiation exposure
  - Dietary iodine content
  - Family history of thyroid cancer:
    - Multiple endocrine neoplasia type 2 (MEN-2)—medullary thyroid cancer
    - Cowden's syndrome—papillary thyroid cancer
    - Gardner's syndrome—papillary thyroid cancer

Anatomy and Patterns of Spread

- Most is commonly spread locally, with extrathyroidal invasion of soft tissue.
- Nodal involvement is common (central compartment, tracheo-esophageal groove, Delphian nodes, cervical nodes, superior mediastinum greater than supraclavicular, retropharyngeal).
- Superior mediastinal nodal involvement is usually associated with extensive neck nodal involvement.
- Common sites for distant metastatic disease include lung and bone.

Presentation

- Typically presents as palpable anterior neck nodule.
- Advanced disease can present with hoarseness from recurrent laryngeal nerve paralysis, breathing, or swallowing difficulties.

Histology

- Most thyroid nodules are benign.
- Pathology:
  - Papillary thyroid cancer accounts for 40% to 90% cases, usually younger women.
  - Follicular thyroid cancer (includes oxyphilic or Hurthle cell variants) accounts for 15% to 40% cases.
  - Medullary thyroid cancer accounts for 2% to 8% cases.
  - Anaplastic thyroid cancer accounts for 1% to 5% cases.
  - Other histologies include sarcomas, malignant hemangioendotheliomas, and lymphomas.

Diagnosis and Workup

- History and physical
- Thyroid ultrasound
- CT neck
  - Avoid iodinated contrast as this will block treatment with I-131 for approximately 6 months.
- Fine needle aspiration biopsy
- Chest x-ray
- Consider preoperative vocal cord examination; if vocal cord paralysis suspected from pressure or invasion of recurrent laryngeal nerve

- Labs including TSH, T3, T4, thyroglobulin
  - For medullary carcinoma, check calcitonin, calcium, CEA, and urine and serum catecholamines.
- Postoperative whole body RAI scan (papillary and follicular thyroid cancer)
- Age, histology, and anatomic extent of disease are of prognostic importance.

Staging (AJCC 7th Edition)

T-stage

Tx	Primary tumor cannot be assessed
T0	No evidence of primary tumor
T1a	Tumor 1 cm or less, limited to the thyroid
T1b	Tumor more than 1 cm but not more than 2 cm, limited to the thyroid
T2	Tumor more than 2 cm but not more than 4 cm, limited to the thyroid
T3	Tumor more than 4 cm in greatest dimension limited to the thyroid, or any tumor with minimal extrathyroid extension
T4a	Tumor of any size extending beyond the thyroid capsule to invade subcutaneous tissues, larynx, trachea, esophagus, or recurrent laryngeal nerve
T4b	Tumor invades prevertebral fascia or encases carotid artery or mediastinal vessels

N-stage

N0	No regional lymph node metastasis
N1a	Metastasis to level VI (pretracheal, paratracheal, and prelaryngeal/Delphian lymph nodes) Regional lymph node metastasis
N1b	Metastasis to unilateral, bilateral, or contralateral cervical (Levels I–V) or retropharyngeal or superior mediastinal lymph nodes (Level VII)

M-stage

M0	No distant metastases
M1	Distant metastases

* All anaplastic carcinomas are considered T4 tumor:
- T4a: Intrathyroidal anaplastic carcinoma
- T4b: Anaplastic carcinoma with gross extrathyroid extension

Group Stage

Papillary or Follicular (Differentiated) UNDER 45 YEARS

	T	N	M
I	Any T	Any N	M0
II	Any T	Any N	M1

(continued)

(continued)

Group Stage

Papillary or Follicular (Differentiated) 45 YEARS AND OLDER

	T	N	M
I	T1	N0	M0
II	T2	N0	M0
III	T3	N0	M0
	T1–3	N1a	M0
IVA	T4a	N0–1b	M0
	T1–3	N1a	M0
IVB	T4b	Any N	M0
IVC	Any T	Any N	M1

Medullary Carcinoma

	T	N	M
I	T1	N0	M0
II	T2–3	N0	M0
III	T1–3	N1a	M0
IVA	T4a	N0–1b	M0
	T1–3	N1a	M0
IVB	T4b	Any N	M0
IVC	Any T	Any N	M1

Anaplastic Carcinoma

	T	N	M
IVA	T4a	Any N	M0
IVB	T4b	Any N	M0
IVC	Any T	Any N	M1

Treatment Overview

- Surgery is the standard primary treatment.
- Extent of initial surgery is controversial, ranging from ipsilateral thyroid lobectomy to total thyroidectomy.
- Extent of neck node removal is controversial.
  - Role of prophylactic or prognostic lymph node dissections is unclear.
  - Modified radical neck dissection is indicated for gross nodal metastases.
- Thyroxine-suppressive therapy of TSH is standard postoperative management for papillary and follicular thyroid cancers.
- Radioactive iodine therapy is used for most follicular thyroid carcinoma, unresectable or residual papillary thyroid carcinoma, and distant metastatic disease.

- EBRT is considered for patients with locally advanced disease with high-risk surgical pathologic features (close/positive margins, extrathyroidal invasion, multiple nodes involved), recurrent or metastatic disease nonresponsive to RAI.
- For differentiated thyroid cancers, role of chemotherapy is limited; doxorubicin is the most active single agent.
- For anaplastic thyroid carcinoma, multimodality therapy with resection, EBRT, and chemotherapy is preferred.

Radiation Therapy Techniques

- Simulation: supine, shoulder pulls, head and shoulder mask
  - Wire surgical scars
- Preoperative diagnostic imaging fused for treatment planning
- Full field IMRT will be used to target volumes
  - Alternative techniques include 3D-conformal planning.
- Postoperative dose is 60 Gy
  - 45 to 50 Gy to thyroid bed and nodal regions (levels II–IV, VI, superior mediastinal nodes)
  - Boost thyroid bed, central nodal compartment, and areas with involved nodes to 60 Gy
  - Escalate dose to 68 to 70 Gy if possible for gross residual disease
- Organs at risk:
  - Spinal cord: max 45 Gy
  - Brachial plexus: max 66 Gy
  - Parotids: combined mean less than 26 Gy, or mean less than 20 Gy in at least one gland
  - Esophagus: mean less than 50 to 60 Gy
  - Mandible: max 70 Gy

6.7   Unknown Head and Neck Primary Site

Epidemiology and Risk Factors

- Approximately 3% of head and neck squamous cell carcinomas metastasize to cervical lymph nodes from an unknown primary site
- Head and neck primary suspected for squamous cell carcinoma or poorly differentiated carcinoma
- Squamous cell carcinoma in the parotid is almost always metastatic from a cutaneous primary
- Adenocarcinoma almost always arises from a primary lesion below clavicles
- Risk factors
  - Depends on suspected primary site

Anatomy and Patterns of Spread

- For level IA involvement, likely primary sites include: mentum, middle 2/3 lower lip, anterior gingiva, and anterior tongue
- For level IB: ipsilateral lips, cheek, nose, medial canthus, oral cavity, and submandibular gland
- For level II: nasopharynx, oropharynx, oral cavity, larynx, hypopharynx, and parotid gland
- For level III: larynx, hypopharynx, thyroid, and infraclavicular primary
- For level IV: infraclavicular primary, thyroid, and esophagus
- For level V: nasopharynx
- For level VI: anterior cervical skin, larynx, and thyroid
- For parotid nodes: skin and oral cavity
- For bilateral nodes: nasopharynx, base of tongue, soft palate, pyriform sinus, and supraglottic larynx
- For Rouviere's node: nasopharynx and pharyngeal wall

Presentation

- Usually presents as an enlarging neck mass
- Often no obvious primary lesion is found

Diagnosis and Workup

- History and physical exam including complete head and neck exam with careful inspection and palpation of oral cavity and anterior oropharynx, examination of the skin of the head and neck region, fiberoptic nasopharyngolaryngoscopy, and palpation of all neck levels
- FNA of lymph node
  - Consider testing for HPV and EBV
- CT head/neck
- Consider MRI
- Chest x-ray
- PET/CT if above workup does not reveal primary
  - Should be performed prior to panendoscopy
- Panendoscopy with directed biopsies of nasopharynx, tonsil, base of tongue, piriform sinuses, and any suspicious lesions
  - Ipsilateral tonsillectomy recommended
- Routine laboratory studies
- Dental evaluation, nutrition evaluation, speech and swallowing evaluation, and audiology testing
  - Consider prophylactic feeding tube placement in patients receiving chemoradiation

Stage

- According to suspected primary site

Treatment Overview

- Primary treatment options include neck dissection or RT followed by evaluation for a neck dissection
- For single positive node without ECE, neck dissection alone is adequate
- For primary RT, include nasopharnyx, oropharynx, and bilateral neck
  - Larynx and hypopharynx can be spared
  - Include oral cavity if level IB involvement
- Concurrent chemotherapy indicated for N2 and N3 disease
  - Preferred concurrent chemotherapy: cisplatin 100 mg/m^2 q21 days × 3 cycles
- For primary nonsurgically treated patients, follow with close follow-up (CT scan of neck 4 to 6 weeks after completion of RT to direct need for modified neck dissection)
  - Most patients with advanced N2–N3 disease should undergo a planned neck dissection as the likelihood of cure is low if a regional recurrence develops

Radiation Therapy Techniques

- Simulation: supine, shoulder pulls, head and shoulder mask
  - Wire lymph nodes, surgical scars
  - Bite block
  - Mouthguards
- Preoperative diagnostic imaging fused for treatment planning
- Full field simultaneous-integrated-boost IMRT will be used to target volumes:
  - Alternative techniques include split-field IMRT (match line just above arytenoids), sequential boost, brachytherapy boost, and 3D-conformal planning.
  - CTV generally includes pharyngeal axis including nasopharynx and oropharynx, and bilateral IB-V and retropharyngeal nodes.
- Dose (conventional fractionation):
  - Gross disease: ≥70 Gy
  - Mucosa: 50 to 60 Gy
  - High-risk nodal stations: 60 to 63 Gy

o   Intermediate risk nodal stations: 50 to 56 Gy
o   Areas at very high risk (ECE, positive margin): 66 Gy
- Organs at risk:
  o   Spinal cord: max 45 Gy
  o   Brainstem: max 54 Gy
  o   Parotids: combined mean less than 26 Gy, or mean less than 20 Gy in at least one gland
  o   Glottic/supraglottic larynx: mean less than 37 Gy
  o   Mandible: max 70 Gy

6.8 Postoperative Head and Neck

- Indications for postoperative RT include: advanced stage (T3–T4), positive or close surgical margins; lymphovascular invasion; perineural invasion; greater than 1 positive node; any single positive node greater than 3 cm; and extracapsular extension.
- Indications for postoperative chemoradiotherapy include: positive surgical margins and extracapsular extension.
- Postoperative RT should begin within 4 to 6 weeks of surgery.
  o   Locoregional control and overall survival better with early RT.
  o   Accelerated fractionation can make up for delay in starting postoperative RT.

Radiation Therapy Techniques

- Simulation: supine, shoulder pulls, neck extension, head and shoulder mask
- Preoperative diagnostic imaging fused for treatment planning
- Full field IMRT will be used to target volumes.
  o   CTV60 will include tumor bed + approximately 1 cm margin.
    ▪   Include surgical clips, scar.
  o   CTV57 will include CTV60 + entire primary operative bed and involved neck nodal levels.
  o   CTV54 will include CTV60 as well as surgically undisturbed sites at risk for microscopic disease.
  o   Consider CTV66 for areas of extracapsular extension or positive/close margin if target can be accurately localized.
  o   PTV will be an additional 5 mm expansion.
- Notes:
  o   For upper level II involvement, extend upper border of level II to include retrostyloid space up to the base of skull.
  o   For contralateral clinically node-negative neck, the uppermost level II nodal target volume should be delineated at the level which the posterior belly of the digastric muscle crosses the jugular vein.
  o   For involvement if IV or V, include the supraclavicular fossa.
  o   When a pathological lymph node abuts or invades a muscle, include the muscle, at least for the entire invaded level.
  o   When a pathological lymph node is located at the boundary with another level, include the adjacent level.
  o   For node positive pharyngeal tumors, include at least lateral retropharyngeal nodes.
  o   Except for well lateralized, early stage, node negative disease, bilateral neck should be covered for oral cavity cancers.

6.9 Eye/Orbit

Epidemiology and Risk Factors

- These are uncommon neoplasms, with approximately 2,500 cases annually in the United States.
- Most common malignancy is metastasis.

- Most common primary malignancies include ocular melanoma (eye) and orbital lymphoma (orbit).
- Risk factors:
  - Uveal melanoma: light eye color, fair skin, UV light exposure, xeroderma pigmentosum, oculodermal melanocytosis, dysokastic nevus syndrome
  - Orbital lymphoma: same as for other non-Hodgkin's lymphomas

Anatomy and Patterns of Spread

- Ocular melanoma:
  - 80% arise in choroid; 10% to 15% in ciliary body; less than 10% in iris
  - Intraocular spread, including vitreous seeding
  - Extrascleral extension
  - Distant metastasis to liver greater than skin, lung
- Orbital lymphoma:
  - Arise in conjunctiva, lacrimal gland, eyelids, uvea, and intraconal and extraconal retrobulbar areas

Presentation

- Ocular melanoma: asymptomatic, visual field distortion, field loss, floaters, flashers, pain, glaucoma
- Orbital lymphoma: orbital mass, proptosis, diplopia, salmon, or flesh-pink colored lesion (conjunctiva)

Histology

- Ocular melanoma: spindle cell (grade 1), mixed cell (grade 2), and epithelioid cell (grade 3)
- Orbital lymphoma: extranodal marginal zone B-cell lymphoma or mucosa-associated lymphoid tissue (MALT)

Diagnosis and Workup

  - History and physical
  - Ocular melanoma: ultrasound, fundus photography, chest x-ray, liver function tests, CBC, LDH, CT chest/abdomen
  - Orbital lymphoma: biopsy of lesion, bone marrow biopsy
- Collaborative Ocular Melanoma Study (COMS) classification:
  - Small: less than 3 mm thick; 5 to 16 mm largest dimension
  - Medium: 3 to 10 mm thick; 5 to 16 mm largest dimension
  - Large: greater than 10 mm thick; greater than 16 mm largest dimension
  - * Size in optic disc diameter: 1 dd = 1.5 mm

Staging (AJCC 7th Edition Staging for Orbital Lymphoma)

T-stage	
Tx	Primary tumor cannot be assessed
T0	No evidence of primary tumor
T1a	Bulbar conjunctiva only
T1b	Palpebral conjunctiva ± fornix ± caruncle
T1c	Extensive conjunctival involvement

(continued)

(continued)

T-stage

T2a	Anterior orbital involvement (± conjunctival involvement)
T2b	Anterior orbital involvement (± conjunctival involvement + lacrimal involvement)
T2c	Posterior orbital involvement (± conjunctival involvement ± anterior involvement and ± any extraocular muscle involvement)
T2d	Nasolacrimal drainage system involvement (± conjunctival involvement but not including nasopharynx)
T3	Lymphoma with preseptal eyelid involvement (defined earlier) 16 ± orbital involvement ± any conjunctival involvement
T4a	Involvement of nasopharynx
T4b	Osseous involvement (including periosteum)
T4c	Involvement of maxillofacial, ethmoidal, and/or frontal sinuses
T4d	Intracranial spread

N-stage

N0	No evidence of lymph node involvement
N1	Involvement of ipsilateral regional lymph nodes*
N2	Involvement of contralateral or bilateral regional lymph nodes*
N3	Involvement of peripheral lymph nodes not draining ocular adnexal region
N4	Involvement of central lymph nodes

M-stage

M0	No evidence of involvement of other extranodal sites
M1a	Noncontiguous involvement of tissues or organs external to the ocular adnexa (e.g., parotid glands, submandibular gland, lung, liver, spleen, kidney, and breast)
M1b	Lymphomatous involvement of the bone marrow
M1c	Both M1a and M1b involvement

*The regional lymph nodes include preauricular (parotid), submandibular, and cervical.

Treatment Overview

- Ocular melanoma:
  - Small
    - Observation
    - If growth: surgery, laser, plaque brachytherapy, proton RT or stereotactic radiosurgery
  - Medium
    - Surgery (enucleation, orbital exenteration, local resection + RT), RT (proton RT, helium, stereotactic radiosurgery, plaque brachytherapy)
  - Large
    - Enucleation

- Orbital lymphoma:
  - Low grade, limited disease: RT alone
  - Intermediate-/high-grade disease: systemic therapy + RT
    - Systemic therapy is CHOP ± R
- Toxicities:
  - Acute: dermatitis, eye irritation
  - Late: cataracts, retinopathy, glaucoma, dry eye

Radiation Therapy Techniques

- Ocular melanoma:
  - I-125 plaque brachytherapy:
    - Field: tumor + 2 mm margin
    - Plaque placed surgically, sutured in place, lead eye shield, 4 to 7 days treatment
    - I-125: minimum tumor dose 85 Gy; dose rate 0.6 to 1.05 Gy/hr
  - Stereotactic radiosurgery:
    - 25 to 40 Gy single fraction to 50% isodose line
- Orbital lymphoma:
  - Radiation dose:
    - Low grade, limited disease: 30 to 30.6 Gy in 17 to 20 fractions
    - Intermediate-/high-grade disease: 40 Gy in 20 fractions
  - Simulation:
    - Supine, head mask
    - Wire lateral canthus
  - Eye shield if tumor coverage is not compromised
  - Anterior lesions: 6 to 9 MeV electrons with 0.5 to 1.0 cm bolus
  - Lacrimal and intra- or extraconal involvement: 3DCRT or IMRT

6.10   Nasal Cavity/Paranasal Sinuses

Epidemiology and Risk Factors

- These are uncommon neoplasms, with approximately 4,500 new cases annually in the United States.
- 55% arise in maxillary sinus, 25% in ethmoid sinus, and 20% in nasal cavity.
- Risk factors:
  - Unclear. Possible chemical/occupational associations (sawmill workers/carpenters).

Anatomy and Patterns of Spread

- Nasal vestibule cancers may spread to nodes 15% of the time.
- Nasal vestibule typically drains to facial/buccinators nodes and submandibular nodes.
- Nasal cavity cancers in olfactory region drain to retropharyngeal nodes.
- Nasal cavity cancers in respiratory region rarely spread to nodes.
- Maxillary sinus cancers, if squamous or undifferentiated, have 30% nodal risk (submandibular, jugulodigastric, jugular, and retropharyngeals).
- Tumors superior–posterior to Ohngren's line (medial canthus to angle of mandible) have poorer prognosis.

Presentation

- Nasal vestibule: ulceration, crusting, scabbing, or minor bleeding
- Nasal cavity: nasal obstruction, discharge, or intermittent epistaxis
- Ethmoid sinus: sinus pain, nasal obstruction, proptosis, or diplopia
- Sphenoid sinus: headache, CN palsy (from cavernous sinus invasion), or retro-orbital pain

- Maxillary sinus: sinus pain, oral cavity ulcer, ill-fitting dentures, nasal obstruction, epistaxis, trismus, headache, proptosis, or diplopia

Histology

- 80% are squamous cell carcinomas.
- Other histologies include sinonasal undifferentiated carcinoma (SNUC), sinonasal neuroendocrine carcinoma (SNEC), adenocarcinoma, rhabdomyarsarcoma, lymphoma, plasmacytoma, melanoma, adenoid cystic carcinoma, and esthesioneuroblastoma (nasal cavity).

Diagnosis and Workup

- History and physical with thorough head and neck examination, including nasal endoscopy and palpation of all neck levels
- Biopsy
- CT head and neck
- Consider MRI skull base
- Consider PET/CT for stage III/IV disease
- Chest x-ray
- Routine laboratory studies

Staging (AJCC 7th Edition)

T-stage	
Tx	Primary tumor cannot be assessed
T0	No evidence of primary tumor
Tis	Carcinoma in situ

Maxillary Sinus

T1	Tumor limited to maxillary sinus mucosa with no erosion or destruction of bone
T2	Tumor causing bone erosion or destruction including extension into the hard palate and/or middle nasal meatus, except extension to posterior wall of maxillary sinus and pterygoid plates
T3	Tumor invades any of the following—bone of the posterior wall of maxillary sinus, subcutaneous tissues, floor or medial wall of orbit, pterygoid fossa, ethmoid sinuses
T4a	Tumor invades anterior orbital contents, skin of cheek, pterygoid plates, infratemporal fossa, cribriform plate, sphenoid or frontal sinuses
T4b	Tumor invades any of the following orbital apex, dura, brain, middle cranial fossa, cranial nerves other than maxillary division of trigeminal nerve (V2), nasopharynx, or clivus

Nasal Cavity and Ethmoid Sinus

T1	Tumor restricted to any one subsite, with or without bony invasion
T2	Tumor invading two subsites in a single region or extending to involve an adjacent region within the nasoethmoidal complex, with or without bony invasion
T3	Tumor extends to invade the medial wall or floor of the orbit, maxillary sinus, palate, or cribriform plate

(continued)

(continued)

T-stage

T4a	Tumor invades any of the following anterior orbital contents, skin of nose or cheek, minimal extension to anterior cranial fossa, pterygoid plates, sphenoid or frontal sinuses
T4b	Tumor invades any of the following orbital apex, dura, brain, middle cranial fossa, cranial nerves other than (V2), nasopharynx, or clivus

N-stage

N0	No regional lymph node metastasis
N1	Metastasis in a single ipsilateral lymph node, 3 cm or less in greatest dimension
N2a	Metastasis in single ipsilateral lymph node more than 3 cm but not more than 6 cm in greatest dimension
N2b	Metastasis in multiple ipsilateral lymph nodes, none more than 6 cm in greatest dimension
N2c	Metastasis in bilateral or contralateral lymph nodes, none more than 6 cm in greatest dimension
N3	Metastasis in a lymph node more than 6 cm in greatest dimension

M-stage

M0	No distant metastases
M1	Distant metastases

Group Stage	T	N	M
0	Tis	N0	M0
I	T1	N0	M0
II	T2	N0	M0
III	T3	N0	M0
	T1–3	N1	M0
IVA	T4a	N0–1	M0
	T1–4a	N2	M0
IVB	Any T	N3	M0
	T4b	Any N	M0
IVC	Any T	Any N	M1

- Kadish Staging System for Esthesioneuroblastoma
  - Stage A   Tumor limited to nasal cavity
  - Stage B   Tumor involving the nasal cavity and paranasal sinuses
  - Stage C   Tumor extends beyond the nasal cavity and paranasal sinuses
  - Stage D   Lymph node or distant metastases

Treatment Overview

- *Nasal cavity/ethmoid sinus*
  - o T1–2: Surgery + postoperative RT (except for T1) (preferred) or definitive RT
  - o T3–4a: Surgery + postoperative RT (preferred) or definitive chemoradiation
  - o T4b or unresectable: definitive chemoradiation
  - o Notes:
    - Consider elective nodal treatment for squamous or undifferentiated tumors (extrapolating from maxillary sinus data).
    - If diagnosed incidentally upon resection of polyps, attempt re-excision to get negative margins.
- *Maxillary sinus*
  - o T1–2N0 (except for adenoid cystic): surgery
    - Postoperative RT for PNI
  - o T1–2N0 (adenoid cystic): surgery
    - Postoperative RT for suprastructure
  - o T3–4N0: surgery + postoperative RT
  - o T4b, Any N: definitive chemoradiation or radiation
  - o T1–4aN+: surgery + postoperative RT
  - o Notes:
    - Re-excision if possible for positive margins.
    - Systemic therapy is a component of care for SNUC.
    - Irradiate neck for T3–4a and node positive.
    - Preferred concurrent chemotherapy: cisplatin 100 mg/m^2 q21 days × 3 cycles.

Radiation Therapy Techniques

- Simulation
  - o Supine, aquaplast, arms down in shoulder pulls, IV contrast, wire all scars, mark canthi. Fill surgical defects with water balloons if present.
- Preoperative diagnostic imaging fused for treatment planning.
- IMRT allows for more dose homogeneity and significantly reduces dose to the spinal cord, allowing for delivery of higher doses without added morbidity.
- Radiation volumes:
  - o Include gross disease, remaining sinus, and portion of adjacent cavities/sinuses
  - o Bilateral neck for greater than T2 esthesioneuroblastoma
  - o Bilateral necks for T3–4 or node positive squamous cell carcinomas
- Radiation dose:
  - o RT alone: 70 Gy in 35 fractions or altered fractionation
  - o Chemoradiation: 70 Gy in 35 fractions
  - o Postoperative radiation: 60 Gy conventionally fractionated

6.11 Ear

Epidemiology and Risk Factors

- Most ear cancers start on the skin of the outer ear.
- Primary cancers of the inner ear are rare.
- Risk factors:
  - o Same as for other cutaneous squamous cell carcinomas
  - o Chronic ear infections

Anatomy and Patterns of Spread

- The ear comprises pinna, external auditory canal, tympanic membrane, and inner ear.
- Lymph node drainage is to parotid, cervical, and postauricular nodes.

Presentation

- Presenting symptoms depend on location of tumor.
  - External ear: persistent lesion
  - Middle ear: bloody discharge, hearing loss, earache
  - Inner ear: headache, hearing loss, tinnitus, dizziness

Histology

- Most are squamous cell carcinomas.
- Other histologies include: basal cell carcinoma, melanoma, and adenocarcinoma.

Diagnosis and Workup

- History and physical exam including complete skin exam, otoscopy, and palpation of regional nodal groups
- Biopsy
- CT head and neck
- Consider MRI
- Routine laboratory studies
- Chest x-ray
- Audiologic testing

Staging

- No site-specific AJCC staging. Use histology appropriate staging.

Treatment Overview

- External ear: primary surgery or RT
  - Surgery preferred for cartilage or auditory canal involvement.
  - Postoperative RT for close/positive margins, greater than 4 cm tumor, or cartilage invasion.
- Middle ear: primary surgery preferred
  - Postoperative RT in almost all cases given high risk of locoregional recurrence.
- Toxicities:
  - Hearing loss
  - Chronic otitis media
  - Cartilage or temporal bone necrosis

Radiation Therapy Techniques

- Simulation: supine, head and shoulder mask
- Use wax bolus to fill external auditory canal and around external ear to improve homogeneity.
- Pinna: orthovoltage x-rays or electrons
- External auditory canal/middle ear: 3D conformal or IMRT
  - Target volume should include ear canal and temporal bone with 2 to 3 cm margin, and ipsilateral preauricular, postauricular, and level II cervical lymph nodes.
- Dose:
  - Pinna: 50 to 60 Gy in 25 to 30 fractions
  - External auditory canal/middle ear: 66 to 70 Gy in 33 to 35 fractions (definitive); 60 Gy in 30 fractions (postoperative)

6.12   Skin—Nonmelanoma

Epidemiology and Risk Factors

- Basal and squamous cell carcinomas of the skin are the most common cancers in the United States with over 1 million new cases annually.
- Basal cell carcinoma is four times more common than squamous cell carcinoma.
- Risk factors:
  - Sun exposure
  - Chemical carcinogen exposure
  - Chronic irritation or inflammation
  - Ionizing radiation
  - Immunodeficiency
  - Genetic predisposition (xeroderma pigmentosum, basal cell nevus syndrome)

Anatomy and Patterns of Spread

- Basal cell carcinomas are generally slow growing over many years.
  - Spread to lymph nodes or distant organs is rare, less than 0.01%.
- Squamous cell carcinomas usually are more aggressive than basal cell carcinomas.
  - Incidence of regional metastasis at diagnosis is 2%; eventually 10% develop regional metastasis.
  - Prognosticators for spread include anatomic site, duration and size of the lesion, depth of dermal invasion, perineural invasion, and degree of differentiation.

Presentation

- Basal cell carcinomas most commonly present on the head and neck region, appearing as an asymptomatic nodule, pruritic plaque, or bleeding sore.
  - Variants include nodular-ulcerative, superficial, morphea-form, sclerosing, infiltrative, and terebrant

Histology

- Squamous cell carcinomas most commonly develop from skin exhibiting solar damage.
  - Less commonly, they arise from a thermal burn scar or chronic ulcer.
  - Actinic keratosis is a precursor of squamous cell carcinomas.
  - Variants include superficial, infiltrative, and spindle cell.

Diagnosis and Workup

- History and physical exam including complete skin exam and palpation of regional nodal groups
- Imaging studies obtained as indicated
- MRI for all patients in whom perineural spread is suspected
- Biopsy

Staging (AJCC 7th Edition Staging—Squamous Cell Carcinoma)

T-stage	
Tx	Primary tumor cannot be assessed
T0	No evidence of primary tumor
Tis	Carcinoma in situ

(continued)

(continued)

T-stage

T1	Tumor 2 cm or less in greatest dimension with less than two high-risk features*
T2	Tumor greater than 2 cm in greatest dimension or tumor any size with two or more high-risk features*
T3	Tumor with invasion of maxilla, orbit, or temporal bone
T4	Tumor with invasion of skeleton (axial or appendicular) or perineural invasion of skull base

N-stage

N0	No regional lymph node metastasis
N1	Metastasis in a single ipsilateral lymph node, 3 cm or less in greatest dimension
N2a	Metastasis in single ipsilateral lymph node more than 3 cm but not more than 6 cm in greatest dimension
N2b	Metastasis in multiple ipsilateral lymph nodes, none more than 6 cm in greatest dimension
N2c	Metastasis in bilateral or contralateral lymph nodes, none more than 6 cm in greatest dimension
N3	Metastasis in a lymph node more than 6 cm in greatest dimension

M-stage

M0	No distant metastases
M1	Distant metastases

*High-Risk Features for the Primary Tumor (T) Staging:

- Depth/Invasion: greater than 2 mm thickness, Clark level Ñ IV, Perineural invasion
- Anatomic Location: Primary site ear, Primary site hair-bearing lip
- Differentiation: Poorly differentiated or undifferentiated

Group Stage	T	N	M
0	Tis	N0	M0
I	T1	N0	M0
II	T2	N0	M0
III	T3	N0	M0
	T1–3	N1	M0
IV	T1–3	N2	M0
	Any T	N3	M0
	T4	Any N	M0
	Any T	Any N	M1

Treatment Overview

- Primary treatment is wide excision with negative margins.
- If clinically lymph node positive, regional lymph node dissection recommended.
- Primary RT given for nonsurgical patients.
- Adjuvant RT recommended for node positive disease, greater than 3 cm primary, perineural invasion, bone/cartilage/muscle invasion, and recurrent disease.
- Adjuvant chemoradiation recommended for positive margins or extracapsular extension.
- A hedgehog pathway inhibitor should be considered for unresectable basal cell carcinomas.

Radiation Therapy Techniques

- Simulation depends on location.
- Superficial/orthovoltage x-rays and electrons are most commonly used.
- Tissue equivalent bolus is used for adequate skin surface dose.
- Use eye shields as needed to protect lens.
- Use wax-covered lead shield as needed to shield teeth, mandible, and nasal cavity.
- Protracted fractionation is associated with improved cosmetic results.
- Primary RT:
  - Less than 2 cm: 64 Gy in 32 fractions; 55 Gy in 20 fractions; 50 Gy in 15 fractions; 35 Gy in 5 fractions.
  - Greater than 2 cm: 66 Gy in 33 fractions; 55 Gy in 20 fractions.
- Adjuvant RT: 50 Gy in 20 fractions; 60 Gy in 30 fractions.
- Primary regional nodal RT: 66 to 70 Gy in 2 33 to 35 fractions.
- Adjuvant regional nodal RT: 56 to 66 Gy in 28 to 33 fractions.

6.13 Skin—Melanoma

Epidemiology and Risk Factors

- There are 76,000 cases annually in the United States. Incidence continues to rise.
- Median age at diagnosis is 59 years.
- Risk factors:
  - History of melanoma, atypical moles, or dysplastic nevi
  - Rarely, familial susceptibility
  - Fair skin and an inability to tan.

Anatomy and Patterns of Spread

- 85% present with localized disease, 10% present with regional disease, and 5% present with metastatic disease.
- Nodal involvement is the strongest prognostic factor.

Presentation

- Typically present with suspicious pigmented lesion

Diagnosis and Workup

- History and physical exam including complete skin exam and palpation of regional nodal groups
- Excisional biopsy of primary with 1 to 3 mm margins to make diagnosis
  - If excisional biopsy not feasible, then full thickness punch biopsy of thickest part is reasonable
- Assessing pathology with Breslow thickness, mitotic rate, and ulceration best predict risk of lymph node metastases

- Sentinel lymph node biopsy:
  - ○ Need not be offered to stage IA patients without adverse features.
  - ○ Indicated for tumor thickness of 0.75 to 1 mm and adverse features such as young age, ulceration, high mitotic rate, positive deep margin can be considered.
  - ○ Indicated for tumor thickness ≥ 1 mm.
  - ○ Note: pure desmoplastic melanomas that have been confirmed as such by dermatopathologist have very low incidence of LN metastases. SLN biopsy is contraindicated in these patients.
- Patients with a positive sentinel node or clinically positive nodes should be considered for nodal dissection.

Stage (AJCC 7th Edition)

T-stage	
Tx	Primary tumor cannot be assessed
T0	No evidence of primary tumor
Tis	Melanoma in situ
T1	<1.0 mm in thickness
T1a	Without ulceration and mitosis <1/mm^2
T1b	With ulceration or mitoses > 1/mm^2
T2	1.01–2.0 mm in thickness
T2a	Without ulceration
T2b	With ulceration
T3	2.01–4.0 mm in thickness
T3a	Without ulceration
T3b	With ulceration
T4	>4.0 mm in thickness
T4a	Without ulceration
T4b	With ulceration
N-stage	
N0	No regional lymph node metastasis
N1	1 node
N1a	Micrometastasis[*]
N1b	Macrometastasis[†]
N2	2–3 nodes
N2a	Micrometastasis[*]
N2b	Macrometastasis[†]
N2c	In transit met(s)/satellite(s) without metastatic nodes

(continued)

(*continued*)

N-stage

N3	Clinical: ≥1 node with in transit met(s)/satellite(s); Pathologic: 4 or more metastatic nodes, or matted nodes, or in transit met(s)/satellite(s) with metastatic node(s)

M-stage

M0	No distant metastases
M1a	Metastases to skin, subcutaneous tissues, or distant lymph nodes
M1b	Metastases to lung
M1c	Metastases to all other visceral sites or distant metastases to any site combined with an elevated serum LDH

*Micrometastases are diagnosed after sentinel lymph node biopsy and completion lymphadenectomy (if performed).

†Macrometastases are defined as clinically detectable nodal metastases confirmed by therapeutic lymphadenectomy or when nodal metastasis exhibits gross extracapsular extension.

Clinical Group Stage	T	N	M
0	Tis	N0	M0
IA	T1a	N0	M0
IB	T1b–2a	N0	M0
IIA	T2b–3a	N0	M0
IIB	T3b–4a	N0	M0
IIC	T4b	N0	M0
III	Any T	N1–3	M0
IV	Any T	Any N	M1

Pathologic Group Stage	T	N	M
0	Tis	N0	M0
IA	T1a	N0	M0
IB	T1b–2a	N0	M0
IIA	T2b–3a	N0	M0
IIB	T3b–4a	N0	M0
IIC	T4b	N0	M0
IIIA	T1–4a	N1a	M0
	T1–4a	N2a	M0
IIIB	T1–4b	N1a	M0
	T1–4b	N2a	M0

(*continued*)

(continued)

Clinical Group Stage	T	N	M
	T1–4a	N1b	M0
	T1–4a	N2b	M0
	T1–4a	N2c	M0
IIIC	T1–4b	N1b	M0
	T1–4b	N2b	M0
	T1–4b	N2c	M0
	Any T	N3	M0
IV	Any T	Any N	M1

Treatment Overview

- Primary treatment is wide excision with or without sentinel node biopsy (see prior section for sentinel lymph node biopsy).

Tumor Thickness	Recommended Clinical Margins
In situ	0.5–1.0 cm
≤1.0 mm	1.0 cm
1.01–2 mm	1–2 cm
2.01–4 mm	2 cm
>4 mm	2 cm

- Adjuvant RT is given in select settings.
- Treatment of the primary site with RT is not typically necessary.
  - Exception is desmoplastic variant with neurotropism. Consider adjuvant treatment in this histology, particularly if margins are questionable.
- Nodal basin irradiation improves locoregional control but not overall survival.
  - Locoregional failure rates after resection and RT are 5% to 10%.
  - Consider adjuvant RT to nodal sites for
    - ≥1 involved parotid node, any size of involvement
    - ≥2 involved cervical nodes or ≥3 cm tumor within a node
    - ≥2 involved axillary nodes or ≥4cm tumor within a node
    - ≥3 involved inguinal nodes or ≥4cm tumor within a node
    - Any ECE
    - In groin consider strongly giving only RT for two of these risk factors if BMI greater than 25.
- In stages IIB and IIC, offer interferon alpha or clinical trial.
- In stage III, offer clinical trial.
- In stage IV, offer systemic therapy including Ipilimumab, Vemurafenib, Dabrafenib, or high-dose IL-2, or clinical trial.

- Consider palliative resection or RT for symptomatic disease.
  - Toxicity:
    - Dermatitis, hematopoetic suppression, but most worrisome lymphedema.
    - Risk of complications significantly related to BMI:
      - BMI of 25 to 30 or greater associated with increased risk.
    - Risk of lymphedema from cervical RT is low.
    - Axillary grade 3 to 4 lymphedema occurred in 8% of TROG patients and the rate of clinically significant edema was 42%.
    - Inguinal lymphedema much more common, with estimates at 4 years of 30% to 50% of grade 3.

Radiation Therapy Techniques

- Simulation depends on location
  - Open neck position for neck
  - Akimbo for axilla
  - Frog legged for inguinal
- Dose: 30 Gy in five fractions biweekly
- Organs at risk:
  - Limit brain, spinal cord, and bowel to less than 24 Gy.

6.14 Salivary Gland

Epidemiology and Risk Factors

- There are approximately 2,500 new cases annually in the United States.
- Incidence is equivalent in males and females.
- Average age at diagnosis is 55 years.
- Salivary glands are composed of two main groups: major and minor.
  - Major salivary glands include parotid, submandibular, and sublingual.
  - Minor salivary glands line the mucosa of the upper aerodigestive tract, with common sites including the hard palate, buccal mucosa, oropharynx, nasal cavity, and paranasal sinuses.
- Parotid gland cancers account for 80% to 90% of all malignant salivary gland tumors.
- 15% to 30% of parotid gland tumors are malignant.
- 50% of submandibular gland tumors are malignant.
- 80% of sublingual gland tumors are malignant.
- The majority of minor salivary gland tumors are malignant.
- Suggested risk factors: nutritional deficiencies (vitamins A and C), exposure to ionizing radiation, UV exposure, genetic predisposition, history of previous cancer of the skin of the face, occupational exposure, viral infection (EBV), and alcohol use.

Anatomy and Patterns of Spread

- Parotid gland is divided into deep and superficial lobes by the facial nerve.
- Parotid glands drain into oral cavity via Stensen's duct.
- Submandibular glands drain into oral cavity via Wharton's duct.
- Sublingual glands drain into oral cavity via Bartholin's duct.
- Most common pattern of spread is by local infiltration and perineural extension.
- Hematogenous spread is more common than regional lymph node metastases:
  - Distant metastases most commonly involve lungs, bones, and liver.
  - Adenoid cystic carcinomas metastasize distantly in approximately 50% cases.
  - Minor salivary gland cancers metastasize distantly in approximately 25% cases.

- Lymph node metastases vary depending on histology, T-stage, site of origin, and grade.
- Lymphatic drainage:
  o Parotid gland: intraparotid, I to III.
  o Submandibular gland: I to III.
  o Sublingual gland: I to III.

Presentation

- Signs and symptoms:
  o Malignant parotid cancers: painless, rapidly enlarging mass; facial weakness, pain, numbness, cranial neuropathy
  o Submandibular gland cancers: mildly tender mass; cranial nerve V, VII (marginal branch), and XII involvement (advanced lesions)
  o Minor salivary gland cancers: symptoms dependent on site of origin

Histology

- Classification of malignant salivary gland tumors:
  o Carcinoma ex pleomorphic adenoma
  o Adenoid cystic carcinoma
  o Mucoepidermoid carcinoma
  o Adenocarcinoma (NOS)
  o Acinic cell carcinoma
  o Squamous cell carcinoma
  o Myoepithelial carcinoma
  o Cystadenocarcinoma
  o Small cell carcinoma
  o Polymorphous low-grade adenocarcinoma
  o Epithelial myoepithelial carcinoma
  o Clear cell carcinoma (NOS)
  o Basal cell adenocarcinoma
  o Salivary duct carcinoma
  o Carcinoma-sarcoma
  o Metastasizing pleomorphic adenoma
  o Large cell undifferentiated carcinoma
  o Lymphoepithelial carcinoma
  o Other rare histologies

Diagnosis and Workup

- History and physical exam including complete head and neck exam including palpation of all neck level and thorough cranial nerve exam
- FNA biopsy of mass
  o Avoid incisional or excisional biopsy because it is associated with higher rate of local recurrence
- CT head and neck and MRI head and neck can be complementary in evaluating tumor depth and local extension
- Chest x-ray
- PET for high-grade aggressive lesions
- Routine laboratory studies
- Dental evaluation, nutrition evaluation, speech and swallowing evaluation, and audiology testing
  o Consider prophylactic feeding tube placement in patients receiving chemoradiation

Staging (AJCC 7th Edition)

T-stage

Tx	Primary tumor cannot be assessed
T0	No evidence of primary tumor
T1	Tumor 2 cm or less in greatest dimension without extraparenchymal extension
T2	Tumor more than 2 cm but not more than 4 cm in greatest dimension without extraparenchymal extension
T3	Tumor more than 4 cm and/or tumor having extraparenchymal extension
T4a	Tumor invades skin, mandible, ear canal, and/or facial nerve
T4b	Tumor invades skull base and/or pterygoid plates and/or encases carotid artery

N-stage

N0	No regional lymph node metastasis
N1	Metastasis in a single ipsilateral lymph node, 3 cm or less in greatest dimension
N2a	Metastasis in single ipsilateral lymph node more than 3 cm but not more than 6 cm in greatest dimension
N2b	Metastasis in multiple ipsilateral lymph nodes, none more than 6 cm in greatest dimension
N2c	Metastasis in bilateral or contralateral lymph nodes, none more than 6 cm in greatest dimension
N3	Metastasis in a lymph node more than 6 cm in greatest dimension

M-stage

M0	No distant metastases
M1	Distant metastases

Group Stage	T	N	M
0	Tis	N0	M0
I	T1	N0	M0
II	T2	N0	M0
III	T3	N0	M0
	T1–3	N1	M0
IVA	T4a	N0–1	M0
	T1–4a	N2	M0

(continued)

(continued)

Group Stage	T	N	M
IVB	Any T	N3	M0
	T4b	Any N	M0
IVC	Any T	Any N	M1

Treatment Overview

- Primary treatment is surgical resection.
  - Exceptions include medically inoperable patients, patients who refuse surgery, distant metastases, unresectable cancers, cancers in which surgical resection would result in significant and unacceptable functional or cosmetic deficits.
- Parotid cancers are typically resected by superficial parotidectomy.
- Deep lobe removal depends on location, extent, and histology.
- Facial nerve is generally preserved unless nerve is grossly encased or involved with cancer.
- Neck dissection indicated for palpable adenopathy or a high-grade primary cancer with aggressive histologic features and high risk of subclinical nodal metastases.
- Primary RT (high-dose conventional EBRT, brachytherapy, neutron beam therapy) can be used for unresectable cancers or for palliation.
- No clear role for chemotherapy in definitive setting.
- Indications for postoperative RT: close/positive margins, high-grade cancer, involvement of skin or bone, involvement of nerve (gross invasion or extensive PNI), tumor extension beyond capsule of gland, lymph node metastases, large tumors requiring radical resection, tumor spillage, recurrent cancer.
- For patients with large primary cancer, high-grade cancer, high-risk histologic features (small cell carcinoma, malignant mixed tumors, mucoepidermoid carcinoma, adenocarcinoma), or high-risk (lymphatic rich) primary tumor site, elective neck dissection or elective neck irradiation is indicated.
- Consider palliative resection or RT for symptomatic disease.

Radiation Therapy Techniques

- Simulation: supine, shoulder pulls, head and shoulder mask
  - Wire lymph nodes, surgical scars, oral commissure
  - Bite block
  - Mouthguards
- Preoperative diagnostic imaging fused for treatment planning
- IMRT is favored for improved homogeneity and reduced dose to contralateral critical structures.
  - Other options include wedge pair or mixed photon/electrons
- Treat primary tumor bed alone for low grade, node-negative patients.
- Consider elective neck RT for high-grade clinically node-negative tumors.
- Treat entire ipsilateral neck RT for node-positive tumors.
- For extensive nerve invasion or adenoid cystic histology, cover nerve pathway up to the base of the skull.
- Radiation dose:
  - Postoperative dose is 60 Gy standard fractionation; consider boost when indicated.
  - Elective neck irradiation dose is 50 to 54 Gy standard fractionation.
  - Definitive dose is at least 66 Gy.

- Organs at risk:
  - Spinal cord: max 45 Gy
  - Brainstem: max 54 Gy
  - Optic chiasm and nerves: max 54 Gy.
  - Temporal brain: max 60 Gy
  - Mandible: max 70 Gy

Chapter 6: Practice Questions

1. Subglottic cancers are what percentage of all larynx cancers?

   A. <5%
   B. 10%
   C. 15%
   D. 20%

2. The primary indication for the use of concurrent chemoradiation for unknown head and neck primary cancer is

   A. Large primary cancer
   B. Primary tumor site
   C. Nodal status
   D. Tumor grade

3. The most frequent site of oral cavity cancer is located at

   A. Lips
   B. Tongue
   C. Floor of mouth
   D. Hard palate

4. Cancer of the inner ear is usually associated with the following signs/symptoms EXCEPT

   A. Bloody discharge
   B. Headache
   C. Hearing loss
   D. Tinnitus

5. Bilateral nodal metastases from nasopharygeal cancer no greater than 2 cm is N staged as

   A. N1
   B. N2
   C. N3a
   D. N3b

6. Which of the following tumors can present with cranial nerve palsies?

   A. Ethmoid sinus
   B. Sphenoid sinus
   C. Maxillary sinus
   D. Nasal cavity

7. Any skin cancer with orbital involvement is T staged as

   A. T3
   B. T4
   C. T4a
   D. T4b

8. Indications for postoperative head and neck radiation include the following EXCEPT

    A. Multiple node positivity
    B. Large nodal size
    C. Extracapsular extension
    D. Tumor grade

9. All these subtypes of oropharynx cancer have a 70% risk of nodal involvement EXCEPT

    A. Soft palate
    B. Base of tongue
    C. Tonsillar pillar
    D. Tonsillar fossa

10. The nodal drainage of the ear is usually to all of the following EXCEPT

    A. Parotid nodes
    B. Cervical nodes
    C. Postauricular nodes
    D. Scalene nodes

11. Nasal cavity tumors that invade the frontal sinuses are best T staged as

    A. T3
    B. T4
    C. T4a
    D. T4b

12. The following are all risk factors for lymphatic spread of oral cavity cancer EXCEPT

    A. Depth of invasion
    B. Primary tumor site
    C. T stage
    D. Grade

13. The least frequently seen subtype of thyroid cancer is

    A. Anaplastic
    B. Medullary
    C. Follicular
    D. Papillary

14. A typical dose for areas of ECE or positive margin in the context of postoperative radiation in oropharynx cancer is

    A. 54 Gy
    B. 57 Gy
    C. 60 Gy
    D. 66 Gy

15. All of the following are associated with the development of thyroid cancer EXCEPT

    A. Radiation exposure
    B. MEN-1 syndrome
    C. Cowden's syndrome
    D. Gardner's syndrome

16. The most frequent histology associated with cancer of the ear is

    A. Basal cell carcinoma
    B. Melanoma
    C. Adenocarcinoma
    D. Squamous cell carcinoma

17. A CTV54 for postoperative head and neck radiation is usually used to

    A. Cover the high-risk tumor bed

    B. Cover the entire operative bed

    C. Cover the involved nodal areas

    D. Cover surgically undisturbed sites at microscopic risk of disease

18. The usual recommended time to start postoperative RT after head and neck surgery is generally

    A. Within a week of surgery

    B. 2 to 3 weeks

    C. 4 to 6 weeks

    D. 8 to 12 weeks

19. All of the following are typical dose fractionation schedules for T1 or T2 radical intent larynx cancer EXCEPT

    A. 66 Gy in 33 fractions

    B. 70 Gy in 35 fractions

    C. 63 Gy in 28 fractions

    D. 60 Gy in 30 fractions

20. Submandibular glands drain into the oral cavity through

    A. Stensen's duct

    B. Wharton's duct

    C. Barholin's duct

    D. Cuvier duct

Chapter 6: Answers

1. A
2/3 of larynx cancers are glottic, 1/3 are supraglottic, and 2% are subglottic.

2. C
Concurrent chemotherapy indicated for N2 and N3 unknown primary head and neck cancer. Preferred concurrent chemotherapy: cisplatin 100 mg/m² q21 days × 3 cycles.

3. A
Distribution of oral cancers by subsite:

Lips	45%
Oral tongue	16%
Floor of mouth	12%
Alveolar ridge	12%
Buccal mucosa	10%
Hard palate	5%

4. A
Presenting symptoms for cancer of the ear depend on location of tumor:
External ear: persistent lesion.
Middle ear: bloody discharge, hearing loss, earache.
Inner ear: headache, hearing loss, tinnitus, dizziness.

5. B
N staging of nasopharynx:
N1: Unilateral metastasis in lymph node(s), 6 cm or less in greatest dimension, above the supraclavicular fossa, and/or unilateral or bilateral, retropharyngeal lymph nodes, 6 cm or less, in greatest dimension
N2: Bilateral metastasis in lymph node(s), 6 cm or less in greatest dimension, above the supraclavicular fossa
N3: Metastasis in a lymph node(s) greater than 6 cm and/or extension to supraclavicular fossa
N3a: Greater than 6 cm in dimension
N3b: Extension to the supraclavicular fossa

6. B
The presentation of sphenoid sinus cancer can include the following:
Headache
CN palsy (from cavernous sinus invasion)
Retro-orbital pain

7. A
T staging of locally advanced skin cancers:
T3: Tumor with invasion of maxilla, orbit, or temporal bone
T4: Tumor with invasion of skeleton (axial or appendicular) or perineural invasion of skull base

8. D
Indications for postoperative RT include:
Advanced stage (T3-T4)
Positive or close surgical margins
Lymphovascular invasion
Perineural invasion
Greater than one positive node
Any single positive node greater than 3 cm
Extracapsular extension

9. A

Clinical nodal involvement at diagnosis
   BOT: 75%
   Tonsillar fossa: 75%
   Tonsillar pillar: 45%
   Soft palate: 45%
   Oropharyngeal wall: 70%

10. D

Anatomy and patterns of spread of cancer of the ear:
   The ear is comprised of pinna, external auditory canal, tympanic membrane, and inner ear.
   Lymph node drainage is to parotid, cervical, and postauricular nodes.

11. C

T staging of advanced nasal cavity tumors:
   T3: Tumor extends to invade the medial wall or floor of the orbit, maxillary sinus, palate, or cribriform plate
   T4a: Tumor invades any of the following: anterior orbital contents, skin of nose or cheek, minimal extension to anterior cranial fossa, pterygoid plates, sphenoid or frontal sinuses
   T4b: Tumor invades any of the following: orbital apex, dura, brain, middle cranial fossa, cranial nerves other than (V2), nasopharynx, or clivus

12. B

Increasing depth of invasion, T-stage, and grade are associated with greater risk of lymph node involvement. Tumor site is associated with nodal levels at risk:
   Upper lip: facial and level IB
   Lower lip: I–III
   Floor of mouth: I–III
   Buccal mucosa: I–III
   Alveolar ridge: levels I–III
   Oral tongue: I–IV

13. A

Pathology of thyroid cancer:
   Papillary thyroid cancer accounts for 40% to 90% cases, usually younger women.
   Follicular thyroid cancer (includes oxyphilic or Hurthle cell variants) accounts for 15% to 40% cases
   Medullary thyroid cancer accounts for 2% to 8% cases
   Anaplastic thyroid cancer accounts for 1% to 5% cases

14. D

Postoperative RT for oropharynx cancer:
   60 Gy to tumor bed + approximately 1 cm margin
   57 Gy to entire primary operative bed and involved neck nodal levels
   54 Gy to intermediate-risk areas outside of operative bed and elective neck
   Consider 66 Gy for areas at very high risk (ECE, positive margin)

15. B

Risk factors for thyroid cancer development:
   Prior ionizing radiation exposure
   Dietary iodine content
   Family history of thyroid cancer
   Multiple endocrine neoplasia type 2 (MEN-2)—medullary thyroid cancer
   Cowden's syndrome—papillary thyroid cancer
   Gardner's syndrome—papillary thyroid cancer

16. D

Most cancers of the ear are squamous cell carcinomas. Other histologies include: basal cell carcinoma, melanoma, and adenocarcinoma.

17. D

Postoperative head and neck radiation:

CTV60 will include tumor bed + ~1 cm margin. Include surgical clips, scar.

CTV57 will include CTV60 + entire primary operative bed and involved neck nodal levels.

CTV54 will include CTV60 as well as surgically undisturbed sites at risk for microscopic disease.

18. C

Postoperative RT should begin within 4 to 6 weeks of surgery. Locoregional control and overall survival better with early RT.

19. D

Dose fractionation schedules for larynx cancer:

T1: 66 Gy in 33 fractions or 63 Gy in 28 fractions

T2: 70 Gy in 35 fractions (6 fractions per week) or 65.25 Gy in 29 fractions

20. B

Parotid glands drain into oral cavity via Stensen's duct. Submandibular glands drain into oral cavity via Wharton's duct. Sublingual glands drain into oral cavity via Bartholin's duct.

Recommended Reading

Adelstein DJ, Li Y, Adams GL, et al. An intergroup phase III comparison of standard radiation therapy and two schedules of concurrent chemoradiotherapy in patients with unresectable squamous cell head and neck cancer. *J Clin Oncol.* 2003;21(1):92-98.

Al-Sarraf M, LeBlanc M, Giri PG, et al. Chemoradiotherapy versus radiotherapy in patients with advanced nasopharyngeal cancer: phase III randomized Intergroup study 0099. *J Clin Oncol.* 1998;16(4):1310-1317.

Ang KK, Harris J, Wheeler R, et al. Human papillomavirus and survival of patients with oropharyngeal cancer. *N Engl J Med.* 2010;363(1):24-35.

Ang KK, Peters LJ, Weber RS, et al. Postoperative radiotherapy for cutaneous melanoma of the head and neck region. *Int J Radiat Oncol Biol Phys.* 1994;30(4):795-798.

Ang KK, Trotti A, Brown BW, et al. Randomized trial addressing risk features and time factors of surgery plus radiotherapy in advanced head-and-neck cancer. *Int J Radiat Oncol Biol Phys.* 2001;51(3):571-578.

Barnes L, Eveson JW, Reichart P, Sidransky D, eds., *World Health Organization Classification of Tumours. Pathology and Genetics of Head and Neck Tumours.* Lyon: IARC Press; 2005.

Barzilai G, Greenberg E, Cohen-Kerem R, Doweck I. Pattern of regional metastases from cutaneous squamous cell carcinoma of the head and neck. *Otolaryngol Head Neck Surg.* 2005;132(6):852-856.

Beitler JJ, Zhang Q, Fu KK. Final results of local-regional control and late toxicity of RTOG 9003: a randomized trial of altered fractionation radiation for locally advanced head and neck cancer. *Int J Radiat Oncol Biol Phys.* 2014;89(1):13-20.

Bernier J, Cooper JS, Pajak TF. Defining risk levels in locally advanced head and neck cancers: a comparative analysis of concurrent postoperative radiation plus chemotherapy trials of the EORTC (#22931) and RTOG (# 9501). *Head Neck.* 2005;27(10):843-850.

Bernier J, Domenge C, Ozsahin M. Postoperative irradiation with or without concomitant chemotherapy for locally advanced head and neck cancer. *N Engl J Med.* 2004;350(19):1945-1952.

Bolek TW, Moyses HM, Marcus RB, Jr. Radiotherapy in the management of orbital lymphoma. *Int J Radiat Oncol Biol Phys.* 1999;44(1):31-36.

Burmeister BH, Mark SB, Burmeister E. A prospective phase II study of adjuvant postoperative radiation therapy following nodal surgery in malignant melanoma: Trans Tasman Radiation Oncology Group (TROG) Study 96.06. *Radiother Oncol.* 2006;81(2):136-142.

Byers RM, Weber RS, Andrews T, McGill D, Kare R, Wolf P. Frequency and therapeutic implications of "skip metastases" in the neck from squamous carcinoma of the oral tongue. *Head Neck.* 1997;19(1):14-19.

Christopherson K, Werning JW, Malyapa RS, Morris CG, Mendenhall WM. Radiotherapy for sinonasal undifferentiated carcinoma. *Am J Otolaryngol.* 2014;35(2):141-146.

Cooper JS, Pajak TF, Forastiere AA, et al. Postoperative concurrent radiotherapy and chemotherapy for high-risk squamous-cell carcinoma of the head and neck. *N Engl J Med.* 2004;350(19):1937-1944.

De Crevoisier R, Baudin E, Bachelot A, et al. Combined treatment of anaplastic thyroid carcinoma with surgery, chemotherapy, and hyperfractionated accelerated external radiotherapy. *Int J Radiat Oncol Biol Phys.* 2004;60(4):1137-1143.

Department of Veterans Affairs Laryngeal Cancer Study Group. Induction chemotherapy plus radiation compared with surgery plus radiation in patients with advanced laryngeal cancer. *N Engl J Med.* 1991;324(24):1685-1690.

Diener-West M, Earle JD, Fine SL, et al. The COMS randomized trial of iodine 125 brachytherapy for choroidal melanoma, III: initial mortality findings. COMS Report No. 18. *Arch Ophthalmol.* 2001;119(7):969-982.

Eisbruch A, Marsh LH, Dawson LA, et al. Recurrences near base of skull after IMRT for head-and-neck cancer: implications for target delineation in high neck and for parotid gland sparing. *Int J Radiat Oncol Biol Phys.* 2004;59(1):28-42.

Forastiere AA, Zhang Q, Weber RS, et al. Long-term results of RTOG 91-11: a comparison of three nonsurgical treatment strategies to preserve the larynx in patients with locally advanced larynx cancer. *J Clin Oncol.* 2013;31(7):845-852.

Grégoire V, Ang K, Budach W, et al. Delineation of the neck node levels for head and neck tumors: a 2013 update. DAHANCA, EORTC, HKNPCSG, NCIC CTG, NCRI, RTOG, TROG consensus guidelines. *Radiother Oncol.* 2014;110(1):172-181.

Grégoire V, Eisbruch A, Hamoir M, Levendag P. Proposal for the delineation of the nodal CTV in the node-positive and the post-operative neck. *Radiother Oncol.* 2006;79(1):15-20.

Hawkins BS; Collaborative Ocular Melanoma Study Group. The Collaborative Ocular Melanoma Study (COMS) randomized trial of pre-enucleation radiation of large choroidal melanoma: IV. Ten-year mortality findings and prognostic factors. COMS report number 24. *Am J Ophthalmol.* 2004;138(6):936-951.

Katz TS, Mendenhall WM, Morris CG, Amdur RJ, Hinerman RW, Villaret DB. Malignant tumors of the nasal cavity and paranasal sinuses. *Head Neck.* 2002;24(9):821-829.

Ko HC, Gupta V, Mourad WF, et al. A contouring guide for head and neck cancers with perineural invasion. *Pract Radiat Oncol.* 2014;4(6):e247-e258.

Le QT, Fu KK, Kroll S, et al. Influence of fraction size, total dose, and overall time on local control of stage T1–T2 glottic carcinoma. *Int J Radiat Oncol Biol Phys.* 1997;39(1):115-126.

Lee N, Harris J, Garden AS, et al. Intensity-modulated radiation therapy with or without chemotherapy for nasopharyngeal carcinoma: radiation therapy oncology group phase II trial 0225. *J Clin Oncol.* 2009;27(22):3684-3690.

Lefebvre JL, Andry G, Chevalier D, et al. Laryngeal preservation with induction chemotherapy for hypopharyngeal squamous cell carcinoma: 10-year results of EORTC trial 24891. *Ann Oncol.* 2012;23(10):2708-2714.

Liebowitz D. Nasopharyngeal carcinoma: the Epstein–Barr virus association. *Semin Oncol.* 1994;21(3):376-381.

Nag S, Quivey JM, Earle JD, et al. The American Brachytherapy Society recommendations for brachytherapy of uveal melanomas. *Int J Radiat Oncol Biol Phys.* 2003;56(2):544-555.

O'Sullivan B, Warde P, Grice B, et al. The benefits and pitfalls of ipsilateral radiotherapy in carcinoma of the tonsillar region. *Int J Radiat Oncol Biol Phys.* 2001;51(2):332-343.

Overgaard J, Hansen HS, Specht L, et al. Five compared with six fractions per week of conventional radiotherapy of squamous-cell carcinoma of head and neck: DAHANCA 6 and 7 randomised controlled trial. *Lancet.* 2003;362(9388):933-940.

Posner MR, Hershock DM, Blajman CR, et al. Cisplatin and fluorouracil alone or with docetaxel in head and neck cancer. *N Engl J Med.* 2007;357(17):1705-1715.

Richter SM, Friedmann P, Mourad WF, et al. Postoperative radiation therapy for small, low-/intermediate-grade parotid tumors with close and/or positive surgical margins. *Head Neck.* 2012;34(7):953-955.

Schwartz DL, Lobo MJ, Ang KK, et al. Postoperative external beam radiotherapy for differentiated thyroid cancer: outcomes and morbidity with conformal treatment. *Int J Radiat Oncol Biol Phys.* 2009;74(4):1083-1091.

Terezakis S, Lee KS, Ghossein RA, et al. Role of external beam radiotherapy in patients with advanced or recurrent nonanaplastic thyroid cancer: Memorial Sloan-Kettering Cancer Center experience. *Int J Radiat Oncol Biol Phys.* 2009;73(3):795-801.

Terhaard CH, Lubsen H, Rasch CR, et al. The role of radiotherapy in the treatment of malignant salivary gland tumors. *Int J Radiat Oncol Biol Phys.* 2005;61(1):103-111.

Tupchong L, Scott CB, Blitzer PH, et al. Randomized study of preoperative versus postoperative radiation therapy in advanced head and neck carcinoma: long-term follow-up of RTOG study 73-03. *Int J Radiat Oncol Biol Phys.* 1991;20(1):21-28.

Yamazaki H, Nishiyama K, Tanaka E, et al. Radiotherapy for early glottic carcinoma (T1N0M0): results of prospective randomized study of radiation fraction size and overall treatment time. *Int J Radiat Oncol Biol Phys.* 2006;64(1):77-82.

Thoracic Malignancies

Tithi Biswas and Neelesh Sharma

7.1   Non-Small Cell Lung Cancer

Epidemiology

- In 2015, an estimated 221,200 new cases will be diagnosed in the United States, second common cancer in both men and women.
- It is the leading cause of death in both sexes with an estimated 158,040 deaths accounting for nearly one-third of all cancer deaths.
- Globally, the reported incidence of lung cancer in 2012 was about 1.8 million with an estimated 1.59 million deaths per year.
- In the United States, the 5-year survival rate is only 17%.
- Smoking is the number one risk factor for developing lung cancer.
- Exposure to asbestos, arsenic, cadmium, chromium, nickel, vinyl chloride, and radon gas are also known carcinogenic to develop lung cancer.
- Lung cancer is still more common among men although the incidence rates are noted to have fallen in the recent decades in several regions of the world.
- It is a disease of old age with median age of diagnosis around 65 years.

Pathology

- Adenocarcinoma is now the most common histologic type followed by squamous cell carcinoma and large cell carcinoma.
- Other less common subtypes are bronchogenic carcinoid, adenosquamous carcinoma.
- Adenocarcinomas are categorized as preinvasive, minimally invasive, and invasive groups.
- Invasive adenocarcinoma is further subdivided into lepidic predominant, papillary, micropapillary, and solid predominant with mucin production.

Genetic Characterization

- In recent years, better understanding of cellular and genetic characteristics of non-small cell lung cancer (NSCLC) has emerged.
- Several driver mutations have been identified particularly for adenocarcinoma histology.
- Such driver mutation has targeted treatment that can yield dramatic results.

See the following table for a complete list of mutations and targeted agents that are available. Not all agents have been proven to have efficacy in NSCLC.

Genetic Alteration	Frequency	Test	Targeted Agents
Nonsquamous			
KRAS mutation	25%	Sequence	None
EGFR mutation	15%	Sequence	Gefitinib, erlotinib, afatinib
EML4-ALK rearrangement	5%–7%	FISH	Crizotinib, ceritinib
ROS1 rearrangement	1%–2%	FISH	Crizotinib
HER-2 mutation	2%–4%	Sequence	Traztuzumab, pertuzumab, lapatinib, afatinib
BRAF mutation	2%–3%	Sequence	Vemurafenib, dabrafenib
RET rearrangement	1%–2%	FISH	Carbozanatinib
MET mutation	1%–2%	Sequence	None
MEK1 mutation	<1%	Sequence	None
PIK3CA mutation	1%–2%	Sequence	None
Squamous			
FGFR1 amplification	20%–25%	FISH	None
FGFR1 mutation	5%	Sequence	None
PIK3CA mutation	5%–10%	Sequence	None
DDR2 mutation	3%–5%	Sequence	Dasatanib
PTEN mutation/deletion	15%–20%	Sequence	None

FISH, fluorescence in situ hybridization.

Screening

- Chest radiograph (CXR) has no role in lung cancer screening.
- Currently, low-dose computed tomographic (LDCT) scan is recommended in healthy current or former smokers (≥30 pack years of smoking, quit <15 years ago), age 55 to 80 years.

Presentation

- Early stage cancers (15% of cases at diagnosis) often are asymptomatic and found incidentally.
- Locally advanced tumors (35%–40%) cause symptoms by local invasion and extension.
- Large central tumors can present with cough, chest pain, dyspnea, or hemoptysis.
- Left-sided tumors can cause hoarseness of voice due to left recurrent laryngeal nerve paralysis.
- Right-sided tumors can cause superior vena cava (SVC) syndrome. 65% to 90% of SVC syndromes are caused by lung cancer. Small cell lung cancer (SCLC) and squamous cell cancers predominate as the cause of SVC among different lung cancer histology.
- Apical tumors can cause classical Pancoast's syndrome due to invasion of lower brachial plexus, sympathetic chain, and satellite ganglion causing lower brachial plexopathy (C8-T1 nerve roots), Horner's syndrome, and first to second rib invasion causing shoulder and chest wall pain.
- Pleural invasion can cause fluid accumulation with dyspnea, cough, or chest pain, and pericardial invasion can present with tamponade when advanced.
- About 30% to 40% of patients with NSCLC present with distant metastasis and related symptoms at diagnosis.
- Most common sites of distant hematogenous spread are central nervous system (CNS), lung, bones, liver, and adrenal glands.
- CNS involvement can present with nonspecific headaches to focal neurologic deficit. Bone involvement can cause focal pain. Liver involvement can present with right upper quadrant pain.

Diagnosis and Workup

- History and physical (H&P) examination: Decreased breath sound from pleural effusion or collapse of a lobe from airway obstruction, focal neurologic deficit due to CNS involvement.
- Imaging: CXR, CT scans of the chest with or without contrast, FDG PET-CT scans, and brain MRI scans with or without gadolinium. If FDG PET is not available, a CT scan of abdomen-pelvis and a bone scan are recommended.
- Mediastinal nodal staging: FDG-PET has better sensitivity (91%), specificity (86%), negative predictive value (95%), and positive predictive value (74%) compared to CT scan (75% sensitivity and 66% specificity).
- Special diagnostic procedures: In otherwise operable candidates, mediastinum should be confirmed with mediastinoscopy to evaluate upper, middle paratracheal and subcarinal lymph nodes.
- The aortopulmonary (AP window) and subaortic region nodes are best evaluated by anterior mediastinoscopy or Chamberlain procedure.
- Video-assisted thoracoscopy has become a valuable adjunct to mediastinoscopy to evaluate paratracheal, subazygos, hilar, and AP window nodal regions.
- Endobronchial ultra sound (EBUS) has become an excellent tool to assess mediastinum and hilar regions except AP window regions.
- Histological confirmation: Every attempt should be made to confirm histological diagnosis with appropriate immunohistochemical staining.
- For peripheral tumors, CT-guided percutaneous biopsy can be done.
- For central or endobronchial tumors, bronchoscopic biopsy is recommended.
- Pulmonary function test (PFT): For evaluation for surgical candidacy in operable tumors is recommended.
- Laboratory tests: Routine complete blood count (CBC) and comprehensive biochemistry profile to complete the workup.

Staging

The most recent (AJCC 7th edition) stage classification of lung cancer is directed by the International Association for the study of Lung Cancer (IASLC). This current stage classification applies for NSCLC as well as for small cell lung cancer and carcinoids.

Stage classification: T, N, M descriptions are given in the following:

Category	Descriptor Definition	Subgroup
T (Primary Tumor)		
T0	No primary tumor	
T1	Tumor ≤3 cm, surrounded by lung or visceral pleura, not more proximal than the lobar bronchus	
T1a	Tumor ≤2 cm	T1a
T1b	Tumor >2 but ≤3 cm	T1b
T2	Tumor >3 but ≤7 cm or tumor with any of the following:	
	Invades visceral pleura, involves main bronchus ≥2 cm distal to the carina, atelectasis/obstructive pneumonia extending to hilum but not involving the entire lung	
T2a	Tumor >3 but ≤5 cm	T2a
T2b	Tumor >5 but ≤7 cm	T2b
T3	Tumor >7 cm	T3 >7

(continued)

(continued)

Category	Descriptor Definition	Subgroup
T (Primary Tumor)		
	or directly invading chest wall, diaphragm, phrenic nerve, mediastinal pleura, parietal pericardium	*T3*
	or tumor in the main bronchus <2 cm distal to the carina	*T3*
	or atelectasis/obstructive pneumonitis of entire lung	
	or separate tumor nodule(s) in the same lobe	*T3*
T4	Tumor of any size with invasion of heart, great vessels, trachea, recurrent laryngeal nerve, esophagus, vertebral body, or carina	*T4*
	or separate tumor nodule(s) in a different ipsilateral lobe	*T4*
N (Regional Lymph Nodes)		
N0	No regional node metastasis	
N1	Metastasis in ipsilateral peribronchial and/or perihilar lymph nodes and intrapulmonary nodes, including involvement by direct extension	
N2	Metastasis in ipsilateral mediastinal and/or subcarinal lymph node(s)	
N3	Metastasis in contralateral mediastinal, contralateral hilar, ipsilateral, or contralateral scalene or supraclavicular lymph node(s)	
M (Distant Metastasis)		
M0	No distant metastasis	
M1a	Separate tumor nodule(s) in a contralateral lobe	*M1a*
	or tumor with pleural nodules or malignant pleural dissemination	
M1b	Distant metastasis	*M1b*

Stage grouping of lung cancer:

T/M	Subgroup	N0	N1	N2	N3
T1	T1a	IA	IIA	IIIA	IIIB
	T1b	IA	IIA	IIIA	IIIB
T2	T2a	IB	IIA	IIIA	IIIB
	T2b	IIA	IIB	IIIA	IIIB
T3	T3 >7 cm	IIB	IIIA	IIIA	IIIB
	T3 invasion	IIB	IIIA	IIIA	IIIB
	T3 satellite	IIB	IIIA	IIIA	IIIB

(continued)

(continued)

T/M	Subgroup	N0	N1	N2	N3
T4	T4 invasion	IIIA	IIIA	IIIB	IIIB
	T4 ipsilateral nodule	IIIA	IIIA	IIIB	IIIB
M	M1a contralateral lung nodule	IVA	IVA	IVA	IVA
		IVA	IVA	IVA	IVA
	M1a Pleura	IVB	IVB	IVB	IVB
	M1b				

Treatment Overview

In NSCLC, stage is the most important prognostic factors and largely determines the appropriate treatment. For treatment decision, a multidisciplinary approach is recommended.

Surgery

- Usually the mainstay of treatment for early stage disease including stage I and stage II cancer.
- Either open thoracotomy or minimally invasive surgery (video-assisted thoracic surgery [VATS]) is done.
- The American College of Chest Physicians (ACCP) lung cancer guidelines suggest minimally invasive VATS or robotic-assisted resection over open thoracotomy.
- Anatomic lobectomy is preferred surgery over limited resection like wedge or segmental resection. Evidence suggests more local recurrence with limited resection but no difference in survival.

Radiation Therapy

- Usually offered for stage III disease with or without chemotherapy (CT) or medically inoperable stage I or II disease.
- For stages II to III disease, fractionated external beam radiation therapy (EBRT) is used.
- For stages II to III definitive radiation therapy (RT), concurrent CT is recommended over sequential CT in otherwise fit patients.
- For stage I medically inoperable peripheral tumors, stereotactic body radiosurgery is recommended (stereotactic body radiation therapy [SBRT]).
- Adjuvant RT is recommended in positive mediastinal nodal disease after surgery.

Chemotherapy

- CT has become an established treatment modality in majority of NSCLC patients. Usually, a platinum-based doublet is recommended regimen for NSCLC.
- CT has been proven to improve survival in adjuvant setting for stage II and stage III resected disease.
- It is recommended in combination with RT for unresectable stage II and stage III disease.
- Concurrent chemoradiation therapy (CRT) is superior to sequential CRT.
- For resected stage IB, adjuvant CT is controversial.
- For stage IV disease, many effective CT regimens are available in the first-line, second-line, or third-line setting.
- In presence of epidermal growth factor receptor (EGFR) mutation or anaplastic lymphoma kinase (ALK) rearrangement, targeted agents like erlotinib and crizotinib, respectively, are recommended as first-line therapy.

Stage Specific Management for NSCLC

- Stages IA to IB:
  - o Surgical resection preferably with an anatomic lobectomy.
  - o No adjuvant therapy for stage IA disease.
  - o Role of adjuvant CT in stage IB is controversial. In primary tumor greater than 4 cm, it may be considered.
- Stages IIA and B:
  - o Surgical resection is preferred treatment followed by adjuvant CT in good performance patients.
  - o No role of adjuvant RT.
- Stage IIIA with positive N2 disease (potentially resectable as judged by single station mediastinal nodal involvement with <3 cm size):
  - o One approach is neoadjuvant CRT in selected good performance patients who are candidates for lobectomy upfront at institution where there is dedicated thoracic surgeon with expertise in lung cancer surgery.
  - o Alternate approach will be definitive concurrent CRT.
- Stage IIIA unresectable disease and IIIB:
  - o Definitive CRT using either weekly low dose CT (carboplatin-paclitaxel) or cisplatin-etoposide (EP) every week 1 and 3.
  - o Consolidative CT in stages IIIA and B is controversial and has not proven to be beneficial. In clinical practice, however, often considered in fit patients.
- Stages IVA and B:
  - o Systemic therapy mostly in good performance status patients.
  - o Radiation therapy only for palliation of symptoms.

Clinical Stage	Surgery	Radiation Therapy	Chemotherapy
IA (medically fit)	Resection	None	None
IB	Resection	None	>4 cm may be considered adjuvantly
I (medically inoperable), peripheral		SBRT	
II	Resection		Adjuvant CT
IIIA (single mediastinal station or <3-cm nodal size)	Neoadjuvant therapy → resection with lobectomy	Neoadjuvant CRT Or Definitive CRT	Neoadjuvant CRT Or Definitive CRT
Stage IIIA inoperable, IIIB		Definitive RT (CRT)	Definitive CT (CRT)
Stage IV			CT

CRT: chemoradiation therapy; CT, chemotherapy; RT, radiation therapy.

Radiation Therapy Technique

Simulation

- CT simulation with appropriate immobilization using Vac bag or alpha cradle in supine position with both arms above head.
- IV contrast is strongly recommended to delineate the lymph nodes.

- 4D CT is recommended when available to assess tumor motion.
- Fusion with FDG PET-CT scan.

Target Delineation

- GTV: Contrast enhanced gross tumor or FDG avid gross tumor.
- CTV: GTV + 0.5-cm margins
- PTV: CTV plus appropriate margin as assessed on 4D CT scan. Motion management is recommended when available and when motion is greater than 1 cm. The treatment machine can be gated with respiration or an ITV-based approach.

External Beam Radiation Therapy

- 3D-CRT: AP-PA and oblique beams to design conformal dose distribution. 6 to 10 MV beams are preferred.
- IMRT or VMAT: inverse planning and can be used when motion assessment is available in selected patient with locally advanced disease. Image guidance is essential.
- Dose: 60 Gy in 30 fractions is standard dose as definitive treatment for locally advanced disease concurrently with CT.
- In neoadjuvant setting: 45 Gy in 25 fractions with concurrent CT.
- 50.4 Gy in 25 fractions in adjuvant setting for positive mediastinal disease.
- 60 Gy in 30 fractions for positive margins and possibly with concurrent CT in medically fit patients.

Stereotactic Body Radiation Therapy

- For medically inoperable peripheral stage I (T1 and selected T2) NSCLC.
- Adequate quality assurance, motion management, and image guidance are essential to do lung SBRT.
- Dose: Optimum dose and fractionation still continues to evolve.
- Based on phase II prospective study, 56 Gy in 3 fractions is dose of choice.
- Other dose and fractionation regimen are also in practice. A biologically equivalent dose (BED) >100 Gy seems to be needed for optimum local control.

Dose Volume Constraints for Normal Tissue for Fractionated Thoracic Radiation Therapy

Organ	RT Dose Constraints
Spinal cord	<45 Gy
Lungs	Mean lung dose <20 Gy
	V20 <35%–40%
	V10 <45%
	V5 <65%
Esophagus	Mean dose 32 Gy
	To keep volume receiving 60 Gy under 20%
Heart	Mean dose <30 Gy
	1/3rd volume <40 Gy
Brachial plexus	Maximum dose <66 Gy

Superior Sulcus Tumor

- Superior sulcus tumors (SSTs) or Pancoast's tumors account for only 3% of all lung cancers.
- SSTs can occur anteriorly where they can invade major blood vessels such as subclavial artery, middle where they can invade brachial plexus, and posteriorly where they invade stellate ganglia or vertebral bodies.

Symptoms:

- Pain in the shoulder and along scapula or vertebral body. The pain can radiate along ulnar distribution of the arm and to the 4th/5th fingers.
- Involvement of the sympathetic chain or the stellate ganglia can cause Horner's syndrome.
- Involvement of first/second rib can cause severe pain.

Workup:

- CT scan of the chest, abdomen, and pelvis; MRI of the chest to assess resectability
- FDG PET scan and MRI brain
- Mediastinoscopy or EBUS to assess mediastinal nodes
- Histological diagnosis with biopsy

Treatment:

- Resectable:
  - Neoadjuvant CRT with cisplatin-EP followed by surgery
- Unresectable:
  - Definitive CRT
- Radiation therapy (RT) dose:
  - 45 Gy for neoadjuvant treatment
  - 60 Gy for definitive treatment

Follow-Up

- First 2 years: Every 4 to 6 months
- 2 to 5 years: Every 6 to 12 months
- After 5 years: Every year
- H&P examination
- Imaging: CT every 4 to 6 months in the first 2 years, then annually

Toxicity

The risk and severity of radiation toxicity are related to the dose and volume of normal tissue that are exposed to RT, to the presence or absence of underlying comorbidities, and the functional organization of the particular organ at risk.

- General acute and late side effects, including fatigue, skin reaction when undergoing RT.
- Radiation pneumonitis (RP) during and after finishing radiation up to 12 to 18 months. Late side effects include pulmonary fibrosis. RP is dose and volume dependent. With mean lung dose of <20 Gy, V20 <30% to 35% the incidence of significant RT pneumonitis is <20%.
- Esophagitis and Esophageal Stenosis. Acute esophagitis is usually the dose limiting toxicity during treatment and occurs in about 18% of cases during concurrent chemo-radiation. Esophageal stenosis or fistula happens in less than 2% of cases.
- Heart: Acute pericarditis can develop during or within several months after finishing treatment. Other late cardiac toxicities are constrictive pericarditis, ischemic heart disease, valvular disease, and conductive defects.

7.2 Small Cell Lung Cancer

Epidemiology

- The incidence of SCLC is declining worldwide and in the United States.
- The Surveillance Epidemiologic and End result (SEER) database reports that SCLC has decreased from about 17% to 13% of all lung cancers in the past 30 years.
- Smoking is the main etiologic factor to cause SCLC accounting for 97% of cases.
- Only, 2% to 3% of patients with SCLC are never smokers.
- The incidence of SCLC peaked when smoking in men had increased. Since the decrease in smoking patterns among men, the incidence of SCLC has declined steadily, whereas in women it peaked later and only recently has declined slightly.

Pathology

- The diagnosis of SCLC is based primarily on light microscopy.
- The appearance is usually dense sheets of small blue cells with scant cytoplasm, fine granular chromatin, inconspicuous nucleoli, and frequent mitosis and necrosis.
- When a component of NSCLC including squamous cell, adenocarcinoma, or large cell carcinoma is present with SCLC, it is usually termed as "combined SCLC."
- In resected specimen, up to 28% of the time, combined SCLC may occur.
- In difficult cases, immunohistochemical stains can be used to confirm diagnosis. Usually, AE1/AE3, which is a marker for carcinoma, and neuroendocrine markers such as synaptophysin, chromogranin, and CD56 are used.
- SCLC has a high proliferative index with Ki-67 of 80% to 100%.

Genetics

- SCLC has been characterized by frequent inactivation of critical tumor suppressor genes including TP53 (75%–90%) and RB1 (60%–90%).
- Several other genetic alterations have been identified in SCLC including amplification of MYC family, inactivation of PTEN (10%), and amplification of FGFR1 (10%).
- The therapeutic implication of most of these genetic alterations in SCLC has not been well understood.

Diagnosis and Workup

- SCLC can present with constitutional symptoms, symptoms due to intrathoracic disease or due to paraneoplastic syndromes.
- The most common symptoms are fatigue, cough, dyspnea, and weight loss.
- Hemoptysis can be present in 14% of cases.
- SVC obstruction can occur in 10% of cases.
- Rarely, SCLC can present as a solitary pulmonary nodule.
- A majority of patients present with metastases. Brain metastasis can be found in 18% of patients at the time of diagnosis.
- The most common paraneoplastic syndrome is syndrome of inappropriate antidiuretic hormone (SIADH) in 75% of cases. Other: Cushing's syndrome (5%).
- Paraneoplastic neurologic syndromes are: subacute peripheral sensory neuropathy, Eaton–Lambert syndrome, cerebellar degeneration, or retinopathy.
- Most endocrine syndromes improve with successful tumor treatment but neurologic syndromes usually do not resolve, even with antitumor treatment.

Similar to NSCLC:

- H&P examination.
- CT scan of the chest with contrast, MRI brain with gadolinium enhancement, and whole body PET scan. PET scan usually replaces bone scan.
- Laboratory tests: CBC, electrolytes, liver and kidney function tests, and lactic dehydrogenase (LDH).

Staging

- The Veterans Administration Lung Study Group (VALSG) had introduced a simple staging system for SCLC.
- This system divides SCLC into limited stage when disease is confined to one hemithorax that can be encompassed in a reasonable radiation field. All other patients are considered as having extensive disease.
- Currently, the use of TNM staging is recommended for localized disease.

Prognostic Factors

- The most important prognostic factor is the stage.
- Other clinical prognostic factors are performance status, and sex.
- Age is usually not prognostic but older patients have limitations in tolerating aggressive treatment.
- Others are elevated LDH, alkaline phosphatase, and possibly presence of paraneoplastic syndromes.

Treatment Overview

General Recommendations: Depends on Stage of the Disease

- Limited stage:
  - All fit patients with performance status of ECOG 0-2 should receive combination CT with concurrent thoracic RT.
  - Patients who achieve response to CRT should receive prophylactic whole brain RT (prophylactic cranial irradiation [PCI]).
- Extensive stage:
  - Systemic CT is the mainstay of treatment. Patients who achieve response may be considered for PCI.
  - There is possible benefit of adding local therapy to intrathoracic disease in responders and may be considered in selected patients.

Chemotherapy

- SCLC is considered to be a systemic disease with extremely high metastatic potential even in limited stage disease.
- CT is the most important therapy in SCLC and combination CT is superior to single agent.
- The EP and cisplatin have been tested in SCLC to produce superior synergistic activity both in preclinical studies and in clinical trials.
- EP is the standard CT for both limited and extensive stage SCLC.
- Carboplatin can be replaced for cisplatin without compromising outcome and less nonhematologic toxicities.
- Usually four to six cycles of CT for all stages of SCLC appear to be optimal. Currently, there is no role of maintenance CT.

Radiation Therapy

- Limited stage:
  - 90% of patients failed locally when treated with CT alone.
  - The meta-analysis showed an additional 5.4% survival benefit in 3 years when thoracic RT was added to systemic therapy.
  - Dose: 45 Gy with 1.5 Gy per fraction twice a day (BID) is the preferable dose fractionation schedule based on the intergroup study.
  - Given the inconvenience of twice a day radiation, it has not been adopted universally.

- o The alternative dose is 60 Gy in 30 fractions.
- o Currently, two randomized studies (one in the United States and the other one in Europe) are comparing 45-Gy BID standard dose to higher single-day fraction dose of 70 and 66 Gy, respectively.
- o Timing of thoracic RT remains controversial. Several meta-analyses suggested benefit of early thoracic RT.
- o The standard is to start thoracic RT during first or second cycle of CT in good performance status patients.
- o With radiation starting early, the controversy regarding radiation volume is less of an issue.
- o To minimize toxicity without compromising local control, currently involved field RT is employed. No elective nodal RT is recommended if the staging is confirmed with modern PET imaging.
- o The reported nodal failure is low if elective nodal irradiation was omitted.
- Extensive disease:
  - o Role of thoracic RT is more controversial in extensive stage disease.
  - o Several clinical studies have shown benefit of improved local control of thoracic disease with addition of thoracic RT following CT but no improvement in survival.
  - o A recent phase III study reported improved survival at 2 years with thoracic RT after CT. At 1 year, there was no improvement and it was the end-point of the study.
  - o There is currently ongoing study by Radiation Therapy Oncology Group (RTOG) comparing consolidative RT to chest and other metastatic sites.
  - o The recommendation is that it may be considered in selected patients who responded well to systemic therapy with good performance status.

Prophylactic Cranial Irradiation

- Brain metastases are detected in at least 18% of SCLC at diagnosis and increase up to 50% to 80% in patients who survive 2 years.
- Based on the meta-analysis, PCI improves survival by 5% in 3 years after CRT.
- PCI is recommended in all limited stage disease that achieves response to initial CRT.
- PCI dose: 25 Gy using 2.5 Gy per fraction.
- PCI is also recommended in extensive stage disease that achieves a response with systemic therapy based on recent EORTC study.

Toxicity of Thoracic Radiation Therapy and Prophylactic Cranial Irradiation

- With BID RT concurrently with CT, rate of grade 2 to 3 esophagitis is higher in the range of 10% to 25%.
- The current dose constraint for esophagus is to keep the mean dose at 32 Gy and to keep the volume of esophagus getting 60 Gy lower.
- RP in SCLC is less well studied. The recent trial reports RP to be in the range of 10%.
- The dose constraint for lung is to keep V20 (volume receiving 20 Gy) under 30% to 35%. When using hyperfractionated regimen, it is to keep V20 under 25%.
- Patients receiving PCI need surveillance for long-term neurotoxicity associated with PCI.
- Current efforts are ongoing to try hippocampal sparing PCI to improve late neurocognitive toxicity.

Outcome

- Since the introduction of EP CT, the median survival of SCLC has improved from 2 months to 7 to 9 months between 1972 and 1990.
- With introduction of thoracic RT and PCI, it has improved only mildly.
- In the SEER program database, OS at 2, 3, and 5 years was 12%, 7%, and 5%, respectively.

Follow-Up

- First 2 years: every 4 months
- 2 to 5 years: every 6 months
- After 5 years: every year

- Imaging: CT scans every 4 to 6 months in the first 2 years, then annually
- Patients who are long-term survivors have significant risk of developing another smoking-related lung malignancy requiring close surveillance

7.3 Thymoma and Thymic Carcinoma

Epidemiology

- Thymic neoplasms are predominantly thymomas (90%) and constitute 30% of all anterior mediastinal masses among adults. Both are epithelial neoplasm with malignant cytologic features in thymic carcinoma.
- SEER data reported that 15 thymomas occur in every 100,000 person-years.
- They are more common in males and in Pacific Islanders and increase in frequency into the eighth decade of life.
- They are often associated with myasthenia gravis (MG); there is no known etiology.
- Thymic carcinoma is a rare, aggressive neoplasm, and has poor prognosis compared to thymoma.
- MG is the most common autoimmune disorder and can be present in 30% to 50% of patients. Younger females and older males are usually affected; the female to male ratio is 2:1.
- Thymic carcinoma has wide variation in age distribution and can be seen between 10 to 76 years of age. It has a slight male preponderance.

Pathology

- Thymomas are grossly lobulated, firm, and may be encapsulated. True thymomas microscopically appear as bland-looking cells compared to thymic carcinoma that has a cytologically malignant appearance.
- Noninvasive thymomas have intact capsule and invasive thymomas invade surrounding structures.
- Both noninvasive and invasive tumors have the potential to spread. Most common sites are pleura, pericardium, and pulmonary nodules. Other extra-thoracic sites including liver, brain, bone, and kidney can occur rarely.
- In 1976, Levine and Rosai proposed classification of thymomas into lymphocytic, epithelial, and mixed.
- Thymic carcinoma: Divided into high-grade and low-grade cancers. Most common histology is squamous cell carcinoma which is low-grade malignancy. Other low-grade histologies are mucoepidermoid and basaloid carcinoma. Some of the high-grade malignancies are lymphoepitheloid carcinoma, small cell, undifferentiated, sarcomatoid, and clear cell carcinomas.
- The median survival for low-grade malignancies ranges from 25.4 months to 6.6 years while for high-grade tumors it ranges from 11.3 to 15 months.
- Currently, World Health Organization (WHO) uses new classification as given in the following:

Tumor Type	Clinicopathologic Classification	Histologic Terminology
A	Benign thymoma	Medullary
B	Category I malignant thymoma	Cortical
B1		Lymphocytic rich; predominantly cortical
B2		Cortical
B3		Well differentiated thymic carcinoma
AB	Benign thymoma	Mixed
C	Category II malignant thymoma	Thymic carcinoma, epidermoid keratinizing and nonkeratinizing carcinoma, lymphoepithelioma-like carcinoma, sarcomatoid carcinoma, clear-cell carcinoma, basaloid carcinoma, mucoepidermoid carcinoma, undifferentiated carcinoma

Diagnosis and Workup

- Meticulous H&P examination.
- Most thymic masses are asymptomatic and are diagnosed incidentally.
- Others may present with chest pain, cough dyspnea. Malignant lesions may present with SVC syndrome, Horner's syndrome, or other neurologic symptoms.
- 71% of patients with thymoma present with variety of autoimmune disorders.
- Imaging studies including contrast enhanced CT scans, MRI scans, and FDG PET scans are useful in assessment of mediastinal masses. High-grade malignancies are associated with higher SUV on PET scan.
- Biopsy: CT or ultrasound-guided biopsy is recommended over fine-needle aspiration and is standard. Anterior parasternal mediastinotomy or a thoracoscopy yields a diagnostic accuracy to almost 100%.

Staging

- In 1981, Masaoka and colleagues have developed a surgical staging system that has been more commonly used in clinical practice due to its simplicity and ease to use for treatment decision.
- The TNM staging is also available but used less commonly in clinical practice.

Masaoka Staging System

Stage	Description	5/10-Year OS (%)
I	Macroscopically completely encapsulated and microscopically no capsular invasion	96/67
II	Macroscopic invasion into surrounding fatty tissue or mediastinal pleura, or	86/60
	Microscopic invasion into capsule	
III	Macroscopic invasion into neighboring organs (pericardium, great vessels, lung)	69/58
IV	Pleural or pericardial dissemination, or	50/0
	Lymphogenous or hematogenous metastasis	

Treatment Overview

- Thymomas are slow growing but are potentially malignant.
- Due to the rarity of this disease, only a few clinical trials are conducted.
- Stage-specific management of thymoma and thymic carcinoma:

Stage	Recommended Treatment
I	Surgery only
II	Surgery. Role of adjuvant RT is controversial. Can be observed if negative margins
III	Complete resection if possible → post-op RT. If unresectable, preop RT or chemo (doxorubicin, cisplatin, ifosfamide based) → surgery. If not candidate for aggressive treatment, RT alone
IV	Combination CT with or without local therapy
Thymic carcinoma	Surgical resection → post-op RT with or without CT

Radiation Therapy Technique

- Simulation: Supine, arms above head on a wing board, Vac bag immobilization.
- Technique: 3D conformal radiation or IMRT.
- Volume: Preop tumor or surgical bed with 2- to 3-cm margins is adequate. Prophylactic supraclavicular and whole mediastinum are not treated.
- Dose: 45 to 50 Gy in the postoperative setting. For gross disease or positive margins, 54 to 60 Gy is recommended.

Radiation Therapy Dose Limitation

- Lungs: Mean lung dose <20 Gy, V20 <35 to 40 Gy
- Spinal cord: 45 Gy
- Heart: Mean heart dose <30 Gy, 1/3 of volume <40 Gy
- Esophagus: Mean dose <32 Gy

Follow-Up

- Late recurrences are seen. Patients need to be followed long term.

7.4   Malignant Pleural Mesothelioma

Epidemiology

- Mesothelioma is a rare cancer with estimated annual incidence of 2,500 cases in the Unites States per year.
- Malignant pleural mesotheli (MPM) occurs mainly in older men (median age, 72 years) and has a median survival of about 1 year.
- Most cases of pleural mesothelioma are linked to asbestos exposure. The latency period between the time of asbestos exposure to development of mesothelioma can be 20 to 40 years.
- While the incidence of mesothelioma is declining in the Unites States due to control of exposure to asbestos, it is increasing in many other places in the world.
- Other etiologic factors leading to mesothelioma include prior ionizing radiation, erionite fibers, BAP1 germline mutations, and DNA tumor virus SV40.

Pathology

- The histologic subtypes of MPM include epithelioid (most common), sarcomatoid, and biphasic (mixed).
- Patients with epithelioid histology have better outcomes than those with either mixed or sarcomatoid histologies.
- It can be difficult to distinguish MPM from benign pleural disease and other malignancies such as metastatic adenocarcinoma or sarcoma.
- A panel of immunohistochemical markers is used to distinguish MPM from lung adenocarcinoma. MPMs typically express Wilms' tumor protein (WT-1), D2-40, and calretinin, and do not express TTF-1 or CEA.

Diagnosis and Workup

- Most patients with MPM present with gradual onset of nonspecific symptoms such as cough, dyspnea, chest pain, weight loss, fever, or night sweats.
- The recommended initial evaluation for suspected MPM includes CT chest with contrast, thoracentesis for cytological assessment, and pleural biopsy.
- In selected patients with potentially resectable disease, MRI may be useful to define the local extent of disease.
- PET/CT is superior to CT alone in assessing mediastinal lymph node involvement and presence of metastatic disease.
- Negative results from cytology and/or pleural biopsy do not exclude the diagnosis of mesothelioma and are often nondiagnostic.

- Surgical intervention (via video thoracoscopic biopsy or open thoracotomy) has a higher diagnostic yield.
- Serum biomarkers do not have an established role in diagnosis. Serum mesothelin-related peptide (SMRP) levels can be used to monitor the disease status.

Category	Descriptor Definition
T (Primary Tumor)	
TX	Primary tumor cannot be assessed
T0	No evidence of primary tumor
T1	Tumor limited to the ipsilateral parietal pleura with or without mediastinal pleura and with or without diaphragmatic pleural involvement
T1a	No involvement of the visceral pleura
T1b	Tumor also involving the visceral pleura
T2	Tumor involving each of the ipsilateral pleural surface (parietal, mediastinal, diaphragmatic, and visceral pleura) with at least one of the following: • Involvement of diaphragmatic muscle Extension of tumor from visceral pleura into the underlying pulmonary parenchyma

T3	Locally advanced but potentially resectable tumor
	• Tumor involving all of the ipsilateral pleural surfaces (parietal, mediastinal, diaphragmatic, and visceral pleura) with at least one of the following:
	  • Involvement of the endothoracic fascia
	  • Extension into the mediastinal fat
	  • Solitary, completely resectable focus of tumor extending into the soft tissues of the chest wall
	  • Nontransmural involvement of the pericardium

T4	T4 locally advanced technically unresectable tumor
	• Tumor involving all of the ipsilateral pleural surfaces (parietal, mediastinal, diaphragmatic, and visceral pleura) with at least one of the following:
	  • Diffuse extension or multifocal masses of tumor in the chest wall, with or without associated rib destruction
	  • Direct transdiaphragmatic extension of tumor to the peritoneum
	  • Direct extension of tumor to the contralateral pleura
	  • Direct extension of tumor to mediastinal organs
	  • Direct extension of tumor into the spine
	• Tumor extending through to the internal surface of the pericardium with or without a pericardial effusion or tumor involving the myocardium

N (Regional Lymph Nodes)	
N0	No regional node metastasis
N1	Metastasis to the ipsilateral bronchopulmonary or hilar lymph nodes
N2	Metastasis in ipsilateral mediastinal and/or subcarinal lymph node(s)
N3	Metastasis in contralateral mediastinal, contralateral internal mammary, ipsilateral, or contralateral supraclavicular lymph node(s)

(continued)

(continued)

M (Distant Metastasis)

M0   No distant metastasis

M1   Distant metastasis

Staging

- Staging is based on International Mesothelioma Interest Group (IMIG) TNM staging system.
- It is difficult to accurately stage patients before surgery.
  - ○ TNM staging system for diffuse MPM:

Treatment Overview

Surgery

- Careful patient assessment is required before surgery to minimize operative morbidity and mortality as well as achieve macroscopic complete resection.
- Surgical options for patients with MPM can include:
  - ○ Pleurectomy/decortication (P/D): Complete removal of the involved pleura and all gross tumors.
  - ○ Radical (or extended) P/D: Resection of diaphragm and pericardium in addition to total pleurectomy.
  - ○ Extrapleural pneumonectomy (EPP): En-bloc resection of involved pleura, lung, ipsilateral diaphragm and pericardium.
- Data from randomized trials are not available to suggest surgery improves survival compared to CT.
- Retrospective studies have demonstrated increased survival for select good risk patients with surgery.
- EPP may be good option for patients with operable early stage disease (confined to pleura), no N2 lymph node involvement, good performance status, and no comorbidities.
- P/D may be better option for patients with operable advanced disease (stages II–III) and/or high risk factors.
- Surgery is not recommended for stage IV MPM and sarcomatoid histology.

Radiation Therapy

- Radiation for MPM is part of multimodality treatment.
- Adjuvant radiation treatment can be done after EPP for patients with good performance status to improve local control.
- Adjuvant radiation is not recommended in the setting of limited or no resection of diseases as it is associated with significant toxicity and does not improve survival.
- Prophylactic radiation to a total dose of 21 Gy (3 × 7 Gy) is recommended to prevent instrument-tract recurrence after pleural intervention.
- Radiation can also be used for palliation of chest pain, bone, and brain mets.

Chemotherapy

- Systemic CT alone is recommended for patients with medically inoperable stages I to IV MPM and those with sarcomatoid histology.
- First-line treatment using cisplatin and pemetrexed is the standard of care for MPM.
- Combined regimen of cisplatin and pemetrexed improved survival compared to cisplatin alone (12.1 vs. 9.3 months).
- Carboplatin and pemetrexed is also acceptable first-line regimen with similar outcomes and is preferred for patients with poor performance status and/or comorbidities.

- In patients who cannot tolerate doublet CT, acceptable first-line single agent options include pemetrexed, vinorelbine.
- Second-line CT options include pemetrexed, gemcitabine, and vinorelbine.
- CT can also be used before or after surgery to improve outcome. Although data from adequately powered randomized trials are not available to support this use.

Radiation Technique

- Simulation: Supine position with arms overhead. Vac bag immobilization.
- Technique: 3D conformal or IMRT technique is used. When using IMRT, careful attention is needed to avoid the contralateral lung getting excessive dose causing fatal RP.
- Volume: The entire hemithorax. Inferiorly, the border needs to extend up to L2 vertebral body to encompass the entire pleural cavity.
- Dose: 50 to 54 Gy using 1.8 Gy per fraction.
- Dose limitation:
  - Spinal cord: 45 Gy
  - Lung (only one lung): Mean lung dose <10 Gy, V20 <10%
  - Heart: Mean dose <30 Gy

7.5 Thoracic Palliation

Airway Obstruction

- Bronchoscopy with stent placement
- Palliative RT: usual schedule is 20 Gy in 5 fractions or 30 Gy in 10 fractions if stage IV disease

SVC Syndrome

- Most frequently seen with lung cancer including both NSCLC and SCLC.
- Always biopsy should be attempted to confirm the diagnosis.
- Radiation dose: depends on stage of the disease. In palliative setting, 30 Gy in 10 fractions is sufficient. In definitive setting, RT can be started with high dose per fraction with 3 to 4 Gy × 2 to 3 fractions and then move to more standard fractionation.

Chapter 7: Practice Questions

1. The following subtype of mesothelioma is the most frequently diagnosed:

   A. Epitheloid
   B. Sarcomatoid
   C. Biphasic
   D. Mixed

2. A typical dose for radical/adjuvant mesothelioma hemithoracic irradiation is

   A. 20 Gy
   B. 30 Gy
   C. 40 Gy
   D. 50 Gy

3. In terms of thoracic palliation, the use of this equivalent dose fractionation schedule (or higher) has been shown to be associated with a small survival impact in good performance status patients

   A. 16 Gy in 2 fractions
   B. 20 Gy in 5 fractions
   C. 30 Gy in 10 fractions
   D. 60 Gy in 30 fractions

4. Distant metastases are usually found in this percentage of non-small cell lung cancer patients at diagnosis

    A. 5% to 10%
    B. 15% to 20%
    C. 30% to 40%
    D. 50% to 60%

5. In the United States, lung cancer is ranked as the following in terms of cancer incidence

    A. First
    B. Second
    C. Third
    D. Fourth

6. The most frequent amplification in squamous lung cancer is

    A. KRAS
    B. EGFR
    C. FGFR1
    D. EML4-ALK

7. A lung cancer patient with contralateral hilar nodes is N staged as

    A. N1
    B. N2
    C. N3
    D. M1

8. The most important prognostic factor for small cell lung cancer is

    A. Stage
    B. Performance status
    C. Sex
    D. LDH level

9. In terms of radical lung RT planning, the total lung V20 dose should be no greater than

    A. 10%
    B. 15%
    C. 25%
    D. 35%

10. The optimal timing for thoracic RT in limited small cell lung cancer is

    A. Prior to CT
    B. At the beginning of CT (i.e., cycle 1/2)
    C. At the end of CT (i.e., cycle 4–6)
    D. After CT

11. Small cell lung cancers account for what percentage of all lung cancers?

    A. 15%
    B. 25%
    C. 35%
    D. 45%

12. The latency period between asbestos exposure and mesothelioma malignancy is approximately

    A. 2 to 4 months
    B. 2 to 4 years
    C. 10 to 12 years
    D. 20 to 40 years

13. All of the following are related to lung cancer development EXCEPT

    A. Heavy metal exposure
    B. Vinyl chloride
    C. Asbestos
    D. Radium gas

14. The estimated 5-year survival of a stage III Masaoka thymoma is approximately

    A. 5%
    B. 50%
    C. 70%
    D. 90%

15. The relative decrease in brain metastases development after the use of prophylactic cranial irradiation in small cell lung cancer is

    A. 5%
    B. 10%
    C. 20%
    D. 50%

16. A mesothelioma with subcarinal node positivity is N staged as

    A. N1
    B. N2
    C. N3
    D. N staging irrelevant

17. A 2-cm primary lung cancer with chest wall invasion is T staged as

    A. T1
    B. T2
    C. T3
    D. T4

18. The usual dose fractionation schedule used for small cell prophylactic cranial irradiation is

    A. 25 Gy in 20 fractions
    B. 25 Gy in 10 fractions
    C. 30 Gy in 10 fractions
    D. 36 Gy in 24 fractions BID

19. According to the Masaoka staging system, a thymoma with invasion into the pericardium is stage

    A. II
    B. IIB
    C. III
    D. IVA

20. The standard radiation dose for stage III unresectable non-small cell lung cancer (NSCLC) treated with concurrent chemoradiation is considered to be

    A. 50 Gy
    B. 60 Gy
    C. 70 Gy
    D. 74 Gy

Chapter 7: Answers

1. A
The histologic subtypes of mesothelioma include epithelioid (most common), sarcomatoid, and biphasic (mixed).

2. D
Typical doses with 3DCRT/IMRT techniques in the adjuvant or radical setting are on the order of 50 to 54 Gy in 1.8 Gy/fraction.

3. C
The use of 30 Gy in 10 fractions is recommended in the American Society for Radiation Oncology (ASTRO) practice guideline.

4. C
About 30% to 40% of patients with non-small cell lung cancer (NSCLC) present with distant metastasis and related symptoms at diagnosis.

5. B
In 2015, an estimated 221,200 new cases will be diagnosed in the United States, second common cancer in both men and women.

6. C
The FGFR1 amplification is seen in approximately 25% of squamous lung cancer cases.

7. C
Metastasis in contralateral mediastinal, contralateral hilar, ipsilateral, or contralateral scalene or supraclavicular lymph node(s) is considered N3 disease.

8. A
The most important prognostic factor is stage. Other clinical prognostic factors are performance status and sex. Age is usually not prognostic but older patients have limitations in tolerating aggressive treatment. Other prognostic factors are elevated LDH, alkaline phosphatase, and possibly presence of paraneoplastic syndromes.

9. D
Lung dose-volume parameters for radical lung planning:
 Mean lung dose <20 Gy
 V20 <35% to 40%

10. B
Timing of thoracic RT remains controversial. Several meta-analyses suggested benefit of early thoracicRT. The standard is to start thoracic RT during first or second cycle of CT in good performance status patients.

11. A
The SEER database reports that small cell lung cancer (SCLC) has decreased from about 17% to 13% of all lung cancers in the past 30 years.

12. D
Most cases of pleural mesothelioma are linked to asbestos exposure. The latency period between the time of asbestos exposure to development of mesothelioma can be 20 to 40 years.

13. D
Smoking is the number one risk factor for developing lung cancer. Exposure to asbestos, arsenic, cadmium, chromium, nickel, vinyl chloride, and radon gas are also known to be carcinogenic to develop lung cancer.

14. C
The 5- and 10-year survival of a stage III Masaoka thymoma is 69% and 58%, respectively.

15. D
The use of prophylactic cranial irradiation (PCI) in limited stage SCLC generally reduces the risk of brain mets in half.

16. B

N (Regional Lymph Nodes) for mesothelioma:

N0 No regional node metastasis

N1 Metastasis to the ipsilateral bronchpulmonary or hilar lymph nodes

N2 Metastasis in ipsilateral mediastinal and/or subcarinal lymph node(s)

N3 Metastasis in contralateral mediastinal, contralateral internal mammary, ipsilateral, or contralateral supraclavicular lymph node(s)

17. C

A lung tumor with chest wall invasion is staged as T3 irrespective of tumor size.

18. B

PCI is recommended in all limited stage disease that achieves response to initial CRT. PCI dose: 25 Gy using 2.5 Gy per fraction.

19. C

Macroscopic invasion into neighboring organs (pericardium, great vessels, and lung) in thymoma is considered to be stage 3.

20. B

Standard dose for NSCLC is 60 Gy in 30 fractions is standard dose as definitive treatment for locally advanced disease concurrently with chemotherapy (CT).

Recommended Reading

Antman KH, Blum RH, Greenberger JS, et al. Multimodality therapy for malignant mesothelioma based on a study of natural history. *Am J Med*. 1980;68:356-362.

Auperin A, Arriagada R, Pignon JP, et al. Prophylactic cranial irradiation for patients with small cell lung cancer in complete remission. PCI Overview Collaborative Group. *N Engl J Med*. 1999;341:476-484.

Bezjak A, Dixon P, Brundage M, et al. Randomized phase III trial of single versus fractionated thoracic radiation in the palliation of patients with lung cancer (NCICCTG SC.15). *Int J Radiat Oncol Biol Phys*. 2002;54:719.

Biswas T, Sharma N, Machtay M. Controversies in the management of stage III non-small cell lung cancer. *Expert Rev Anticancer Ther*. 2014;14(3):333-347.

Bonner JA, Sloan JA, Shanahan TG, et al. Phase III comparison of twice-daily split-course irradiation versus once-daily irradiation for patients with limited stage small cell lung carcinoma. *J Clin Oncol*. 1999;17:2681-2691.

Cao CQ, Yan TD, Bannon PG, et al. A systematic review of extrapleural pneumonectomy for malignant pleural mesothelioma. *J Thorac Oncol*. 2010;5:1692-1703.

Carbone M, Kratzke RA, Testa JR. The pathogenesis of mesothelioma. *Semin Oncol*. 2002;29:2-17.

de Graaf-Strukowska L, van der Zee J, van Putten W, et al. Factors influencing the outcome of radiotherapy in malignant mesothelioma of the pleura: a single-institution experience with 189 patients. *Int J Radiat Oncol Biol Phys*. 1999;43:511-516.

De Ruysscher D, Pijls-Johannesma M, Vansteenkiste J, et al. Systematic review and meta-analysis of randomised, controlled trials of the timing of chest radiotherapy in patients with limited-stage, small cell lung cancer. *Ann Oncol*. 2006;17:543-552.

Detterbeck FC. Clinical value of the WHO classification system of thymoma. *Ann Thorac Surg*. 2006;81:2328-2334.

Emami B, Lyman J, Brown A, et al. Tolerance of normal tissue to therapeutic irradiation. *Int J Radiat Oncol Biol Phys*. 1991;21:109-122.

Engels EA, Pfeiffer RM. Malignant thymoma in the United States: demographic patterns in incidence and associations with subsequent malignancies. *Int J Cancer*. 2003;105:546-551.

Falkson CB, Bezjak A, Darling G, et al. The management of thymoma: a systematic review and practice guideline. *J Thorac Oncol*. 2009;4:911-919.

Fried DB, Morris DE, Poole C, et al. Systematic review evaluating the timing of thoracic radiation therapy in combined modality therapy for limited-stage small cell lung cancer. *J Clin Oncol*. 2004;22:4837-4845.

Furuse K, Fukuoka M, Kawahara M. Phase III study of concurrent versus sequential thoracic radiotherapy in combination with mitomycin, vindesine, and cisplatin in unresectable stage III non-small cell lung cancer. *J Clin Oncol*. 1999;17:2692-2699.

Gandara DR, Chansky K, Albain KS, et al. Long-term survival with concurrent chemoradiation therapy followed by consolidation docetaxel in stage IIIB non-small cell lung cancer: a phase II Southwest Oncology Group Study (S9504). *Clin Lung Cancer*. 2006;8:116-121.

Ginsberg RJ, Rubinstein LV. Randomized trial of lobectomy vs. limited resection for T1N0 non-small cell lung cancer. *Ann Thorac Surg*. 1995;60:615-623.

Govindan R, Page N, Morgensztern D, et al. Changing epidemiology of small cell lung cancer in the United States over the last 30 years: analysis of the surveillance, epidemiologic, and end results database. *J Clin Oncol.* 2006;24:4539-4544.

Howlader N, Noone AM, Krapcho M, et al. *SEER Cancer Statistics Review, 1975–2010.* Bethesda, MD: National Cancer Institute; 2013. http://seer.cancer.gov/csr/1975_2011/

Hsu CP, Chan CY, Chen CL, et al. Thymic carcinoma: ten years' experience in twenty patients. *J Thorac Cardiovasc Surg.* 1994;107:615-620.

Jeremic B, Shibamoto Y, Nikolic N, et al. Role of radiation therapy in the combined-modality treatment of patients with extensive disease small cell lung cancer: a randomized study. *J Clin Oncol.* 1999;17:2092-2099.

Kelsey CR, Werner-Wasik M, Marks LB. Stage III lung cancer: two or three modalities? The continued role of thoracic radiotherapy. *Oncology (Williston Park).* 2006;20:1210-1219; discussion 1219, 1223, 1225.

Law MR, Hodson ME, Heard BE. Malignant mesothelioma of the pleura: relation between histological type and clinical behaviour. *Thorax.* 1982;37:810-815.

Lung Cancer Study Group. Effects of post-operative mediastinal radiation on completely resected stage II and stage III epidermoid cancer of the lung. *N Engl J Med.* 1986;315:1377-1381.

Machtay M. Pulmonary complications of anti-cancer treatment. In Abeloff M, ed. *Clinical Oncology.* 3rd ed. London: Churchill Livingston; 2003.

Machtay M, Hsu C, Komaki R, et al. Effect of overall treatment time on outcome after concurrent chemoradiation for locally advanced non-small cell lung carcinoma: analysis of the Radiation Therapy Oncology Group (RTOG) experience. *Int J Radiat Oncol Biol Phys.* 2005;63:667-671.

Marino P, Preatoni A, Cantoni A. Randomized trials of radiotherapy alone versus combined chemotherapy and radiotherapy in stages IIIa and IIIb non-small cell lung cancer: a meta-analysis. *Cancer.* 1995;76:593-601.

Masaoka A, Monden Y, Nakahara K, et al. Follow-up study of thymomas with special reference to their clinical stages. *Cancer.* 1981;48:2485-2492. [PMID: 7296496]

Mornex F, Resbeut M, Richard P, et al. Radiotherapy and chemotherapy for invasive thymomas: a multicentric retrospective review of 90 cases. *Int J Radiat Oncol Biol Phys.* 1995;32:651-659.

Murray N, Coy P, Pater JL, et al. Importance of timing for thoracic irradiation in the combined modality treatment of limited-stage small cell lung cancer. The National Cancer Institute of Canada Clinical Trials Group. *J Clin Oncol.* 1993;11:336-344. [PMID: 8381164]

O'Rourke N, Garcia JC, Paul J, et al. A randomised controlled trial of intervention site radiotherapy in malignant pleural mesothelioma. *Radiother Oncol.* 2007;84:18-22.

Park K, Sun J-M, Kim S-W, et al. Phase III trial of concurrent thoracic radiotherapy with either the first cycle or the third cycle of cisplatin and etoposide chemotherapy to determine the optimal timing of thoracic radiotherapy for limited-disease small cell lung cancer. *J Clin Oncol.* 2012;30:abstract 7004.

Patchell RA, Tibbs PA, Walsh JW, et al. A randomized trial of surgery in the treatment of single metastases to the brain. *N Engl J Med.* 1990;322:494-500.

Pfister DG, Johnson DH, Azzoli CG, et al. American Society of Clinical Oncology treatment of unresectable non-small cell lung cancer guideline: Update 2003. *J Clin Oncol.* 2004;22:330-353.

Pignon J, Arriagada R, Ihde D, et al. A meta-analysis of thoracic radiotherapy for small cell lung cancer. *N Engl J Med.* 1992;327:1618-1624.

PORT Meta-Analysis Group. Postoperative radiotherapy in non-small cell lung cancer: Systematic review and meta-analysis of individual patient data from nine randomised controlled trials. *Lancet.* 1998;352:257-263.

Roach MR, Gandara DR, Yuo HS, et al. Radiation pneumonitis following combined modality therapy for lung cancer: Analysis of prognostic factors. *J Clin Oncol.* 1995;13:2606-2612.

Rodrigues G, Lock M, D'Souza D, et al. Prediction of radiation pneumonitis by dose-volume histogram parameters in lung cancer. A systematic review. *Radiother Oncol.* 2004;71:127-138.

Rojas AM, Lyn BE, Wilson EM, et al. Toxicity and outcome of a phase II trial of taxane-based neoadjuvant chemotherapy and 3-dimensional, conformal, accelerated radiotherapy in locally advanced non-small cell lung cancer. *Cancer.* 2006;107:1321-1330.

Rossi A, Di Maio M, Chiodini P, et al. Carboplatin- or cisplatin-based chemotherapy in first-line treatment of small cell lung cancer: the COCIS meta-analysis of individual patient data. *J Clin Oncol.* 2012;30:1692-1698.

Rusch VW, Giroux D, Kennedy C, et al. Initial analysis of the international association for the study of lung cancer mesothelioma database. *J Thorac Oncol.* 2012;7:1631-1639.

Ryu JS, Choi NC, Fischman AJ, et al. FDG-PET in staging and restaging non-small cell lung cancer after neoadjuvant chemoradiotherapy: correlation with histopathology. *Lung Cancer.* 2002;35:179-187.

Santoro A, O'Brien ME, Stahel RA, et al. Pemetrexed plus cisplatin or pemetrexed plus carboplatin for chemonaive patients with malignant pleural mesothelioma: results of the International Expanded Access Program. *J Thorac Oncol.* 2008;3:756-763.

Simpson JR, Francis ME, Perez-Tamayo R, et al. Palliative radiotherapy for inoperable carcinoma of the lung: final report of a RTOG multi-institutional trial. *Int J Radiat Oncol Biol Phys.* 1985;11:751-758.

Slotman B, Faivre-Finn C, Kramer G, et al. Prophylactic cranial irradiation in extensive small cell lung cancer. *N Engl J Med.* 2007;357:664-672.

Slotman BJ, Faivre-Finn C, van Tinteren H, et al. Randomized trial on thoracic radiotherapy (TRT) in extensive-stage small cell lung cancer. *J Clin Oncol.* 2014;32:5s.

Stahel RA, Weder W, Felip E. Malignant pleural mesothelioma: ESMO clinical recommendations for diagnosis, treatment and follow-up. *Ann Oncol.* 2009;20:73-75.

Suster S, Rosai J. Thymic carcinoma: a clinicopathologic study of 60 cases. *Cancer.* 1991;67:1025-1032.

Timmerman RD, Kavanagh BD, Cho LC, et al. Stereotactic body radiation therapy in multiple organ sites. *J Clin Oncol.* 2007;25:947-952.

Turrisi AT, 3rd, Kim K, Blum R, et al. Twice-daily compared with once-daily thoracic radiotherapy in limited small cell lung cancer treated concurrently with cisplatin and etoposide. *N Engl J Med.* 1999;340:265-271. [PMID: 9920950]

Ung YC, Yu E, Falkson C, et al. The role of high-dose-rate brachytherapy in the palliation of symptoms in patients with non-small cell lung cancer: a systematic review. *Brachytherapy.* 2006;5:189-202.

Vallieres E, Shepherd FA, Crowley J, et al. The IASLC Lung Cancer Staging Project: proposals regarding the relevance of TNM in the pathologic staging of small cell lung cancer in the forthcoming (seventh) edition of the TNM classification for lung cancer. *J Thorac Oncol.* 2009;4:1049-1059.

van Meerbeeck JP, Kramer GW, Van Schil PE, et al. Randomized controlled trial of resection versus radiotherapy after induction chemotherapy in stage IIIA-N2 non-small cell lung cancer. *J Natl Cancer Inst.* 2007;99:442-450.

Vogelzang NJ, Rusthoven JJ, Symanowski J, et al. Phase III study of pemetrexed in combination with cisplatin versus cisplatin alone in patients with malignant pleural mesothelioma. *J Clin Oncol.* 2003;21:2636-2644.

Wakelee HA, Stephenson P, Keller SM, et al. Postoperative radiotherapy (PORT) or chemoradiotherapy (CPORT) following resection of stages II and IIIA non-small cell lung cancer (NSCLC) does not increase the expected risk of death from intercurrent disease (DID) in Eastern Cooperative Oncology Group (ECOG) trial E3590. *Lung Cancer.* 2005;48:389-397.

Warde P, Payne D. Does thoracic irradiation improve survival and local control in limited-stage small cell carcinoma of the lung? A meta-analysis [see comments]. *J Clin Oncol.* 1992;10:890.

Breast Cancer

Allison M. Quick and Julia White

8.1 Breast Cancer

Epidemiology and Risk Factors

- Breast cancer is the most common malignancy in women in the United States with approximately 230,000 new cases of invasive breast cancer per year.
- Breast cancer is the second leading cause of cancer-related death in women, with approximately 39,000 deaths annually.
- Risk factors for breast cancer:
  - Female sex
  - Age greater than 50
  - BRCA 1 or 2 mutation or other inherited genetic conditions such as Li-Fraumeni or Cowden syndrome
  - Family history of breast or ovarian cancer
  - Late parity (>30 years of age) or nulliparity
  - Early menarche and/or late menopause
  - Hormone replacement therapy with estrogen and progestin
  - Obesity
  - Prior chest radiation
  - Prior history of atypical ductal hyperplasia or lobular carcinoma in situ
- Protective factors:
  - Breast feeding for greater than 1 year
  - Oopherectomy

Anatomy and Patterns of Spread

- The breast tissue is located on the anterior chest wall over the pectoralis muscle between the second and sixth rib from the sternum to the mid-axillary line.
  - The pectoralis minor (pec minor) arises from the third, fourth, and fifth rib and inserts into the coracoid process.
- The anatomical borders of the breast are as follows:
  - Medial: Sternum
  - Lateral: Mid-axillary line
  - Cranial: second rib
  - Caudal: sixth rib
- The breast is composed of mammary gland, fat, blood vessels, nerves, and lymphatics.
- The Cooper's ligaments are fibrous septa connecting skin to the deep fascia over the pectoralis muscles.

- Primary breast cancers can spread locally to involve surrounding breast tissue, nipple/areola complex, skin, pectoralis muscles, and ribs.
- Breast cancer spreads lymphatically, primarily through the axillary nodes.
  - o Axillary levels
    - ■ Level 1: lymph nodes that are located lateral to pec minor
    - ■ Level 2: lymph nodes that are located between the medial and lateral border of pec minor and the interpectoral nodes (i.e., Rotters' nodes)
    - ■ Level 3: lymph nodes located medial to the medial margin of pec minor
  - o The risk of axillary nodal involvement increases as the size of the primary tumor increase:

T-Stage	Incidence of Positive Axillary Nodes
T1a	5%
T1b	10%
T1c	20%
T2	40%
T3	75%
T4	85%

- Additional lymphatic drainage occurs through the internal mammary nodes and through the transpectoral nodes to the supraclavicular nodes.
  - o The internal mammary nodes within the first three intercostal spaces along the edge of the sternum are at highest risk when the primary breast cancer is located in the medial, central, or lower breast and in the setting of known axillary nodal metastases.
  - o The supraclavicular lymph nodes are located in the supraclavicular fossa bordered by the clavicle and subclavian vein inferiorly, the internal jugular vein medially, and the omohyoid laterally.

Presentation

- Abnormal screening mammogram
- Palpable breast or axillary mass
- Bloody nipple discharge
- Skin or nipple changes

Diagnosis and Workup

- History and physical
- Bilateral diagnostic mammogram with ultrasound as necessary
  - o BIRADS categories:

Category	Assessment	Recommendations
0	Incomplete	Need additional imaging
1	Negative	Routine screening

(continued)

(continued)

Category	Assessment	Recommendations
2	Benign	Routine screening
3	Probably benign	6-month follow-up mammogram
4	Suspicious abnormality	Biopsy recommended
5	Highly suspicious of malignancy	Biopsy and treatment as necessary
6	Known biopsy proven malignancy	Treatment as indicated

- Breast MRI if indicated
  - o Use of MRI is controversial and has not been shown to reduce positive margins, re-excision, or local control in patients receiving breast conservation therapy.
  - o American Cancer Society guidelines for screening breast MRI
    - History of BRCA 1 or 2 mutation
    - Prior chest radiation between 10 to 30 years of age
    - First degree relative with BRCA mutation, Li Fraumeni, or Cowden disease
    - Multifocal or multicentric breast cancer to determine extent of disease and screen contralateral breast
    - Intent for neoadjuvant chemotherapy
    - Axillary nodal adenocarcinoma or Paget's disease with no mammographic evidence of breast primary
    - Consider for dense breast tissue and personal history of ductal carcinoma in situ, lobular carcinoma in situ, atypical ductal hyperplasia, or atypical lobular hyperplasia
- Biopsy
  - o Core needle biopsy done stereotactically in case presenting with microcalcifications on mammography, with ultrasound for those with masses or MRI guidance when detected only on this imaging modality to determine:
    - Histology
      - Noninvasive
        - DCIS
          - Comedo
          - Noncomedo (cribriform, micropapillary, papillary, solid)
          - Grade: low, intermediate, high
        - LCIS
      - Invasive
        - Invasive ductal carcinoma (85%)
        - Invasive lobular carcinoma
        - Others: Tubular, Medullary, Mucinous
    - Estrogen and progesterone hormone receptor and Her2neu status
      - Estrogen (ER) and Progesterone (PR) receptor positivity: ~65% to 70%
      - Her2 positivity: ~15% to 20%
      - Triple negative (ER, PR, and HER2 all negative): ~ 10% to 15%
      - Molecular subtypes
        - Luminal A: ER/PR + Her2neu –
        - Luminal B: ER/PR + Her2neu +

- - Basal like: ER/PR – Her2neu – (triple negative)
  - Her2neu+: ER/PR – Her2neu +
  o Fine needle aspiration of suspicious axillary nodes
- Routine labs with CBC, chemistries, and LFTs with alkaline phosphatase
- Preoperative chest x-ray
- Routine staging scans with CT chest, abdomen, and pelvis and nuclear bone scan for clinical Stage III or for Stages I to IIB if signs or symptoms present
- CT chest to assess disease presence and extent in the regional nodal sites if neoadjuvant chemotherapy planned
- Genetic counseling if high risk for hereditary breast cancer
- Fertility counseling if premenopausal

Staging

Primary Tumor (T) Staging (AJCC 7th Edition)

Tx	Primary tumor cannot be assessed	T2	>2 cm but ≤5 cm
T0	No evidence of primary tumor	T3	>5 cm
Tis (DCIS)	Ductal Carcinoma in situ	T4	Tumor extension to chest wall and/or skin (ulceration or skin nodules)
Tis (LCIS)	Lobular Carcinoma in situ	T4a	Extension to chest wall, not including only pectoralis muscle invasion
T1	Tumor size ≤ 2 cm	T4b	Skin ulceration and/or ipsilateral nodules and/or edema (including peau d'orange) of the skin that do not meet criteria for T4d
T1mi	≤1 mm	T4c	T4a and T4b
T1a	>1 mm but ≤5 mm	T4d	Inflammatory carcinoma*
T1b	>5 mm but ≤1 cm		
T1c	>1 cm but ≤2 cm		

*Clinical syndrome of breast erythema and edema (peau d'orange) of a third or more of the breast. The tumor is often present in the dermal lymphatics of the involved skin but this pathologic finding is not required or sufficient by itself for diagnosis.

Regional Lymph Nodes (N) Staging (AJCC 7th Edition)

Clinical		Pathologic (pN)	
NX	Regional nodes not assessed	pNX	Regional nodes not assessed
N0	No regional node metastasis	pN0	No regional node metastasis
N1	Metastasis to movable ipsilateral level I, II axillary nodes	pN1	
N2		pN1mi	Micrometastases (>0.2 mm and/or more than 200 cells, but not greater than 2.0 mm)

(continued)

Regional Lymph Nodes (N) Staging (AJCC 7th Edition) (*continued*)

Clinical		Pathologic (pN)	
N2a	Metastasis to ipsilateral level I, II axillary nodes that are clinically fixed or matted	pN1a	Metastases in 1–3 axillary nodes, at least one greater than 2.0 mm
N2b	Metastases in clinically detected ipsilateral internal mammary nodes in the *absence* of clinically evident axillary node metastases	pN1b	Metastases in internal mammary nodes with micro or macrometastases detected by sentinel node biopsy
N3		pN1c	Metastases in 1–3 axillary nodes and in internal mammary nodes with micro or macrometastases detected by sentinel node biopsy
N3a	Metastases in ipsilateral infraclavicular (level III) axillary lymph node(s)	pN2	
N3b	Metastases in ipsilateral internal mammary node(s) and level I, II axillary lymph nodes	pN2a	Metastases in 4–9 axillary nodes (at least one tumor deposit >2.0 mm)
N3c	Metastases in ipsilateral supraclavicular lymph node(s)	pN2b	Metastases in clinically detected internal mammary nodes in the *absence* of axillary node metastases
		pN3	
		pN3a	Metastases in ≥10 axillary nodes or to the infraclavicular (level III) nodes
		pN3b	Metastases in clinically detected ipsilateral internal mammary nodes in the presence of ≥1 positive axillary nodes; or >3 axillary nodes and internal mammary nodes with micro or macrometastases detected by sentinel node biopsy
		pN3c	Metastasis in ipsilateral supraclavicular nodes

Distant Metastasis (AJCC 7th Edition)

M0	No clinical or radiographic distant metastases
M1	Distant metastases

Anatomic Stage (AJCC 7th Edition)

Stage 0	Tis	N0	M0
Stage IA	T1	N0	M0

(continued)

Anatomic Stage (AJCC 7th Edition) (*continued*)

Stage IB	T0	N1mi	M0
	T1	N1mi	M0
Stage IIA	T0	N1	M0
	T1	N1	M0
	T2	N0	M0
Stage IIB	T2	N1	M0
	T3	N0	M0
Stage IIIA	T0	N2	M0
	T1	N2	M0
	T2	N2	M0
	T3	N1	M0
	T3	N2	M0
Stage IIIB	T4	N0	M0
	T4	N1	M0
	T4	N2	M0
Stage IIIC	Any T	N3	M0
Stage IV	Any T	Any N	M1

8.2   DCIS and Early-Stage Breast Cancer (Stages I and II)

Treatment Overview

- Patients with DCIS can be treated with breast conservation therapy or mastectomy.
  - Mastectomy has slightly higher local control rates than breast conservation therapy depending on characteristics of DCIS but survival is greater than 98% for both treatment options.
  - The goal of treatment for DCIS is to prevent the first invasive breast cancer.
- Patients with early-stage breast cancer can be treated with breast conservation therapy or mastectomy with no local-regional recurrence or survival difference between the treatments.
- Contraindications for breast conservation therapy requiring radiation therapy (RT):
  - Absolute
    - Pregnancy
    - Diffuse suspicious or malignant appearing microcalcifications/multicentric disease
    - Widespread disease that cannot be excised through a single incision to obtain negative margins and acceptable cosmetic outcome
    - Persistently positive margin after re-excision
  - Relative
    - Prior radiation to chest wall or breast
    - Active connective tissue disease involving skin, particularly scleroderma and lupus with skin manifestations
    - Large tumors in a small breast that would leave patient with a poor cosmetic outcome
- Chemotherapy and/or endocrine therapy may be indicated depending on stage and ER/PR and Her2 status.

8.3   DCIS

- Surgical management: Lumpectomy without axillary staging or total mastectomy
  - A sentinel node biopsy is often done when a mastectomy is performed in order to spare the patient a full lymph node dissection if invasive disease is found in the mastectomy specimen.
- Adjuvant whole breast radiation after lumpectomy to reduce risk of noninvasive and invasive ipsilateral in breast recurrence
  - NSABP B17: Lumpectomy alone versus lumpectomy + RT in women with DCIS
    - RT reduced rate of in breast recurrence from 35% to 19.8% at 15 years. Both invasive (19.6%–10.7%) and noninvasive (15.4%–9%) recurrences were reduced
    - No OS benefit
    - Comedo necrosis was independent risk factor for ipsilateral breast recurrence
  - Four other randomized clinical trials and a meta-analysis confirm the efficacy of breast RT in reducing local-regional recurrence risk
  - Boost: No randomized data on use of boost to lumpectomy cavity
- Lumpectomy alone without radiation an option, especially with low-intermediate risk DCIS
  - Low to intermediate-risk DCIS has approximately 6% risk of ipsilateral breast recurrence at 5 years and 14% risk ipsilateral breast recurrence at 12 years with lumpectomy alone based on ECOG 5194
  - Low–intermediate grade DCIS, less than 25 mm in size still benefit from RT, based on Radiation Therapy Oncology Group (RTOG) 9804 where at 7 years the risk of in breast recurrence from lumpectomy alone was 6.7% and for those treated with post lumpectomy breast RT less than 1%
  - DCIS Recurrence score, a commercially available multigene assay, is prognostic for all and invasive recurrences post lumpectomy for DCIS and may be helpful for clinical decision making
- Consider Tamoxifen for 5 years, for hormone receptor-positive DCIS, for an additional 30% reduction in local ipsilateral recurrence risk; also reduces risk of contralateral breast cancer
  - NSABP B24: Lumpectomy + RT ± 5 years of Tamoxifen
    - Tamoxifen reduced ipsilateral invasive (9%–6.6%) and noninvasive (7.6%–6.7%) breast recurrence and contralateral invasive or noninvasive cancer (8.1%–4.9%)
- Anastrozole was shown to be superior than Tamoxifen for postmenopausal women less than 60 years of age with ER- or PR-positive DCIS treated with lumpectomy and adjuvant radiation on NSABP B-35 (presented in abstract only)

8.4   Invasive Breast Cancer

- Surgical management:
  - Lumpectomy or total mastectomy with axillary staging
    - Radical mastectomy does not provide survival or local control benefit over total mastectomy based on NSABP B-04.
    - Mastectomy and breast conservation therapy have equivalent overall survival rates.
      - NSABP B-06: Modified radical mastectomy (total mastectomy + ALND) versus lumpectomy + ALND + RT versus lumpectomy + ALND
        - No OS difference between three arms
      - More modern studies also support equivalent local-regional control and overall survival between breast conservation therapy and mastectomy.
  - Axillary staging
    - For pathologically node-negative women SLN biopsy alone is sufficient and ALND can be omitted.
      - NSAPB B-32: Clinically node-negative patients randomized to SLN biopsy (with ALND if sentinel node positive) versus SLN biopsy + ALND
        - No OS, PFS, or DFS difference

- For pathologically positive nodes:
  - If treated with lumpectomy and sentinel node biopsy, axillary lymph node dissection can be omitted if patient had one to two positive axillary nodes, whole breast radiation is planned, and patient did not receive neoadjuvant chemotherapy.
    - ACOSOG Z0011: Women with clinical T1 to 2, N0 women s/p lumpectomy and SLN biopsy with one to two positive sentinel nodes randomized to ALND or no further axillary treatment followed by whole breast radiation ± systemic therapy
    - No difference in local or regional recurrence
      - 5-year axillary recurrence: 0.9% with ALND and 0.5% with sentinel lymph node biopsy (SLNB).
  - If these criteria are not met, ALND or axillary radiation is recommended.
    - Axillary node dissection includes removal of axillary levels I and II.
    - Axillary radiation is equivalent to axillary node dissection for patients with early-stage breast cancer treated with lumpectomy or mastectomy and found to have positive axillary nodes on sentinel node biopsy based on the EORTC AMAROS trial.
    - 5-year axillary recurrence rates were 0.43% after dissection versus 1.19% (0.31–2.08) after axillary RT.
    - Axillary radiation results in less lymphedema.
- Adjuvant radiation:
  - Radiation after lumpectomy decreases local recurrence by about 2/3 compared to lumpectomy alone.
    - NSABP B-06: Local recurrences were 39% with lumpectomy alone and 14% with the addition of radiation.
    - Modern data show much lower local recurrence rates for patients treated with breast conservation therapy.
  - Early Breast Cancer Trialists' Collaborative Group (EBCTCG) meta-analysis of patients treated with breast conservation therapy with or without adjuvant RT did show reduction in local recurrence and breast cancer death with the addition of radiation.
    - One breast cancer death was avoided by year 15 for every four local recurrences avoided at year 10.
  - Lumpectomy cavity boost:
    - Indications:
      - Age < 50
      - High grade
      - Positive lymph nodes
      - Close or positive margins
    - EORTC 22881-10882: Lumpectomy + ALND and 50 Gy whole breast radiation ± 16 Gy boost to lumpectomy cavity:
      - Boost reduced local recurrence from 10% to 6%
      - Strongest reduction in women less than 40 years of age (23.9% vs. 13.5%)
      - Higher fibrosis rate with boost (4.4% vs. 1.6%)
  - Lumpectomy alone + endocrine therapy without radiation can be considered for the following:
    - pT1, N0
    - ER and/or PR positive and committed to 5 years of antiendocrine therapy
    - Age between 65 and 70 years
    - Negative margins
      - Prime II: Women 65 years and older with hormone receptor positive, pT1-2 (<3 cm) N0M0 breast cancer s/p lumpectomy with negative margins ± adjuvant whole breast radiation
        - Local recurrence 1.3% with radiation and 4.1% without radiation at 5 years
        - No OS difference

- CALGB 9343: Women 70 years and over with clinical T1N0M0, ER-positive breast cancer s/p lumpectomy + Tamoxifen ± whole breast radiation
  - In breast cancer recurrence was 2% with Tamoxifen and RT and 9% with Tamoxifen alone
  - No OS or time to mastectomy difference
- ○ Hypofractionation:
  - ■ The American Society for Radiation Oncology (ASTRO) Task Force Guidelines:
    - Evidence supports hypofractionated whole breast radiation for the following:
      - Age 50 and older
      - pT1-2 N0 treated with lumpectomy
      - No chemotherapy given
      - Dose homogeneity within ±7% in central axis
  - ■ Canadian trial:
    - Women s/p lumpectomy with negative margins, pT1-2, and separation <25 cm randomized to
      - 50 Gy in 25 fractions versus 42.6 Gy in 16 fractions (2.66 Gy)
      - No boost
      - 10-year risk of local recurrence 6.7% in standard arm versus 6.2% in hypofractionation arm
      - No difference in cosmetic outcome
  - ■ START B (UK):
    - 40 Gy /15 fx (2.67 Gy/fx) versus 50 Gy/25 fx
    - Similar local control and late toxicity affects in both groups
- ○ Partial breast radiation:
  - ■ NSABP B 39/RTOG 0413: Whole breast radiation versus partial breast radiation for Stages 0, I, or II breast cancer resected by lumpectomy; closed to accrual; results pending
  - ■ ASTRO "suitable" criteria for partial breast radiation:
    - Patient factors
      - Age 50 or greater
      - No BRCA mutation
      - No neoadjuvant chemotherapy
    - Pathologic factors
      - Tumor 2 cm or less (pT1)
      - Node negative (pN0)
      - At least 2-mm margin
      - No LVSI
      - ER +
      - Unifocal/unicentric
      - Invasive ductal or favorable subtype
      - No pure DCIS or extensive intraductal component
- ○ Regional nodal radiation:
  - ■ Indicated for four or more positive nodes
  - ■ Controversial in setting of one to three positive nodes
    - NCIC-CTG MA.20: Women with positive nodes or high-risk features (T3 or <10 nodes dissected with either grade 3 histology, ER negativity, or LVSI) but node-negative s/p lumpectomy and SLNB or ALND and whole breast radiation with or without regional nodal radiation
      - Regional nodal radiation
        - Ipsilateral internal mammary nodes in first three intercostal spaces
        - Supraclavicular
        - Axillary nodes
      - Regional nodal radiation improved disease-free survival but with no OS difference.
        - Higher rates of lymphedema (8.4% vs. 4.5%) and pneumonitis (1.2% vs. 0.2%) in nodal radiation arm.

- Systemic therapy/endocrine therapy:
  - o Chemotherapy indications:
    - Triple negative breast cancer greater than 5 mm
    - Her2 amplified breast cancers greater than 5 mm
      - Trastuzumab is given following doxorubicin and cyclophosphamide and concurrently with taxane and then continued for a total duration of 1 year
    - ER- and/or PR-positive breast cancer
      - If node negative and tumor greater than 5 mm, perform 21-gene assay (Oncotype)
        - Low recurrence score (<18): Endocrine therapy alone
        - Intermediate recurrence score (18–30): Endocrine therapy ± chemotherapy
        - High recurrence score (≥31): Endocrine therapy and chemotherapy
      - If node positive, endocrine therapy and chemotherapy
        - SWOG RxPONDER (S1007) trial: Patients with one to three positive nodes randomized to endocrine therapy ± chemotherapy based on results of 21-gene assay; results pending
    - Consider neoadjuvant chemotherapy if T2 or T3 and otherwise a candidate for breast conservation therapy
      - Axillary evaluation with ultrasound should be performed prior to neoadjuvant therapy with FNA or core needle biopsy of suspicious nodes.
        - For patients with clinical Stage II breast cancer who have a mastectomy, who are initially clinically node positive (with positive biopsy), and achieve a complete pathologic response in the axillary nodes at the time of surgery, benefit of postmastectomy radiation may be minimal and is subject of ongoing clinical trial. If patient has residual nodal disease after neoadjuvant chemotherapy, postmastectomy radiation is indicated.
      - Place clips in tumor bed for accurate localization if complete radiographic/clinical response to chemotherapy.
  - o Endocrine therapy:
    - Adjuvant Tamoxifen or aromatase inhibitor (AI) if ER and/or PR positive for minimum of 5 years
      - NSABP B-14: Women with ER-positive invasive breast cancer s/p lumpectomy or mastectomy with negative pathologic lymph nodes randomized to 5 years of Tamoxifen or placebo
        - Tamoxifen improved disease-free survival (by approximately 30%), distant disease-free survival, and overall survival compared to placebo
        - No additional benefit beyond 5 years was seen
      - NSABP B-21: Following lumpectomy + ALND, patients with invasive breast cancer 1 cm or less randomized to (a) Tamoxifen (b) radiation + placebo, or (c) radiation + Tamoxifen
        - Risk of in-breast recurrence at 8 years
          - Tamoxifen: 16.5%
          - RT + Placebo: 9.3%
          - RT+ Tamoxifen: 2.8%
    - AIs improved disease-free survival compared to Tamoxifen for postmenopausal women with hormone receptor-positive breast cancer.
    - AI (exemestane) with ovarian suppression improved disease-free survival and reduced recurrences compared to Tamoxifen and ovarian suppression for premenopausal women with hormone-positive early-stage breast cancer (TEXT and SOFT trials).

Radiation Therapy Techniques

- Whole breast radiation
  - o CT simulation for treatment planning
  - o Patient in supine or prone position
  - o Both arms above head in breast board, vac fix, alpha cradle, or other immobilization device

- o Radio-opaque markers placed along lumpectomy scar, palpable breast tissue from 2 o'clock to 10 o'clock, and superior border of breast
- o Traditional clinical borders of breast for 2D RT
  - Superior: inferior clavicle (1 cm above breast tissue)
  - Inferior: 1 to 2 cm below breast tissue
  - Lateral: mid-axillary line
  - Medial: midline
- o Anatomic boundaries for Breast clinical target volume (CTV) Contouring for 3DCRT (from http://www.rtog.org/CoreLab/ContouringAtlases/BreastCancerAtlas.aspx)
  - Cranial: clinical border and second rib insertion
  - Caudal: clinical border and loss of CT breast tissue
  - Anterior: skin
  - Posterior: excludes pectoralis muscles and chest wall
  - Lateral: mid axillary line excluding latissimus dorsi (lat dorsi)
  - Medial: sternal-rib junction
- o Target volumes
  - Lumpectomy
    - GTV = scar, seroma and/or surgical clips
    - CTV = GTV + 1 cm
    - PTV = CTV + 0.7 cm
    - PTV eval = PTV cropped 5 mm from skin surface
  - Breast
    - CTV = All palpable breast tissue and CT glandular breast tissue; lumpectomy CTV; and clinical and anatomic boundaries
    - PTV = CTV + 0.7 cm
    - PTV eval = PTV cropped 5 mm from skin surface
- o Organs at risk
  - Lung
  - Heart
  - Thyroid
  - Contralateral breast
- o Dose: 50 Gy in 25 daily fractions
  - Consider 42.5 Gy in 16 fractions if criteria for hypofractionation are met
- o Boost: 10 to 16 Gy in 2 Gy fractions using photons or electrons depending on depth of lumpectomy cavity
- o Dosimetry
  - Tangential opposing fields to cover breast PTV
  - Options to achieve dose homogeneity in breast tissue and spare OARs
    - Wedges or compensators
    - Field in field segments (forward planned)
    - IMRT
    - Prone positioning
- o Dose volume histograms (DVH) parameters
  - Breast PTV eval: 95% receives 95% prescription dose
  - Lumpectomy PTV eval: 100% receives 95% to 100% of prescription dose
  - Volume of breast at final boost dose is 30%
  - Ipsilateral lung: V20 ≤ 10%
    - Hypofractionation: V16 ≤ 15%
  - Heart: V25 less than 5%; mean dose less than 5 Gy; max dose 40 Gy
    - Hypofractionation: V20 ≤ 5%; mean less than 2 Gy; max 35 Gy

- Partial breast radiation
  - Radiation to lumpectomy cavity alone with margin
    - APBI: post lumpectomy in 5 to 8 treatment days, often 4 to 10 fractions, can be BID
    - Intra op PBI: single dose treatment post lumpectomy intraoperatively prior to closure of the cavity
  - Techniques
    - Brachytherapy
      - Interstitial brachytherapy
        - CT simulation
        - Plan number of catheters based on CTV
          - CTV = tumor bed + 1 to 2 cm margin for subclinical disease
          - CTV = PTV = PTV eval
        - Catheters placed percutaneously under ultrasound, fluoroscopic, or CT guidance
        - Catheters then loaded with radioactive source
          - Typically Ir192 for high dose rate (HDR)
        - Prescription
          - 34 Gy BID in 10 fractions
      - Intracavitary brachytherapy
        - Single lumen or multilumen catheter balloon placed into lumpectomy cavity and inflated
        - CT simulation
          - Balloon should be at least 7 mm from the skin surface
        - CTV = tumor bed + 1 cm = PTV = PTV eval
        - Iridium (Ir) 192 HDR
        - 34 Gy BID × 10 fractions
          - Prescribed to 1 cm from balloon surface
      - External beam radiation (3DCRT or intensity-modulated radiation therapy [IMRT])
        - CT based planning
        - Contour whole breast and lumpectomy
          - Lumpectomy cavity/whole breast reference must be 30% or less
        - Contour lung, thyroid, heart
        - CTV = tumor bed + 1.5 cm
        - PTV = CTV + 1 cm
        - PTV eval = excludes chest wall and cropped 5 mm inside skin
        - Dose = 38.5 Gy BID × 10 fractions
      - Intraoperative radiation
        - Single fraction delivered to tumor bed at time of lumpectomy
        - 20 Gy × 1 (TARGIT Trial)

8.5   Locally Advanced Breast Cancer (Stages IIIA, B, and C)

Treatment Overview

- Systemic therapy: often performed prior to surgical management for locally advanced breast cancer
  - Neoadjuvant chemotherapy
    - There is no difference in recurrence or survival if chemotherapy is given preoperatively or postoperatively for patients with operable breast cancer (NSABP B18).
    - The addition of docetaxel (T) to AC preoperatively increased pCR rate (26% vs. 13%).
      - Patients with pCR had improved survival compared to those without pCR.
    - It can be used to downsize primary to allow for breast conservation therapy if mastectomy indicated due to primary tumor size.
  - Adjuvant
    - The addition of paclitaxel to doxorubicin and cyclophosphamide (AC) improves disease-free and overall survival for node-positive breast cancer.

- o   Endocrine therapy
  - ▪   Typically it is started after chemotherapy for hormone receptor-positive patients.
- o   Targeted therapy
  - ▪   Herceptin is indicated for Her2neu positive breast cancer.
    - –   Given following AC and concurrently with weekly taxane
    - –   Continues every three weeks after systemic therapy completed for total duration of one year
- •   Surgery
  - o   Mastectomy with sentinel node biopsy or ALND if node positive
  - o   Lumpectomy if a candidate for breast conservation therapy with sentinel node biopsy or axillary node dissection
- •   Radiation
  - o   Postmastectomy RT to chest wall and regional lymphatics including undissected axilla, supraclavicular nodes, and internal mammary nodes
    - ▪   Indications:
      - –   Four or more positive nodes
      - –   Many one to three node-positive cases
      - –   Any Stage III breast cancer
      - –   Role of PMRT in the setting of pT1-2 breast cancer with one to three continues to evolve
        - •   Consider PMRT for one to three nodes with the following risk factors
          - •   LVSI
          - •   Gross extranodal extension
          - •   Greater than 20% ratio of positive nodes to number of nodes removed
          - •   Grade 3 histology
          - •   ER negative tumor
          - •   Young age/premenopausal status
          - •   Positive margins
      - –   British Columbia Trial
        - •   Premenopausal women s/p modified radical mastectomy with positive lymph nodes randomized to cyclophosphamide, methotrexate, 5-FU (CMF) versus. CMF + PMRT
          - •   PMRT improved OS at 20 years from 37% to 47% and reduced local recurrence from 26% to 10%
      - –   Danish trials
        - •   DBCG 82b
          - •   Premenopausal women with positive axillary nodes, tumor size greater than 5 cm, or skin or pectoral fascia invasion randomized to modified radical mastectomy followed by CMF with or without PMRT
          - •   PMRT decreased local failure at 10 years from 32% to 9%
          - •   PMRT improved OS at 10 years from 45% to 54%
        - •   DBCG 82c
          - •   Postmenopausal women with same entry criteria
          - •   Randomized to modified radical mastectomy and Tamoxifen × 1 year with or without PMRT
          - •   PMRT reduced local recurrence at 10 years from 35% to 8% and improved OS 36% to 45%
      - –   EBCTCG meta-analysis
        - •   Postmastectomy radiation for node-positive patients
          - •   Reduced local recurrence rates from 29% to 7% at 5 years
          - •   Improved 15-year breast cancer mortality by approximately 5%
          - •   Benefit seen in all node-positive patients, regardless of number of positive nodes
    - ▪   Consider chest wall boost if T4 disease or close (≤2 mm)/positive margin
  - o   If treated with lumpectomy, RT to whole breast and regional lymphatics including undissected axilla, supraclavicular nodes, and internal mammary nodes followed by boost to lumpectomy cavity

- o Current recommendations for PMRT following neoadjuvant chemotherapy:
  - All clinical Stage III patients at diagnosis should receive PMRT regardless of pathologic nodal status.
  - Omission of radiation for those who were node positive initially and post NAC have pathologically negative nodes is currently being investigated.

Radiation Therapy Technique

- CT simulation for treatment planning
  - o Images obtained from above mandible to below chest wall and including entire lung
- Patient in supine position on breast board, wing board, or other immobilization device
- Radio-opaque markers placed along mastectomy scar and chest wall from 2 o'clock to 10 o'clock, including postoperative changes and prior approximate location of breast tissue
- Chest wall
  - o Traditional borders for 2D RT
    - Superior: bottom of clavicular head
    - Interior: 1 to 1.5 cm below inframammary fold of opposite breast
    - Medial: mid axillary line
    - Lateral: sternum
    - Anterior: flash over chest wall
- Regional nodes
  - o Traditional borders for 2D RT
    - Medial: pedicle of vertebral bodies
    - Lateral: 1 cm medial to humeral head at coracoid process
    - Superior: below cricoid cartilage
    - Inferior: bottom of clavicular head
- Anatomic borders (from http://www.rtog.org/CoreLab/ContouringAtlases/BreastCancerAtlas.aspx) for delineating target volumes for 3DCRT or IMRT treatment planning
  - o Chest wall
    - Cranial: bottom of clavicular head
    - Caudal: clinical reference and/or loss of contralateral breast on CT
    - Anterior: skin
    - Posterior: rib-pleural space interface
    - Lateral: mid axillary line, excluding latissimus dorsi (lat dorsi)
    - Medial: sternal-rib junction
  - o Axillary nodes
    - Axillary level I:
      - Cranial: axillary vessels cross lateral edge of pec minor
      - Caudal: pectoralis major insertion into ribs
      - Anterior: anterior surface of pec major and lat dorsi
      - Posterior: anterior surface of subscapularis
      - Lateral: medial border of lat dorsi
      - Medial: lateral border of pec minor
    - Axillary level II:
      - Cranial: axillary vessels cross medial edge of pec minor
      - Caudal: axillary vessels cross lateral edge of pec minor
      - Anterior: anterior surface of pec minor
      - Posterior: ribs and intercostal space
      - Lateral: lateral border of pec minor
      - Medial: medial border of pec minor
    - Axillary level III:
      - Cranial: insertion of pec minor at coracoid process
      - Caudal: axillary vessels cross medial edge of pec minor

- Anterior: posterior surface of pec major
- Posterior: ribs and intercostal space
- Lateral: medial border of pec minor
- Medial: thoracic inlet

o Supraclavicular nodes
  - Cranial: below cricoid cartilage
  - Caudal: bottom of clavicular head
  - Anterior: sternocleidomastoid muscle (SCM)
  - Posterior: anterior scalene muscle superiorly and the junction of the first rib and clavicle inferiorly
  - Lateral: lateral to SCM
  - Medial: excludes thyroid and trachea

o Internal mammary nodes
  - Cranial: superior aspect of medial first rib
  - Caudal: cranial aspect of fourth rib

o Target volumes
  - Mastectomy scar
    - Scar: contoured from radio-opaque wire placed along incision and any postoperative changes deep to the wire
    - Scar CTV: scar + 1 cm
      • Limit expansion posteriorly at anterior surface of ribs and at skin
      • Should not cross midline unless clinically indicated
    - Scar PTV: CTV + 7 mm
    - Scar PTV eval: PTV cropped 3 mm from skin surface and posteriorly excludes lung and heart; should not cross midline unless clinically indicated
  - Chest wall
    - CTV: mastectomy scar CTV, clinical extent of chest wall, postoperative changes on CT, and anatomical borders; limited by skin anteriorly and ribs posteriorly
    - PTV: CTV + 7 mm
    - PTV eval: PTV cropped 3 mm from skin surface and posteriorly to the posterior rib surface; should not cross midline
  - Axilla
    - CTV: Undissected axilla; typically level III and some of level II unless axillary node dissection not performed
    - PTV: CTV + 5 mm; excludes ipsilateral lung
  - Supraclavicular
    - CTV: anatomical borders
    - PTV: CTV + 5 mm; excludes thyroid, trachea, esophagus, vertebral body and ipsilateral lung
  - Internal mammary
    - CTV: internal mammary vessels in first three intercostal spaces
    - PTV: CTV + 5 mm without anterior or posterior expansion

o OARs
  - Ipsilateral lung
  - Contralateral lung
  - Heart
  - Contralateral breast
  - Thyroid
  - Spinal cord

- Dose
  o 50 Gy in 2 Gy fractions to chest wall, axillary, supraclavicular, and internal mammary nodes
  o Chest wall boost to 10 to 16 Gy in 2 Gy fractions if indicated for T4 disease or close/positive margin

- Dosimetry
  - Chest wall
    - Tangential opposing fields to cover chest wall PTV
    - Options to achieve dose homogeneity and spare OARs
      - Wedges or compensators
      - Field in field segments (forward planned)
      - IMRT
    - Bolus: 5 mm over chest wall every day or 1 cm over chest wall every other day
  - Axillary and Supraclavicular nodes
    - Mono-isocentric technique
      - Single isocenter placed at junction of chest wall and nodal fields
      - Tangential fields for chest wall and made nondivergent superiorly at isocenter
      - Nodal fields are treated with a nondivergent anterior oblique field at isocenter with gantry rotated approximately 15° to contralateral side to avoid spinal cord
        - Matched inferior border to superior nondivergent border of chest wall tangents
        - An opposing posterior or posterior oblique field to improve dose homogeneity of axillary and supraclavicular target volumes recommended
    - Dual isocenter technique
      - Required if field size greater than 20 cm
      - Supraclavicular field set up the same as mono-isocentric technique
      - Tangents
        - Couch kick approximately 5° away from collimator to prevent divergence into SC field
          - Couch kick: arctan (1/2 tangent field length/SAD)
        - Rotate collimator slightly to avoid overlap on skin
  - Internal mammary nodes
    - Treatment techniques
      - Deep/partially wide tangents
        - Include three upper intercostal spaces in tangents with heart and lung blocked below IM nodes
      - Medial tangent (photon field) matched to electron field to treat IMN (Kuske technique)
        - Match at skin
        - Angle electron approximately 5° less than medial tangent
      - IMRT for left sided cancer for cardiac sparing
- DVH analysis:
  - Target dose goals (50 Gy/25 fraction prescription dose):
    - Chest wall PTV eval: 95% receives ≥ 47.5 Gy
    - Scar PTV eval: 95% to 100% received full dose
    - SCL PTV: 95% receives ≥ 47.5 Gy; dmax less than 52 Gy
    - Axilla PTV: 95% receives ≥ 45 Gy
  - OARs
    - Ipsilateral lung: V20 less than 35%
    - Heart: V25 heart less than 5%, mean heart dose less than 500 cGy

Toxicity for Breast and Post Mastectomy Radiation

- Acute
  - Radiation dermatitis
  - Fatigue
- Late
  - Altered breast cosmesis
    - Effects on reconstructed breast if present

- o Soft tissue fibrosis of chest wall muscles
- o Reduced arm range of motion
- o Lymphedema
  - ▪ Approximately 5% after SNLB, 10% with ALND, and up to 20% with ALND and regional nodal radiation
- o Pneumonitis
- o Rib fracture
- o Cardiotoxicity
- o Brachial plexopathy
- o Second malignancy

Follow-Up

- DCIS
  - o H & P every 6 months for 5 years, then annually
  - o Annual mammogram
- Invasive breast cancer
  - o H & P every 3 months for 5 years, then annually
  - o Annual mammogram
  - o No routine staging scans performed in the absence of symptoms
  - o Annual gynecologic exam if on Tamoxifen
  - o Bone density test at baseline and every 2 years if on AI

8.6   Inflammatory Breast Cancer

- Presentation of rapid erythema, swelling, and Peau d'orange of a third or more of the breast
- Mammography typically shows diffuse skin thickening throughout the breast with underlying mass
- Work-up includes skin biopsy and biopsy of breast mass
  - o Hallmark Pathology: dermal lymphatic invasion of involved skin
    - ▪ NOT required or alone sufficient for diagnosis; the diagnosis is clinical after biopsy-proven invasive breast cancer
- Metastatic workup required including CT chest, abdomen, and pelvis, and Nuclear bone scan
- Treatment: Neoadjuvant chemotherapy followed by mastectomy and postmastectomy radiation to chest wall and regional nodes including axilla, supraclavicular, and internal mammary nodes
- If patient progresses on neoadjuvant chemotherapy, patient can be treated with alternative systemic therapy and/or preoperative RT

8.7   Breast Cancer During Pregnancy

- First trimester at diagnosis
  - o Discuss termination of pregnancy
  - o Mastectomy + axillary staging with adjuvant chemotherapy if indicated in second trimester
    - ▪ Blue dye contraindicated for sentinel node biopsy
    - ▪ Radiolabeled colloid appears safe
  - o RT and/or endocrine therapy if indicated to begin postpartum
- Second trimester/early third trimester at diagnosis
  - o Mastectomy or lumpectomy with axillary staging
  - o Alternatively, neoadjuvant chemotherapy with surgery postpartum
  - o RT and/or endocrine therapy if indicated to begin postpartum
- Late third trimester
  - o Mastectomy or lumpectomy with axillary staging
  - o Adjuvant chemotherapy, RT and/or endocrine therapy if indicated to begin postpartum

8.8   Locally Recurrent or Metastatic Breast Cancer

- Local recurrence only (breast or chest wall)
  - o Mastectomy if prior breast conservation therapy with radiation
  - o Chest wall recurrence after prior mastectomy
    - Surgical resection alone if prior radiation
    - If no prior radiation, surgical resection followed by postmastectomy radiation to chest wall and regional nodes
    - The addition of systemic therapy in addition to local-regional treatment has demonstrated improve overall survival (Calor Trial)
- Regional recurrence
  - o Axillary: resection if feasible followed by RT to chest wall and regional nodes if no prior radiation
  - o Supraclavicular and/or internal mammary: RT to chest wall and regional nodes with boost to positive node(s) if no prior radiation
- Metastatic disease
  - o Systemic therapy indicated
    - Hormone receptor positive: Endocrine therapy (typically first line) or chemotherapy if endocrine refractory
    - Chemotherapy for triple negative or Her2 positive; Targeted anti-Her2 therapy for Her2 positive
    - Zometa, pamidronate, or denosumab if bone metastases present
  - o Role of radiation is palliative
    - Brain metastases
      - Stereotactic radiation for limited number of brain metastases
      - Whole brain RT for diffuse brain metastases or leptomeningeal disease
    - Bone metastases
    - Other sites of disease causing pain/discomfort/bleeding
    - No clear role for selective internal radiation therapy (SBRT) for oligometastatic disease at this time

Chapter 8: Practice Questions

1. All of the following are "suitable" criteria for partial breast irradiation EXCEPT

   A. Age 60 or greater
   B. No BRCA mutations
   C. Close or negative margin
   D. No lymphovascular invasion

2. According to the EBCTCG meta-analysis for postmastectomy node-positive breast cancer patients receiving RT, there was the following absolute percentage improvement in 15-year breast cancer survival of

   A. 0%
   B. 5%
   C. 10%
   D. 15%

3. T4 breast tumors have what risk of axillary node positivity?

   A. 20%
   B. 40%
   C. 75%
   D. 85%

4. A typical single dose used for partial breast intraoperative irradiation as per the TARGIT trial is

    A. 12 Gy
    B. 16 Gy
    C. 20 Gy
    D. 24 Gy

5. An inflammatory breast carcinoma is best T staged as

    A. T3
    B. T4
    C. T4i
    D. T4d

6. In terms of mammogram screening, a BIRADS 5 category finding is associated with

    A. Probably benign
    B. Suspicious abnormality
    C. Highly suspicious of malignancy
    D. Known biopsy proven malignancy

7. The following are known risk factors for breast cancer EXCEPT

    A. Obesity
    B. Late menarche
    C. Late menopause
    D. Late parity

8. The additional risk of lymphedema associated with regional radiation of the breast is approximately

    A. 1%
    B. 5%
    C. 10%
    D. 20%

9. The hallmark of inflammatory breast cancer is

    A. Dermal invasion
    B. Poorly differentiated tumor
    C. Triple negative disease
    D. Lymphatic invasion

10. The maximum ipsilateral lung dose for a regional breast irradiation technique should be limited to the following:

    A. V20 < 15%
    B. V20 < 20%
    C. V20 < 25%
    D. V20 < 35%

11. Axillary lymph nodes that are located medial to the medial margin of the pectoralis minor muscle are

    A. Level 1
    B. Level 2
    C. Level 3
    D. Not axillary in origin

12. All of the following are forms of noncomedo DCIS EXCEPT

    A. Solid
    B. Cribriform
    C. Papillary
    D. Cystic

13. The ACOSOG Z0011 breast cancer trial found what magnitude of axillary recurrence between ALND and SLNB?

    A. No difference
    B. 0.4%
    C. 1.0%
    D. 1.9%

14. The following are clinical borders of the breast EXCEPT

    A. Medial: sternum
    B. Lateral: mid-axillary line
    C. Cranial: first rib
    D. Caudal: sixth rib

15. According to the NSABP B06 trial, local recurrence is reduced by what absolute percentage with the use of adjuvant radiation?

    A. 5%
    B. 15%
    C. 25%
    D. 50%

16. A typical hypofractionation schedule used for whole breast RT is

    A. 30 Gy in 5 fractions
    B. 40 Gy in 10 fractions
    C. 42.5 Gy in 16 fractions
    D. 45 Gy in 15 fractions

17. The lymphedema risk after axillary lymph node dissection (ALND) is

    A. 0%
    B. 5%
    C. 10%
    D. 20%

18. According to the British Columbia trial assessing postmastectomy regional radiation therapy for breast cancer demonstrated an absolute percentage survival improvement at 20 years of

    A. 0%
    B. 5%
    C. 10%
    D. 20%

19. According to the EORTC 22881-10882 trial, the use of a 16 Gy boost to lumpectomy cavity after 50 Gy of whole breast radiation was associated with what absolute percentage reduction in local recurrence?

    A. 0%
    B. 4%
    C. 8%
    D. 12%

20. The NSABP B-06 was a clinical trial assessing

    A. Primary RT
    B. Adjuvant RT
    C. Chemotherapy
    D. Hormonal therapy

Chapter 8: Answers

1. C
Margins should be 2 mm or greater for partial breast irradiation.

2. B
EBCTCG meta-analysis of postmastectomy radiation for node-positive patients demonstrated reduced local recurrence rates from 29% to 7% at 5 years and improved 15-year breast cancer mortality by approximately 5%.

3. D
T-stage incidence of positive axillary nodes:

T1a	5%
T1b	10%
T1c	20%
T2	40%
T3	75%
T4	85%

4. C
Intraoperative radiation, single fraction delivered to tumor bed at time of lumpectomy, 20 Gy × 1 (TARGIT Trial).

5. D
T Staging of breast carcinoma:

T4	Tumor extension to chest wall and/or skin (ulceration or skin nodules)
T4a	Extension to chest wall, not including only pectoralis muscle invasion
T4b	Skin ulceration and/or ipsilateral nodules and/or edema (including peau d'orange) of the skin that do not meet criteria for T4d
T4c	T4a and T4b
T4d	Inflammatory carcinoma

6. C
BIRADS category assessment:

0	Incomplete
1	Negative
2	Benign
3	Probably benign
4	Suspicious abnormality
5	Highly suspicious of malignancy
6	Known biopsy proven malignancy

7. B
Risk factors for breast cancer:

Female sex

Age > 50

BRCA 1 or 2 mutation or other inherited genetic conditions such as Li-Fraumeni or Cowden syndrome

Family history of breast or ovarian cancer

Late parity (>30 years of age) or nulliparity

Early menarche and/or late menopause

Hormone replacement therapy with estrogen and progestin

Obesity

Prior chest radiation

Prior history of atypical ductal hyperplasia or lobular carcinoma in situ

8. B
Regional nodal radiation improved disease-free survival but with no OS difference. Higher rates of lymphedema (8.4% vs. 4.5%) and pneumonitis (1.2% vs. 0.2%) in nodal radiation arm.

9. A

Hallmark pathology for inflammatory breast cancer is dermal lymphatic invasion of involved skin.

10. D

Ipsilateral lung for regional breast irradiation: V20 greater than 35%

11. C

Axillary levels

 Level 1: lymph nodes located lateral to pec minor

 Level 2: lymph nodes located between the medial and lateral border of pec minor and the interpectoral nodes (i.e., Rotters' nodes)

 Level 3: lymph nodes located medial to the medial margin of pec minor

12. D

Noncomedo DCIS: cribriform, micropapillary, papillary, and solid

13. B

ACOSOG Z0011: Women with clinical T1-2, N0 women s/p lumpectomy and SLN biopsy with 1-2 positive sentinel nodes randomized to ALND or no further axillary treatment followed by whole breast radiation ± systemic therapy. No difference in local or regional recurrence. 5-year axillary recurrence: 0.9% with ALND and 0.5% with SLNB.

14. C

The clinical borders of the breast are as follows:

 Medial: sternum

 Lateral: mid-axillary line

 Cranial: second rib

 Caudal: sixth rib

15. C

NSABP B-06: Local recurrences 39% with lumpectomy alone and 14% with the addition of radiation.

16. C

Typical conventionally fractionated dose: 50 Gy in 25 daily fractions. Consider 42.5 Gy in 16 fractions if criteria for hypofractionation are met.

17. C

Lymphedema risk is approximately 5% after SNLB, 10% with ALND, and up to 20% with ALND and regional nodal radiation.

18. C

The British Columbia Trial assessed premenopausal women s/p modified radical mastectomy with positive lymph nodes randomized to CMF versus. CMF + PMRT. PMRT improved OS at 20 years from 37% to 47% and reduced local recurrence from 26% to 10%.

19. B

NSABP B-06: Local recurrences 39% with lumpectomy alone and 14% with the addition of radiation.

20. B

NSABP B-06: Modified radical mastectomy (Total mastectomy + ALND) versus lumpectomy + ALND + RT versus lumpectomy + ALND. No OS difference between three arms.

Recommended Reading

DCIS

Allred DC, Anderson SJ, Paik S, et al. Adjuvant tamoxifen reduces subsequent breast cancer in women with estrogen receptor-positive ductal carcinoma in situ: a study based on NSABP protocol B-24. *J Clin Oncol.* 2012;30(12):1268-1273.

McCormick B, Winter K, Hudis C, et al. RTOG 9804: a prospective randomized trial for good-risk ductal carcinoma in situ comparing radiotherapy with observation. *J Clin Oncol.* 2015;33(7):709-715.

Solin LJ, Gray R, Hughes LL, et al. Surgical excision without radiation for ductal carcinoma in situ of the breast: 12-year results from the ECOG-ACRIN E5194 study. *J Clin Oncol.* 2015;33(33):3938-3944.

Wapnir IL, Dignam JJ, Fisher B, et al. Long-term outcomes of invasive ipsilateral breast tumor recurrences after lumpectomy in NSABP B-17 and B-24 randomized clinical trials for DCIS. *J Natl Cancer Inst.* 2011;103(6):478-488.

Oncotype

Paik S, Shak S, Tang G, et al. A multigene assay to predict recurrence of tamoxifen-treated, node-negative breast cancer. *New Engl J Med.* 2004;351(27):2817-2826.

Sparano JA, Gray RJ, Makower DF, et al. Prospective validation of a 21-gene expression assay in breast cancer. *New Engl J Med.* 2015;373(21):2005-2014.

Early-Stage Invasive Breast Cancer

Bartelink H, Maingon P, Poortmans P, et al. Whole-breast irradiation with or without a boost for patients treated with breast-conserving surgery for early breast cancer: 20-year follow-up of a randomised phase 3 trial. *Lancet Oncol.* 2015;16(1):47-56.

Clarke M, Collins R, Darby S, et al. Effects of radiotherapy and of differences in the extent of surgery for early breast cancer on local recurrence and 15-year survival: an overview of the randomised trials. *Lancet.* 2005;366(9503):2087-2106.

Darby S, McGale P, Correa C, et al. Effect of radiotherapy after breast-conserving surgery on 10-year recurrence and 15-year breast cancer death: meta-analysis of individual patient data for 10,801 women in 17 randomised trials. *Lancet.* 2011;378(9804):1707-1716.

Donker M, van Tienhoven G, Straver ME, et al. Radiotherapy or surgery of the axilla after a positive sentinel node in breast cancer (EORTC 10981-22023 AMAROS): a randomised, multicentre, open-label, phase 3 non-inferiority trial. *Lancet Oncol.* 2014;15(12):1303-1310.

Fisher B, Anderson S, Bryant J, et al. Twenty-year follow-up of a randomized trial comparing total mastectomy, lumpectomy, and lumpectomy plus irradiation for the treatment of invasive breast cancer. *New Engl J Med.* 2002;347(16):1233-1241.

Fyles AW, McCready DR, Manchul LA, et al. Tamoxifen with or without breast irradiation in women 50 years of age or older with early breast cancer. *New Engl J Med.* 2004;351(10):963-970.

Giuliano AE, Hunt KK, Ballman KV, et al. Axillary dissection vs no axillary dissection in women with invasive breast cancer and sentinel node metastasis: a randomized clinical trial. *JAMA.* 2011;305(6):569-575.

Haviland JS, Owen JR, Dewar JA, et al. The UK Standardisation of Breast Radiotherapy (START) trials of radiotherapy hypofractionation for treatment of early breast cancer: 10-year follow-up results of two randomised controlled trials. *Lancet Oncol.* 2013;14(11):1086-1094.

Hughes KS, Schnaper LA, Bellon JR, et al. Lumpectomy plus tamoxifen with or without irradiation in women age 70 years or older with early breast cancer: long-term follow-up of CALGB 9343. *J Clin Oncol.* 2013;31(19):2382-2387

Kunkler IH, Williams LJ, Jack WJ, Cameron DA, Dixon JM. Breast-conserving surgery with or without irradiation in women aged 65 years or older with early breast cancer (PRIME II): a randomised controlled trial. *Lancet Oncol.* 2015;16(3):266-273.

Romestaing P, Lehingue Y, Carrie C, et al. Role of a 10-Gy boost in the conservative treatment of early breast cancer: results of a randomized clinical trial in Lyon, France. *J Clin Oncol.* 1997;15(3):963-968.

Smith BD, Arthur DW, Buchholz TA, et al. Accelerated partial breast irradiation consensus statement from the American Society for Radiation Oncology (ASTRO). *J Am Coll Surg.* 2009;209(2):269-277.

Veronesi U, Cascinelli N, Mariani L, et al. Twenty-year follow-up of a randomized study comparing breast-conserving surgery with radical mastectomy for early breast cancer. *New Engl J Med.* 2002;347(16):1227-1232.

Whelan TJ, Olivotto IA, Parulekar WR, et al. Regional nodal irradiation in early-stage breast cancer. *New Engl J Med.* 2015;373(4):307-316.

Whelan TJ, Pignol JP, Levine MN, et al. Long-term results of hypofractionated radiation therapy for breast cancer. *New Engl J Med.* 2010;362(6):513-520.

Endocrine/Systemic Therapy

Cuzick J, Sestak I, Baum M, et al. Effect of anastrozole and tamoxifen as adjuvant treatment for early-stage breast cancer: 10-year analysis of the ATAC trial. *Lancet Oncol.* 2010;11(12):1135-1141.

Early Breast Cancer Trialists' Collaborative Group (EBCTCG). Effects of chemotherapy and hormonal therapy for early breast cancer on recurrence and 15-year survival: an overview of the randomised trials. *Lancet.* 2005;365(9472):1687-1717.

Fisher B, Dignam J, Bryant J, Wolmark N. Five versus more than five years of tamoxifen for lymph node-negative breast cancer: updated findings from the National Surgical Adjuvant Breast and Bowel Project B-14 randomized trial. *J Natl Cancer Inst.* 2001;93(9):684-690.

Mamounas EP, Bryant J, Lembersky B, et al. Paclitaxel after doxorubicin plus cyclophosphamide as adjuvant chemotherapy for node-positive breast cancer: results from NSABP B-28. *J Clin Oncol.* 2005;23(16):3686-3696.

Pagani O, Regan MM, Walley BA, et al. Adjuvant exemestane with ovarian suppression in premenopausal breast cancer. *New Engl J Med.* 2014;371(2):107-118.

Rastogi P, Anderson SJ, Bear HD, et al. Preoperative chemotherapy: updates of National Surgical Adjuvant Breast and Bowel Project Protocols B-18 and B-27. *J Clin Oncol.* 2008;26(5):778-785.

Romond EH, Perez EA, Bryant J, et al. Trastuzumab plus adjuvant chemotherapy for operable HER2-positive breast cancer. *New Engl J Med.* 2005;353(16):1673-1684.

Locally Advanced Breast Cancer

McGale P, Taylor C, Correa C et al. Effect of radiotherapy after mastectomy and axillary surgery on 10-year recurrence and 20-year breast cancer mortality: meta-analysis of individual patient data for 8135 women in 22 randomised trials. *Lancet.* 2014;383(9935):2127-2135.

Overgaard M, Hansen PS, Overgaard J, et al. Postoperative radiotherapy in high-risk premenopausal women with breast cancer who receive adjuvant chemotherapy. Danish Breast Cancer Cooperative Group 82b Trial. *New Engl J Med.* 1997;337(14):949-955.

Overgaard M, Jensen MB, Overgaard J, et al. Postoperative radiotherapy in high-risk postmenopausal breast-cancer patients given adjuvant tamoxifen: Danish Breast Cancer Cooperative Group DBCG 82c randomised trial. *Lancet.* 1999;353(9165):1641-1648.

Ragaz J, Jackson SM, Le N, et al. Adjuvant radiotherapy and chemotherapy in node-positive premenopausal women with breast cancer. *New Engl J Med.* 1997;337(14):956-962.

Bone/Sarcoma

Christie Binder, Simon Brown, and Arthur Y. Hung

9.1 Osteosarcoma: Most Common Primary Malignant Bone Tumor

- Arises in the metaphysis of long bones (i.e., distal femur proximal tibia and proximal humerus).
- Usually around age 20, second incidence wave age 60 to 80 years.
- Younger patients tend to have extremity disease while older patients have more craniofacial disease.
- Five-year survival in 1960s was greater than 20%; primarily treated with limb amputation while most died of lung metastases.
- Currently 5-year survival about 60% with addition of chemotherapy, improved surgical techniques, surgical devices, and diagnostic methods.
- Three major therapeutic options: surgery, chemotherapy, and palliative RT.
- Local recurrence is directly correlated to the surgical margins and degree of tumor necrosis following chemotherapy.
- Metastatic osteosarcoma overall survival ranges from 10% to 50%. Overall poor prognosis.
- No benefit for prophylactic pulmonary irradiation for patients.
- Interferons (IFNs), granulocyte-macrophage colony stimulating factor (GM-CSF), SRc, mTor, Hedgehog (Hh), insulin like growth factor-R (IGF-R), human epidermal growth factor receptor 2 (HER-2), vascular endothelial growth factor (VEGF), and Receptor activator of nuclear factor kappa-B ligand (RANKL) are currently under investigation as markers for treatment for osteosarcoma.

Surgery

- Goal is complete tumor removal with wide margin for local control and improved overall survival.
- Amputation was the main and standard therapy option before 1970s. Survival ranged 5% to 23%.
- Now 90% of patients undergo wide resection with limb-sparing surgery (LSS).
- Limb-salvage surgery is the gold standard in osteosarcoma treatment.
- No difference in survival rate with amputation versus LSS, but there is a high trend of local recurrence with LSS. Picci et al. (JCO, 1993;11(9):1763–1769) noted 7% versus 2.4% in patients with high-grade osteosarcoma.
- Recommended only under conditions that safe surgical margins can be achieved.
- If tumor is unable to be resected with appropriate margins, amputation is considered.
- Complications of amputation are wound necrosis, infection, overgrowth of bone in children, neuroma, stump pain, and phantom limb pain.
- Resection is determined by Enneking's surgical-staging system of bone sarcoma.
  - ○ Intracompartmental: tumors are confined within the cortex of the bone.
  - ○ Extracompartmental: tumor extends beyond bone cortex.

Stage	Grade	Site (1)	Metastasis
IA	Low grade	T1—intracompartmental	M0 (none)
IB	Low grade	T2—extracompartmental	M0 (none)
IIA	High grade	T1—intracompartmental	M0 (none)
IIB	High grade	T2—extracompartmental	M0 (none)
III	Metastatic	T1—intracompartmental	M1 (regional or distant)
III	Metastatic	T2—extracompartmental	M1 (regional or distant)

- Options available for reconstruction after limb salvage tumor resection include endoprosthetic reconstruction, autografts, allografts, and rotationplasty.
- Endoprosthetic reconstruction:
  - Disadvantages such as infection, loosening of prosthesis, joint stiffness, limb shortening or lengthening and implant fracture. Infection rates are 11% for adults and 20% for children.
- Autografts reconstruction:
  - Tumor-bearing bone removed, sterilized by extracorporeal irradiation, or pasteurization and reimplanted into place to replace bone defect; difficult for lower lib reconstruction due to decreased ability to sustain body weight.
- Allograft reconstruction:
  - Although bone bank has, in children, several advantages such as biological integration and joint preservation compared with metal implants, its complications include infection, fracture, nonunion of the host-allograft junction, usually within first 3 years of surgery.
- Rotationplasty can be usually applied to tumors located in the femur or proximal tibia especially in patients with remaining growth potential. Disadvantage is a cosmetic problem, which can be unacceptable especially to adolescents and females.
- Lung metastasectomy has been shown to increase or prolong survival in osteosarcoma patients with lung metastasis. Five-year survival of patients with complete lung metastasectomy was 12% to 23%, whereas that of patients without aggressive surgical resection was 2.6%, thus should be performed to prolong survival of the patients whenever possible.

Chemotherapy

- This is the most common treatment.
- Current standard protocol for multiagent chemo is doxorubicin, cisplatin, methotrexate (MTX) (MAP), ± ifosfamide.
- Meta-analysis demonstrated that multiagent regimens have significantly better outcomes than two drug regimens.
- There is no significant difference between MAP ± ifosfamide.
- Neoadjuvant chemotherapy can induce tumor necrosis in primary tumor, facilitate surgical resection, and eradicate micrometastases; patients do better with neoadjuvant chemotherapy.
- Degree of tumor necrosis is a prognostic factor.
- Tumor necrosis is assessed as grade 1 (no necrosis), 2 (50%–95%), 3 (>95% but <100%), and 4 (100%).
- Liposomal muramyl tripeptide phosphatidylethanolamine (L-MTP-PE) is the first new drug approved for treatment of nonmetastatic osteosarcoma in the last 30 years. L-MTP-PE with MAP and ifosfamide significantly improved the 6-year overall survival of patients with primary osteosarcoma from 70% to 78%.
  - This combination is expected to become a "routine" agent.

Radiation Therapy

- This is used when margins are close, margins are positive, and with subtotal resection, no resection, or palliation.
- Consider using protons when high doses cannot be used with photons due to normal tissue constraints:
  o Can do part with photons and part with protons.
- With high dose radiation therapy (RT), extent of resection does not correlate with outcome: similar overall survival (OS), disease free survival (DFS), and local control at 5 years for gross total resection + RT versus subtotal resection + RT.
- Five-year local control—72%, 5-year OS—67%, 5-year DFS—65%, 5-year distant metastases—26%.
- Risk factors: ≥ grade 2 disease and treatment length.
- Grades 3 and 4 toxicities are seen in 24% to 30.1%.
- RT is more effective after response to chemotherapy or good resection.
- No definite dose–response but patients who received greater than 55 Gy did better; microscopic disease is generally given 60 to 68 Gy, negative margins 55 to 60 Gy, and gross residual disease greater than 68 Gy.

9.2 Ewing's Sarcoma

General

- Aggressive and rare sarcoma of bone and soft tissue.
- Peak incidence in adolescents and young adults.
- Radiosensitive.
- Most patients die from metastases.
- Distant recurrence is more common than local failure.

Prognosis

- Current 5-year OS for localized disease is 65% to 75%.
- Current 5-year OS for metastatic disease to lungs is only 50%.
- Current 5-year OS for metastatic disease not limited to the lungs is less than 30%.
- Long-term survival after recurrence is less than 24% and worse for distant recurrence.
- Factors that generally affect prognosis: local versus metastatic, site of metastasis, age greater than 14 years, bone marrow involvement, adequacy of local control of primary, and adequacy of systemic control for metastases.
- Local disease prognostic factors: primary tumor volume greater than 200 mL or 8 cm in diameter, histologic response seen after chemotherapy in resection patients.
- Minimal residual disease (MRD)—tumor cells in bone marrow or blood—not yet widely accepted but patients with MRD behave like metastatic patients; could be detecting metastatic disease before it is clinically/ radiographically apparent.

Molecular Studies

- Disease is caused by translocation between EWS gene on chromosome 22 and an ETS-type gene.
- Treatments under research: targeting the EWS-FL1 fusion oncogene, IGF1-R, osteoclast function, PARP1, PKC-beta, CD99, GD-2, and VEGF.

Treatment

- Multidisciplinary approach is best.
- Intensive neoadjuvant chemotherapy followed by local control with surgery ± RT or radiation only.

Surgery

- Resection (marginal or wide resection) is preferred because it has better local control than definitive RT (HR of 2.41 for RT vs. surgery).
- Overall survival and distance recurrence are similar for definitive RT versus surgery.
- Intralesional or debulking resection has no advantage over definitive RT and should, therefore, not be performed.

Radiation Therapy

- Definitive RT is advised only for inoperable tumors with a recommended dose of 54 to 55 Gy with 2 cm margin.
- Postoperative RT is recommended if resection is not complete; if resection is adequate there is no current evidence for post-op RT although there may be a role if histologic response is poor or there is marrow involvement.
- Preoperative RT can be considered when it would help with surgical margins or would reduce tumor volume to gain less postsurgical side effects; this is given with chemotherapy if indicated.
- RT may improve response to neoadjuvant chemotherapy in poorly responsive patients.
- GTV1 = volume occupied at diagnosis by visible or palpable disease including enlarged lymph nodes (if tumor has a "pushing" effect on body cavities, GTV1 excludes the prechemotherapy volume where that volume extends into the cavity).
- CTV1 = GTV1 + 1 cm and sites with potential occult tumor involvement including drainage for clinically or pathologically involved lymph nodes; if N0 then no drainage is irradiated.
- PTV1 = CTV1 surrounded by a geometric margin to account for variability in setup, breathing or motion during treatment (photons) OR clinical target volume (CTV) (brachytherapy) OR CTV plus margins dependent on each beam (protons); minimum of 0.5 cm margin.
- GTV2 = residual visible or palpable tumor following induction chemotherapy with or without surgery. For unresected tumors, GTV2 includes the pretreatment abnormalities in bone and the gross residual tumor in soft tissue after induction chemotherapy. For partially resected tumors, GTV2 includes residual abnormalities in bone and the gross residual tumor in soft tissue and the tumor bed harboring microscopic residual tumor. For tumors with microscopic residual and greater than 90% necrosis, this is the postinduction chemotherapy target volumes determined on preoperative imaging.
- CTV2 = GTV2 + 1 cm and areas at risk for microscopic disease including lymph nodes adjacent to the gross target volume (GTV) when appropriate.
- PTV2 = CTV2 surrounded by a geometric margin to account for variability in setup, breathing or motion during treatment (photons) OR CTV2 (brachytherapy) OR CTV2 plus margins dependent on each beam (protons); minimum of 0.5 cm margin.
- Use 1.8 Gy fractions.
- Definitive RT = 45 Gy to PTV1 with a 10.8 Gy boost to PTV2.
- Pre-op RT = 36 Gy to PTV1.
- Post-op RT to gross residual disease = 45 Gy to PTV1 with a 10.8 Gy boost to PTV2.
- Post-op RT to microscopic disease, greater than 90% necrosis = 50.4 Gy to PTV2.
- Post-op RT to microscopic disease, less than 90% necrosis = 50.4 Gy to PTV1.

Chemotherapy

- In Europe, induction chemo is VIDE (vincristine, ifosfamide, dactinomycin, and etoposide).
- In North America, induction chemo is VDC-IE (vincristine, dactinomycin, cyclophosphamide, ifosfamide, and etoposide).
- Recurrent disease is treated with high-dose chemotherapy; however, no good regimen has been established and prognosis is poor.

Side Effects

- RT greater than growth impairment, secondary malignancy, (RT dose dependent, less likely if dose <48 Gy, 20-year risk of any secondary malignancy is 9.2% and risk of secondary sarcoma is 6.5%).
- Patients with primary malignant bone tumors, cumulative incidence of second solid malignancy was 1.4% at 10 years with a poor 5-year overall survival of less than 40%.
- Surgery greater than endoprosthetic infections, endoprosthetic replacements in children, and bone-healing difficulties.

9.3   Extremity Soft-Tissue Sarcomas

General

- These tumors form a diverse and complex tumor group that arise from the connective tissue of any organ or at any anatomic location of the body.
- The majority occur in the muscle groups of the extremities with thigh being the most common site.
- They account for less than 1% of all malignancies and approximately 40% of all newly diagnosed soft-tissue sarcoma will die from the disease.
- Some genetic syndromes are associated with soft-tissue sarcomas, for example, Li Fraumeni syndrome and Neurofibromatosis type I.
- Other etiologic factors are ionizing RT, chemical exposures, chronic soft-tissue injury, or chronic lymph edema.

Prognosis

- Tumor sizes greater than 10 cm, high grade, and deep origin are associated with worse prognosis.
- Positive margins are associated with an increased risk of local recurrence.

Anatomy

- Distal to the medial border of the scapula in the upper extremity and the iliac crest in the lower extremity.

Treatment

- Primary treatment is LSS when possible with RT for high-risk cases.
- Though not always indicated, the addition of adjuvant chemotherapy increases disease-free and overall survival.
- LSS + adjuvant RT versus amputation has no difference in disease-free survival or overall survival.
- LSS alone has a 30% to 50% local control rate; the addition of adjuvant RT increases this to 90% but with no effect on overall survival.
- Postoperative versus preoperative RT has no difference in regional or distant failure or progression-free survival.
- Preoperative RT may have a slight overall survival benefit over postoperative RT after 2.5 years.
- There is no clear benefit for a postoperative boost if preoperative RT has been given.
- Adjuvant RT may be excluded if low risk of local recurrence, early stage disease, small size, superficial location, low grade, potential for good surgical margins, and ability to salvage if recurrence/metastasis occurs.

Toxicity

- Acutely, RT leads to decreased strength, decreased range of motion, skin toxicity, and edema.
- Wound-healing complications are more common for tumor sizes greater than 10 cm.

- Preoperative RT leads to an increased risk of wound-healing complications, almost exclusively in the lower extremity.
- Preoperative has more short-term morbidity but better long-term function.
- Postoperative RT has greater acute skin toxicity.
- Postoperative RT increases the risk of chronic fibrosis, joint stiffness, edema, and bone fractures, likely due to the increased field size and dose.
- Risk of bone fracture is dose dependent; keep V40 less than 64%, mean less than 37 Gy, max less than 59 Gy.

RT Techniques

- Preoperative RT uses a smaller field and lower dose than postoperative RT.

Postoperative Volumes and Dosing

- Surgical bed + 1.5 cm radial margin and 4 cm cranio-caudal margin.
- Surgical bed 45 to 50.4 Gy in 1.8 to 2 Gy fractions.
- Tumor bed + 1.5 cm radial margin and 2 cm cranio-caudal margin; 45 to 50.4 Gy in 1.8 to 2 Gy fractions PLUS boost to the tumor bed of 10 to 16 Gy.
- Treat after recovery from surgery, about 6 weeks.

Preoperative Volumes and Dosing

CTV = GTV + 1.5 to 2 cm radial margin and 4 cm cranio-caudal margin + peritumoral edema; 50 Gy in 25 fractions.

- Surgery 4 to 6 weeks after RT.
- Intensity modulated radiation therapy (IMRT) potentially superior to conventional techniques to cover target while protecting normal tissue; lower local recurrence with IMRT, and significant reduction of late toxicities.
- Brachytherapy—contraindicated as primary adjuvant treatment if (a) CTV cannot be adequately covered by implant geometry, (b) critical anatomic structures would receive a meaningful dose, (c) there is positive margins, and (d) there is skin involvement.
- Exact role of brachytherapy is unclear, but evidence is suggestive that it should not be used in upper extremity or proximal limbs and may be less efficacious that IMRT.
- There is no role for heavy particles in soft tissue sarcoma (STS).
- There is no evidence that hyper- or hypofractionation offers a benefit.
- The addition of intraoperative RT may improve local control but further investigation is needed.
- There may be need to replan during treatment if there is greater than 1 cm increase in tumor size.

9.4   Retroperitoneal Sarcoma

General

- Soft-tissue sarcomas are uncommon: 15% of all sarcomas; less than 1% of adult malignant tumors.
- 10% to 15% of soft-tissue sarcomas are retroperitoneal sarcoma (RPS).
- Overall 5-year survival is 50% to 60%.
- Local recurrence is the most common form of relapse and cause of death.
- 5-year distant recurrence rate is 13% to 34%.
- 3/4 RP masses are malignant.
- There are more than 50 types and subtypes of RPS arising from adipose, muscle, connective, vascular, deep skin, and bone; malignant peripheral nerve sheath tumors are classified under sarcoma as well.
- Risk factors include genetic alterations and exposure to RT or chemicals.
- They are the largest tumors found in the human body.

- Due to location and the fact they are slow growing, they rarely cause signs or symptoms until a significant size; thus a majority of tumors are greater than 5 to 10 cm at presentation.

Clinical Presentation

- Average age at presentation is mid-50s.
- Increasing abdominal girth, pain, palpable mass, and compression symptoms.

Anatomy

- Anteriorly bordered by the peritoneal extensions anchoring the transverse colon, small bowel, ascending and descending colon, part of the duodenum, part of the liver, and part of the pancreas.
- Can be divided into perirenal (anterior and posterior) and pararenal.
- Contains vital organs (pancreas, kidneys, adrenals part of the duodenum, and the ascending and descending colon), greater abdominal vessels, abdominal lymphatics, six major nerves, the autonomic lumbar chains, and fasciae.
- Primary RPS originates in the RP space but not from the RP organs.

Histology

- Grade is based on differentiation, mitotic rate, and necrosis.
- There is no single agreed-upon grading system.
- Liposarcoma and leiomyosarcoma are the most common variants in RPS.
- There are four major liposarcomas—atypical/well-differentiated, dedifferentiated, myxoid, and pleomorphic.
- Well-differentiated and dedifferentiated are the most common RPS liposarcomas.
- Well-differentiated retroperitoneal liposarcomas have a long, indolent course.
- Dedifferentiated liposarcomas have areas of high-grade poorly differentiated sarcoma and are more likely to metastasize.

Genetics

- CINSARC expression is a prognostic marker.
- Well-differentiated RPS has supernumary rings and/or giant rod chromosomes with amplifications from 12q13 to 15 regions; most common are MDM2, CDK-4, HMGA2, and TSPAN31 with coamplification of MDM2 and CDK-4 being most likely.
- Dedifferentiated RPS has supernumary rings and/or giant rod chromosomes with amplifications from 12q13 to 15 regions; most common are MDM2, CDK-4, HMGA2, and TSPAN31.
- Dedifferentiated RPS shows more complex chromosomal aberrations than well-differentiated.
- c-Jun in the JNK pathway is implicated in the transition from well-differentiated to dedifferentiated.

Prognosis

- Overall survival is influenced by extent of resection, tumor size, histological grade, and stage at presentation.
- Local control is influenced by extent of resection, tumor grade.
- Tumor grade is the most important prognostic factor.
- Tumors are benign, intermediate (locally aggressive), intermediate (rarely metastasizing), and malignant.

Staging

- CT or MRI of the abdomen and pelvis with contrast.
- Positron emission tomography (PET) scan.
- Biopsy is important in patients at risk for incomplete resection and if pre-op external beam radiation therapy (EBRT) is planned.

Simulation

- Contrast enhanced CT simulation ≤ 3-mm slices.
- Four DCT if target is above the iliac crest.
- May need to replan during treatment if greater than 1 cm increase in tumor size.

Treatment Overview

- Treatment at a multidisciplinary center with sarcoma specialists is recommended.
- Surgery is the primary treatment; complete macroscopic resection with negative margins is best; incomplete resection should be performed only for symptomatic relief.
- No randomized trial of surgery versus surgery + pre-op EBRT has been done (European Organisation for Research and Treatment of Cancer [EORTC] has one in process), but data from pre-op EBRT + surgery versus historical data from surgery suggests only that pre-op EBRT for intermediate or high-grade RPS leads to better local control, disease-free survival, and overall survival.
- Pre-op EBRT is favored over post-op because (a) tumor is more easily definable, (b) the tumor displaces critical structures, (c) RT dose needed before surgery is less because the tumor is better vascularized and oxygenated, and (d) there is decreased risk of intraoperative tumor seeding.
- Pre-op RT is possible if the tumor can be macroscopically resected, no urgent surgery is needed, EBRT can be delivered with acceptable normal tissue constraints, and disease is localized.
- IMRT is generally preferred.
- Preoperative boost dose with dose painting is not recommended as standard practice.
- Intraoperative electron radiation therapy (IOERT) + EBRT + surgery may lead to better local control for primary disease, but the addition of IOERT has no overall survival benefit and has high toxicity.
- IOERT only at experienced centers.
- Surgery 4 to 6 weeks after EBRT.
- Systemic therapy is not as common but anthracylcines and alkylating agents are first line.
- Well-differentiated and dedifferentiated respond poorly to chemotherapy.
- Systemic therapies targeting MDM2 and CKD4 are under investigation.

Dosing

- 50.4 Gy in 1.8 Gy fractions or 50 Gy in 2 Gy fractions.
- ≥ 95% of the planning target volume (PTV) should receive greater than 95% of the prescription dose.
- 99% to 100% of the CTV should receive greater than 95% of the prescription dose.

Guidance

- If greater than 1 cm tumor motion, then respiratory control is recommended.
- Volumetric soft-tissue imaging 2 to 5 ×/week and orthogonal kV imaging otherwise.

Toxicities

- IOERT—gastrointestinal (GI) (N/V, pain, bowel dysfunction, proctitis, obstruction, and fistula) and neural toxicities (pain or neuropathy).
- EBRT—depends on location of tumor; special care must be taken when kidneys or liver are involved to ensure that some functioning kidney and liver tissue remains after surgery and RT.

Patterns of Spread

- Local recurrence is the most common form of relapse.
- Distant disease occurs in 20% to 25% of patients and is usually by hematogenous spread.
- Most common sites of spread are lung and liver.

9.5   Bone Metastases

General

- 50% to 80% of patients experience some improvement in pain.
- 20% to 50% of patients have complete relief of their pain.
- Patients with moderate pain respond better than those with severe pain.
- Pain relief may be from impact on osteoclasts and RANK signaling in normal tissue more than from decreased tumor burden.
- Bone metastasis is more common from lung, prostate, and breast.
- For pain, both long acting and short acting, opioids are used for baseline and breakthrough pain control, respectively.
- Bowel regimen is indicated if chronic opiate use; constipation is seen in 25% to 50% of these patients.
- 8 Gy × 1 can be used for pain relief unless contraindicated.

Radiation Therapy Oncology Group (RTOG) 9714 Phase III Randomized Trial

- 8 Gy × 1 versus 3 Gy × 10 for patients with painful bony metastasis from prostate or breast primaries (w/no current or impending pathological fracture).
- No difference in pain relief and narcotic use, complete and partial response, survival, and rate of pathological fracture at 3 months.
- More acute toxicity with 30 Gy.
- More retreatment with 8 Gy.

ASTRO Recommendations

- 8 Gy ×1 noninferior to 3 Gy ×10, 4 Gy ×6, 4 Gy × 5 in providing pain relief.
- Higher retreat rate with single fractionation treatment versus fractionated RT 20% versus 8% because of recurrent pain.
- No difference in long-term toxicity between 8 Gy × 1 and prolonged RT courses for uncomplicated, painful bone metastasis.
- Single dose contraindicated if previously irradiated, pathologic fracture, and spinal cord or cauda equine involvement.
- Radionucleotides for patients with numerous osteoblastic bony mets that don't fit into a single RT field.
- Repeat treatment generally okay, suggests to sum biologically effective doses from initial and repeat treatment to estimate risk of RT myelopathy if spinal cord involved.
- Surgery and systemic pharmaceuticals do not obviate the need for RT.
- Longer RT reschedules 30 Gy in 10 fx most commonly used postsurgery because intent is to eradicate microscopic disease rather than relieve symptoms through partial tumor regression.
- Bisphosphonates with concurrent EBRT thought to palliate pain while promoting reossification of damaged bone no difference in pain relief with mild acute toxicity.

9.6   Malignant Cord Compression

General

- MRI and myelography are definitive diagnostic tests for cord compression.
- Bony compression is a negative predictive outcome for RT.
- Malignant spinal cord metastasis (MSCC) occurs in 5% to 14% of cancer patients.
- Initiate definitive treatment within 24 hours of diagnosis of metastatic spinal cord compression.
- When MSCC is suspected, start steroids immediately (Dy).
- Rate of ambulation higher with use of corticosteroids although they are not needed if patient has good motor function (Dy).
- Generally, RT recommended for radiosensitive tumors and limited survival and surgery for unstable disease for patients with longer survival and good performance status (Dy).

Dexamethasone

- Randomized control trial of 57 patients for high-dose dexamethasone + RTx or RT only: patients with dexamethasone had significantly more gain of function and more durable gain of function with minimal toxicity; 96 mg IV bolus + 96 mg PO × 3 days + 10-day taper.
- Corticosteroids are unnecessary for patients with good motor function.
- A potential contraindication to corticosteroid therapy is a young patient with an undiagnosed mass; corticosteroids may cause an oncolytic effect on lymphomas and thymomas delaying diagnosis.

Functional Outcomes

A predictive score model has been developed to predict post-RT ambulation that has been validated with prospective data:

- Based on primary tumor type, interval between tumor diagnosis and MSCC (≤ or > 15 months), visceral mets at time of RT, motor function prior to RT (ambulatory, ambulatory w/assistance, nonambulatory, and parapalegia), and time developing motor deficits prior to RT (1, 2, >2 weeks)
- Score ranges from 21 to 44.
- Groups are predictive of postRT ambulation and 6-month survival rates.
- Three groups:
  - ○ Group 1 (21–28) = worst prognosis and short course of palliative RT for pain is recommended.
  - ○ Group 2 (29–37) = trend that laminectomy + stabilization + RT is best.
  - ○ Group 3 (38–44) = best prognosis and RT alone provides good control.

Surgery + RT versus RT Alone (Patchell Study)

- Primary end point of the study was the ability to walk after treatment.
- Randomized control trial—direct decompressive surgery + RT versus RT alone started 24 hours after randomization.
- Surgery = direct decompressive surgery (resection of tumor and stabilization if needed).
- RT = 30 Gy in 10 fractions.
- Selective patients—symptomatic for less than 48 hours, single area, not radiosensitive, no preexisting or concomitant neuro problems, expected survival greater than 3 months, acceptable surgical candidates.
- Initial surgical decompression had more patients regain ability to walk and retain this longer than RT alone.
- Frankel Grade(s) are: A (Complete paralysis), B (Sensory function only below the injury level), C (Incomplete motor function below injury level), D (fair to good motor function below injury level), E (normal function).
- Percentage of patients with Frankel scores at or above study entry was significantly higher in the surgery group than the RT group.
- Patients significantly retained the ability to walk and were more likely to regain ability to walk with surgery.
- Initial surgery reduced steroid and opiate requirements.
- Initial surgery led to increased survival time.
- No increase in morbidity or mortality was seen.
- Surgery did not result in prolonged hospitalization.

9.7 Heterotopic Ossification

General

Definition: benign condition of abnormal formation of mature lamellar bone in soft tissues.

- **It** often contains bone marrow.
- It is a form of dystrophic soft-tissue calcification.
- It can occur near any major joint or in soft tissue not surrounding a joint after trauma (contusion or abdominal wounds).

Presentation

- Most often it is asymptomatic, detected as incidental finding on imaging.
- Symptoms include pain, decreased range of motion (ROM), loss of function of joint, or warmth, mild edema, and erythema if heterotopic ossification (HO) is superficial.

Imaging

- Bone scan can detect HO in 3 weeks.
- Plain films can detect HO in 4 to 6 weeks.

Risk Factors

- A history of previous HO most important
- Male
- Type of surgery
- Type of injury
- Skeletal hyperostosis
- Hypertrophic OA
- Ankylosing spondylitis

Pathophysiology

- Caused by:
  - o Trauma—fractures, dislocations, operative procedures, and severe burns.
  - o Most commonly after hip fracture and open reduction and internal fixation (ORIF) or total hip arthroplasty.
  - o Neurologic injury—spinal trauma, head injuries, less common conditions (encephalitis, meningitis, myelitis, tetanus, brain tumors, epidural abscess, and SAH).
  - o Hip and then elbow and shoulder are the most common locations.
  - o Genetic disorders—fibrodysplasia ossifcans progressiva (FOP), progressive osseous heteroplasia (POH, dermal HO), Albright's hereditary oseodystrophy (AHO and PHO related to GNAS1 mutations, dermal and subcutaneous HO).
  - o Inappropriate differentiation of pluripotent mesenchymal stem cells into osteoblastic stem cells in response to an imbalance in local or systemic factors (e.g., BMP-4, prostaglandin-E2).
  - o Need osteogenic precursor cells, inducing agents, and an appropriate environment.

Grading

- Brooker grades for hip HO based on degree of HO (good picture in Balboni review):
  - o I—islands of bone within soft tissue
  - o II—bone spurs from the pelvis or proximal femur with greater than 1 cm between
  - o III—bone spurs from the pelvis or proximal femur with less than 1 cm between
  - o IV—bone ankylosis of the hip

Brooker grades III and IV are clinically significant.

Treatment Overview

- If HO is present, surgical excision of HO followed by prophylaxis.
- To prevent HO, RT or non-steroidal anti inflammatory drugs (NSAIDs) are recommended.
- RT is slightly more effective in preventing clinically significant (Brooker 3, 4) HO.
- There is no difference between RT and NSAIDS for asymptomatic HO.
- 6 Gy is equivalent to NSAIDS.

Radiation Therapy

- RT reduces osteoprogenitor cell population and differentiation.
- Post-op RT is more effective than pre-op RT.
- Give RT less than 72 hours post-op; 7 to 8 Gy × 1 is a good average dose.
- There is dose response relationship present between RT dose and efficacy.
- Hip field includes the region medial to center of hip between the lesser trochanter and ischial ramus, the area lateral to the center of the hip between the greater trochanter and the ilium, and the region surrounding the prosthetic femoral neck.
- Shield testis.
- There is less than 1% risk of grades III or IV HO after RT.

NSAIDs

- NSAIDs inhibit induction of local and systemic factors.
- Indomethacin is most commonly used.
- Other agents include diclophenac, diclophenac–colestyramine, and acetylsalicylic acid (less effective).
- Selective NSAIDs are best due to less GI effects.
- 3% risk of grades III or IV HO after NSAIDs.

Toxicity

- Indomethacin has been found to increase the rate of bone nonunion after fracture; however, the risk of nonunion in patients treated with RT can be minimized with appropriate shielding.
- NSAIDs can have GI side effect.
- RT side effects are acute (wound healing problems) or chronic (trochanteric nonunion, secondary malignancy, and testicular dose).

Chapter 9: Practice Questions

1. The main advantage of preoperative radiation therapy (RT) over postoperative RT in extremity soft tissue sarcoma (STS) is potentially

    A. Local failure
    B. Regional failure
    C. Distant failure
    D. Longer term survival

2. In terms of osteosarcoma, the difference in overall survival between amputation and limb-sparing surgery (LSS) is

    A. 3 months
    B. 6 months
    C. 12 months
    D. No difference in overall survival

3. Surgical staging of a high-grade intracompartmental nonmetastatic osteosarcoma is

    A. IB
    B. IIA
    C. IIB
    D. III

4. Preoperative dose for retroperitoneal sarcoma (RPS) is generally

    A. 40 Gy
    B. 45 Gy
    C. 50 Gy
    D. 55 Gy

5. Spinal cord compression can occur in what percentage of cancer patients?

    A. <0.1%
    B. 1%
    C. 10%
    D. 20%

6. Complete relief from bone pain with the use of palliative RT occurs

    A. <5%
    B. 20% to 50%
    C. 60% to 70%
    D. 80% to 90%

7. According to the American Society for Radiation Oncology (ASTRO) bone mets guideline, the retreatment rate of fractionated RT is

    A. 4%
    B. 8%
    C. 15%
    D. 20%

8. General contraindications for single-fraction radiation therapy (RT) to the bone include the following EXCEPT

    A. Cervical metastases
    B. Previous RT
    C. Spinal cord compression
    D. Pathological fracture

9. Distant metastases occur in what percentage of retroperitoneal sarcomas (RPSs)?

    A. 5%
    B. 15%
    C. 25%
    D. 35%

10. The following factor is prognostic for an increase in local recurrence:

    A. Tumor size
    B. Deep origin
    C. High grade
    D. Positive margin

11. All of the following are prognostic for extremity soft-tissue sarcoma outcome EXCEPT

    A. tumor size
    B. deep origin
    C. high grade
    D. positive margin

12. The 5-year survival associated with metastatectomy of lung mets from osteosarcoma is approximately

    A. 2%
    B. 5%
    C. 15%
    D. 30%

13. Overall survival for retroperitoneal sarcoma (RPS) is associated with the following EXCEPT

    A. Extent of resection
    B. Tumor location
    C. TUMOR size
    D. Grade

14. The 5-year overall survival for adult Ewing's sarcoma with lung metastases only is

    A. 70%
    B. 50%
    C. 30%
    D. 10%

15. RT dose for heterotopic bone prophylaxis is generally in the range of

    A. 5 Gy
    B. 7 Gy
    C. 10 Gy
    D. 15 Gy

16. Wound healing for extremity soft tissue sarcoma (STS) is potentially inferior in patients with all of the following EXCEPT

    A. Preoperative RT
    B. Lower extremity
    C. Large tumors
    D. Higher age

17. Typical 5-year survival rate for adult osteosarcoma is

    A. 20%
    B. 40%
    C. 60%
    D. 80%

18. The local control of limb-sparing surgery (LSS) alone is approximately

    A. 40%
    B. 60%
    C. 75%
    D. 90%

19. Ewing's sarcoma is associated with a translocation of the EWS gene on chromosome

    A. 12
    B. 15
    C. 22
    D. 1

20. A typical dose that is given for preoperative Ewing's sarcoma is

    A. 20 Gy
    B. 36 Gy
    C. 45 Gy
    D. 54 Gy

Chapter 9: Answers

1. D

Postoperative versus preoperative RT has no difference in regional or distant failure or progression-free survival. Preoperative RT may have a slight overall survival benefit over postoperative RT after 2.5 years.

2. D

There is no difference in survival rate with amputation versus limb-sparing surgery (LSS), but there is a high trend of local recurrence with LSS.

3. B

All high-grade tumors are Stage II with intracompartmental resections denoted with A (extracompartmental resections are B).

4. C

Dosing for retroperitoneal sarcoma (RPS): 50.4 Gy in 1.8 Gy fractions or 50 Gy in 2 Gy fractions.

5. C

MSCC can occur in 5% to 14% of cancer patients.

6. B

50% to 80% of patients experience some improvement in pain. 20% to 50% of patients have complete relief of their pain.

7. B

American Society for Radiation Oncology (ASTRO) recommendations for bone mets:

    8 Gy ×1 noninferior to 3 Gy ×10, 4 Gy × 6, 4 Gy × 5 in providing pain relief.

    higher retreat rate with single fractionation treatment versus fractionated RT 20% versus 8% because of recurrent pain

    No difference in long-term toxicity between 8 Gy × 1 and prolonged RT courses for uncomplicated, painful bone mets.

8. A

Single dose is contraindicated if there is previously irradiated, pathologic fracture, and spinal cord or cauda equina involvement.

9. C

Local recurrence is the most common form of relapse. Distant disease occurs in 20% to 25% of patients and is usually hematogenous spread with the most common sites of spread being lung and liver.

10. D

Positive margins are associated with an increased risk of local recurrence.

11. D

Prognosis of extremity STS:

    Tumor size greater than 10 cm

    High grade

    Deep origin

12. C

Lung metastasectomy has been shown to increase or prolong survival in osteosarcoma patients with lung metastasis. Five-year survival of patients with complete lung metastasectomy was 12% to 23%, whereas that of patients without aggressive surgical resection was 2.6%; thus it should be performed to prolong survival of the patients whenever possible.

13. B

Overall survival for retroperitoneal sarcoma (RPS) is influenced by extent of resection, tumor size, histological grade, and stage at presentation.

14. B

Prognosis of Ewing's sarcoma:

    Current 5-year overall survival (OS) for localized disease is 65% to 75%.

    Current 5-year OS for metastatic disease to lungs only is 50%.

15. B

Radiation therapy (RT) for prophylaxis:

Reduces osteoprogenitor cell population and differentiation.

Post-op RT is more effective than pre-op RT.

Give RT less than 72 hours post-op; 7 to 8 Gy ×1 is a good average dose.

16. D

Wound-healing complications are more common for tumor sizes greater than 10 cm. Preoperative RT leads to an increased risk of wound-healing complications, almost exclusively in the lower extremity.

17. C

Five-year survival for osteosarcoma is about 60% with addition of chemotherapy, improved surgical techniques, surgical devices, and diagnostic methods.

18. A

Limb sparing surgery (LSS) alone has a 30% to 50% local control rate; the addition of adjuvant RT increases this to 90% but with no effect on overall survival.

19. C

Ewing's sarcoma disease is caused by translocation between EWS gene on chr 22 and an ETS-type gene.

20. B

A preoperative dose of 36 Gy is typically used for Ewing's sarcoma.

Recommended Reading

Ando K, Heymann M-F, Stresing V, et al. Current therapeutic strategies and novel approaches in osteosarcoma. *Cancers (Basel)*. 2013;5(2):591-616.

Baldini EH, Wang D, Haas RL, et al. Treatment guidelines for preoperative radiation therapy for retroperitoneal sarcoma: preliminary consensus of an international expert panel. *Int J Radiat Oncol Biol Phys*. 2015;92(3):602-612.

Ciernik IF, Niemierko A, Harmon DC, et al. Proton-based radiotherapy for unresectable or incompletely resected osteosarcoma. *Cancer*. 2011;117(19):4522-4530.

DeLaney TF, Park L, Goldberg SI, et al. Radiotherapy for local control of osteosarcoma. *Int J Radiat Oncol Biol Phys*. 2005;61(2):492-498.

Dunst J, Ahrens S, Paulussen M, et al. Second malignancies after treatment for Ewing's sarcoma: a report of the CESS-studies. *Int J Radiat Oncol Biol Phys*. 1998;42(2):379-384.

Dy SM, Asch SM, Naeim A, et al. Evidence-based standards for cancer pain management. *J Clin Oncol*. 2008;26(23):3879-3885.

Hartsell WF, Scott CB, Bruner DW, et al. Randomized trial of short- versus long-course radiotherapy for palliation of painful bone metastases. *J Natl Cancer Inst*. 2005;97(11):798-804.

Kan SL, Yang B, Ning GZ, et al. Nonsteroidal anti-inflammatory drugs as prophylaxis for heterotopic ossification (HO) after total hip arthroplasty: a systematic review and meta-analysis. *Medicine (Baltimore)*. 2015;94(18):e828. doi:10.1097/MD.0000000000000828.

Kuttesch JF Jr, Wexler LH, Marcus RB, et al. Second malignancies after Ewing's sarcoma: radiation dose-dependency of secondary sarcomas. *J Clin Oncol*. 1996;14(10):2818-2825.

Lutz S, Berk L, Chang E, et al. Palliative radiotherapy for bone metastases: an ASTRO evidence-based guideline. *Int J Radiat Oncol Biol Phys*. 2011 Mar 15;79(4):965-976. doi:10.1016/j.ijrobp.2010.11.026. Epub 2011 Jan 27.

Pakos EE, Ioannidis JP. Radiotherapy vs. nonsteroidal anti-inflammatory drugs for the prevention of heterotopic ossification after major hip procedures: a meta-analysis of randomized trials. *Int J Radiat Oncol Biol Phys*. 2004 Nov 1;60(3):888-895.

Patchell RA, Tibbs PA, Regine WF, et al. Direct decompressive surgical resection in the treatment of spinal cord compression caused by metastatic cancer: a randomised trial. *Lancet*. 2005 Aug 20–26;366(9486):643-648.

Rades D, Douglas S, Huttenlocher S, et al. Validation of a score-predicting post-treatment ambulatory status after radiotherapy for metastatic spinal cord compression. *Int J Radiat Oncol Biol Phys*. 2011 Apr 1;79(5):1503-1506. doi: 10.1016/j.ijrobp.2010.01.024. Epub 2010 June 3.

Rosenberg SA, Tepper J, Glatstein E, et al. The treatment of soft-tissue sarcomas of the extremities: prospective randomized evaluations of (1) limb-sparing surgery plus radiation therapy compared with amputation and (2) the role of adjuvant chemotherapy. *Ann Surg.* 1982 Sep;196(3):305-315.

Schwarz R, Bruland O, Cassoni A, et al. The role of radiotherapy in oseosarcoma. *Cancer Treat Res.* 2009;152:147-164. doi:10.1007/978-1-4419-0284-9_7.

Sørensen S, Helweg-Larsen S, Mouridsen H, Hansen HH. Effect of high-dose dexamethasone in carcinomatous metastatic spinal cord compression treated with radiotherapy: a randomized trial. *Eur J Cancer.* 1994;30A(1):22-27.

Yang JC, Chang AE, Baker AR, et al. Randomized prospective study of the benefit of adjuvant radiation therapy in the treatment of soft tissue sarcomas of the extremity. *J Clin Oncol.* 1998;16(1):197-203.

10

Central Nervous System

Stephanie E. Weiss

10.1　Primary Malignancies

10.1.1 Grade II Astrocytoma, Oligodendroglioma, and Oligoastrocytoma

Epidemiology

- Incidence is approximately 2,000/yr.
- They account for approximately 15% of all primary brain tumors.
- The female to male ratio is 2–3 to 1.
- Astrocytoma is greater than oligodendroglial histology.
- Incidence of oligodendroglial histology is increasing.
- They are slightly more common in Caucasians, males.
- Age range of occurrence is 35 to 45 years.
- Seizure is common: approximately 80% and is a favorable prognostic factor.
- Astrocytoma of optic structures is associated with NF-1.
- Many will progress to high-grade lesions with or without treatment.

Pathology

- Astrocytomas
  - Fibrillary most common
  - Gemistocytic may be more aggressive
  - Protoplasmic have better prognosis
  - Common molecular modifications: inactivation of TP53, IDH1 greater than IDH2 mutations
- Oligodendrogliomas
  - Have "chicken wire" vasculature and "fried egg" cell appearance
  - Codeletion of 1p/19q in 40% to 80% of tumors; is predictive and prognostic; often occur with IDH1/2 mutations
- Oligoastrocytomas
  - Mixed histologic variant
  - Prognosis may be relative to histologic mix

Risk Stratification

- *High-risk*: ≥3 of the following: Tumor ≥6 cm, tumor crossing mid-line, age ≥40, astrocytoma histology, and neurologic deficit
- *RTOG 98-02* high risk: age ≥40 and/or less than gross total resection

Presentation

- Frequently seizure approximately 80%—a favorable prognostic feature. May be any neurologic symptom and referable to location: Headache, nausea, altered mental status, diplopia, visual field deficit, motor or sensory deficit, aphasia, cranial nerve deficit coordination, or gait disturbance.

Diagnosis and Workup

- History and physical examination: Mental status, cranial nerve exam, motor, and sensory exam, cerebellar exam, assess for presence of expressive and/or receptive aphasia. Complete respiratory, cardiovascular, and lower extremity exam to rule out common comorbidities.
- Imaging: Pre- and postoperative MRI with T1 ± C, T2 and flair, thin slice volumetric MRI +/C with 3D reconstruction. Post-op MRI should be within 72 hours of surgery. Except low signal intensity *without enhancement* on T1 weighted images. Expect high signal on T2/flair imaging. Calcifications (high T1, low T2/flair signal) may be present (more frequently associated with 1p/19q deleted oligodendroglioma).
- Surgery:
  - Tissue diagnosis required; maximal safe resection recommended. Extensive surgery likely predicts better overall survival. *Subtotal resection considered a high-risk feature in RTOG 98-02.*
  - If biopsy only, surgeon should attempt to sample any regions suspicious for high grade on imaging (i.e., enhancement) to limit sampling error in grading.

Treatment Overview

- Surgery:
  - Probably therapeutic: Extent of resection has been shown in sub-group and retrospective analysis to be predictive of OS.
  - Consider at recurrence if there has been durable long-term PFS.
- Chemo-Radiation therapy (RT):
  - Adjuvant: For high-risk patients
    - RTOG 98-02 definition: Subtotal resection and/or age ≥40 years.
    - EORTC/RTOG 04-24 definition.
    - Patients with ≥3 of the following: Tumor crossing midline, age ≥40 years, tumor ≥6 cm, preoperative neurologic deficit (not seizure), astrocytoma histology.
  - At recurrence in previously untreated disease

Disease-Specific Management

	Management
Seizure	Levetiracetam 500 mg po bid
Symptomatic edema	Dexamethasone 4 mg po qid and with taper as tolerated GI prophylaxis while on steroid
PJP prophylaxis	Double-strength sulfamethoxazole and trimethoprim or atovaquone: 1,500 mg po QD or pentamidine 300 mg by inhalation q4 wks
Lower extremity swelling	Lower extremity ultrasound to rule out DVT
Respiratory symptoms	Consider pulmonary embolus Other common respiratory and cardiovascular morbidities

Radiation Therapy Technique

- Simulation:
    CT simulation with thermoplastic mask for immobilization in supine position, neck in neutral position. Fusion with T1 with pre- and postoperative T2/flair and T1 + C sequences.
- Target delineation:
    - Radiation therapy
        - 5,040 cGy–5,400 cGy in 180 cGy fractions, single course.
        - GTV: T2/Flair signal intensity including surgical bed.
        - CTV: GTV + 2 cm. May shave of natural anatomic boundaries such as bone.
        - PTV: CTV + 0.5 cm (or machine set-up tolerance).
        - There is no role for dose-escalation.
- Chemotherapy:
    - Post-RT adjuvant PCV × 6 (Procarbazine 60 mg/m^2; CCNU 110 mg/m^2; VCR 1.4 mg/m^2) based on RTOG 98-02.
                or
    - Concomitant Temozolomide 75 g/m^2 followed by adjuvant TMZ (150–200 mg/m^2) × up to12 cycles based on RTOG 04-24.

Dose Constraints Based on TD 5/5 (Emami et al., 1991) and QUANTEC (Mayo et al., 2010)

Organ-at-Risk (OAR)	Dose Constraint (1.8–2 Gy/fx)
Optic nerves and chiasm	<54 Gy
Retina	45–50 Gy
Brainstem	54 Gy (whole brainstem)
	59 Gy (1–10 mL)
Cochlea	≤45 Gy mean dose

Outcomes

- Low-risk patients with no postoperative adjuvant tx *(RTOG 98-02)*
    - 2-year PFS: 82%   2-year OS: 99%
    - 5-year PFS: 48%   5-year OS: 93%
- High-risk patients *with* postoperative adjuvant PCV-RT *(RTOG 98-02)*
    - 5-year PFS: 61%   5-year OS: 72%
    - 10-year PFS: 50%   10-year OS: 60%
- High-risk patients *with* postoperative adjuvant TMZ-RT *(RTOG 04-24)*
    - 3-year PFS: 59.2%   3-year OS: 73%

High Risk Variable	RTOG 98-02	RTOG 04-24[t]
Astrocytoma histology	–	+
Age ≥ 40	+	+
Preoperative neurologic deficit	–	+
Size ≥ 6 cm	–	+
Tumor crossing midline[*]	–	+
Subtotal resection[*]	+	–

[*]By definition tumor crossing midline will not be totally resectable.
[t]RTOG 0424 required ≥3 features to be called high risk.

Toxicity

- Fatigue, hair loss, skin irritation/dryness, thrush, and edema with symptoms referable to tumor location such as weakness, numbness, gait disturbance, and aphasia. These may potentially require an increase in steroids: headache, nausea, and stuffiness in ear. Seizures and bleeding are rare.
- Late complications: Mild to moderate long-term neurocognitive effects are common; severe neurocognitive effects rare. Optic neuropathy, radiation necrosis, and hypopituitarism can occur if the pituitary gland is in the field or receives high dose. Secondary malignancy is rare but known effect. However, transition of low-grade glioma to high grade is not related to radiation therapy.
- Chemotherapy toxicity:
  - Temozolomide: acute pancytopenia, nausea, vomiting, infertility, and constipation particularly with odansetron GI prophylaxis.
  - PCV: Pancytopenia, nausea, vomiting, fatigue, mouth ulcers, GI upset, peripheral neuropathy, liver, and renal dysfunction.

Follow-Up

- Initially q3 months with MRI T1 ± Contrast, T2/flair
- MRI every 3 to 6 months for 5 years, then annually
- History and physical examination: mini-mental status with neurologic history and physical

10.1.2 Ependymoma

Epidemiology

- It accounts for approximately 2% of adult primary brain tumors.
- In *adults*, only 25% occur in the brain; 75% in the spine.
- Risk factors are unclear.
- "Classic" ependymoma:
  - Male = Female
  - Predilection for the ventricle
  - CSF dissemination less than 10%
    - Infratentorial: 9%
    - Supratentorial: 1.5%
- Subependymoma:
  - Rare
  - Fourth or lateral ventricle
  - Male more than female

Pathology

- "Classic" ependymoma: Typically grade II or Grade III
  - Controversy regarding any difference in prognosis by grade
  - Nestin expression may better correlate with poor prognosis
- Subependymoma:
  - Slow growing and histologically benign

Presentation

- Posterior fossa tumors: increased intracranial pressure: headache, nausea, vomiting, ataxia, vertigo, and papilledema
- Cranial nerve deficit, especially CN nerves VI to X
- Seizures, neurologic deficit referable to region of involvement
- If CSF dissemination may have findings related to level of cord involvement

Diagnosis and Workup

- History and physical examination:
  - Cranial nerves, motor, sensory, cerebellar, reflexes, pain, incontinence, and Brown-Sequard Syndrome
- Imaging:
  - Pre- and postoperative (within 72 hours) MRI brain:
    - Classic ependymoma: T1: hypo intense; prominent gadolinium uptake. Often cystic and with calcifications. Calcification in fourth ventrial highly suggestive but not pathognomonic of classic ependymoma. T2: hyper intense.
    - Subependymoma: MRI; ventricular predilection, isointense on T1, hyper intense on T2. Nonenhancing with contrast, well circumscribed nodular tumor, ventricular predilection, isointense on T1, hyper intense on T2.
  - MRI spine:
    - Exclude metastatic disease (up to 10%).
- CSF:
  - Important for posterior fossa and anaplastic tumors.
  - *Ideally from lumbar site preoperatively or if not done/contraindicated 2 to 3 weeks postoperatively.*
  - 1/3 of patients with mets identified with CSF.

Treatment Overview

- Surgery: Maximal safe resection indicated
  - No randomized trials. Observational trials suggest GTR have more favorable prognosis.
- Radiation therapy:
  - Adjuvant: Warranted in cases of subtotal resection of grade II or grade III lesion based on nonrandomized data.
  - Retrospective data in patients GTR and wide clear margin of resection of grade II ependymoma and no spinal metastasis may not need RT, particularly if supratentorial. However, this is controversial. Relapse may subject patient to further workup and reoperation to achieve maximal control.
  - Offered for all patients with grade III even after GTR.
  - If evidence of metastasis in CNS neuraxis, craniospinal RT warranted.
  - No clear role for RT after GTR of subependymoma.
- Chemotherapy:
  - No routine role; controversial. Some retrospsective evidence suggests in setting of STR outcomes comparable to GTR + RT.

Radiation Therapy Technique

- Simulation: CT simulation with thermoplastic mask in supine position
- Fuse with pre- and postsurgical MRI (flair, T1 ± C)
- Target delineation:
  - GTV: Surgical bed and any residual disease based on MR post-op imaging
  - CTV: GTV + 1.5 cm
  - PTV: CTV + 0.5 cm or per machine specific set-up error
- Dose:
  - Limited Field
    - PTV: 50 to 54 Gy in1.8 Gy Fractions
  - Craniospinal
    - Whole brain and spine to bottom of thecal sac:
      - 36 Gy/1.8 Gy/fractions
    - Boost brain primary to 54 Gy/1.8 Gy as in limited field.

Outcomes

- 10-year actuarial OS:
  - GTR + RT: 83%
  - GTR alone: 67%
  - SRT + RT: 43%
- **Toxicity**
  - Brain: Fatigue, hair loss, skin irritation/dryness, thrush, and edema with symptoms referable to tumor location such as weakness, numbness, gait disturbance, and aphasia. These may potentially require increase in steroids: headache, nausea, and stuffiness in ear. Seizures and bleeding are rare.
  - Late complications: Mild to moderate long-term neurocognitive effects are common; severe neurocognitive effects are rare. Optic neuropathy, radiation necrosis and hypopituitarism can occur if gland is in the field. Secondary malignancy is rare but known effect. However, transition of low-grade glioma to high grade is not related to radiation therapy.
  - If Cranio-spinal: Increased risk of neuro-cognitive and pituitary deficit; Lhermitt's sign—Typically occurs 3 to 4 months after RT. Electrical shock-like paresthesia or numbness from the neck to the extremities upon neck flexion. Transient demyelination. Rare: Radiation myelopathy (RM). Occurs at least 6 to 12 months. Irreversible. Diagnosis by exclusion.

Follow-Up

- If no metastasis: Initially at 3 months with brain MRI T1 ± Contrast, T2/flair. Then MRI every 6 months for 2 years. Then every 6 to 12 months.
- If metastasis at presentation: Follow with brain and spine MRI.
- History and physical examination: Full neurologic history with mini-mental status and physical with attention to endocrine function if pituitary in or near field.

10.1.3 High-Grade Glioma

Epidemiology

- It is the most common primary in older population.
- It presents with headaches in 1/2 of patients.
- Etiology is unknown. There may be some familiar cases.
- Role of cell phone use, head injury, N-Nitroso compounds, occupational exposure are controversial.
- May be secondary to low-grade glioma or de novo. Secondary tumors occur in younger population. Often there is a more favorable prognosis. It usually involves a different genetic pathway.

Pathology

- Glioblastoma (GBM)
  - Grade IV Astrocytoma
  - *Microvascular proliferation and pesudopalisading necrosis are pathologic hallmarks*
  - May contain oligodendroglial subtypes
  - MGMT-methylation prognostic for more favorable survival. May be predictive for better response to Temozolomide
  - IDH1 and IDH2 mutations more common in secondary GBM. Favorable prognostic marker
- Grade III Astrocytoma
  - Increased atypia, mitotic activity compared to LGG
  - GFAP protein +

- Grade III Anaplastic oligodendroglioma
  - Increased atypia, mitotic activity compared to LGG
  - "Chicken wire" vasculature, perinuclear halos, and "fried egg" appearance
  - 1p/19q codeletion favorable prognostic feature and predictive of better response to both chemo and radiation therapy
- Grade III Anaplastic oligoastrocytoma
  - Have pathologic and molecular features of both astrocytoma and oligodendroglioma
  - Controversial if prognosis is relative to proportion of the histologic mix

Presentation

- May be any focal neurologic deficit or symptoms of mass effect. Dependent upon location and size of lesions. Headache in about half of patients. Seizure presented in about 50% of Grade III lesions, and about 25% of Grade IV.

Diagnosis and Workup

- History and physical examination: Mental status, cranial nerve exam, motor, and sensory exam, cerebellar exam, assess for presence of expressive and/or receptive aphasia. Complete respiratory, cardiovascular, and lower extremity exam to rule out common comorbidities.
- Imaging: Pre- and postoperative MRI with T1 ± C, T2 and flair, thin slice volumetric MRI ± C with 3D reconstruction. Post-op MRI should be within 72 hours of surgery. Hypo intense on T1 and enhances heterogeneously with contrast. Increased T2/flair signal abnormality. Occasionally grade III lesions will have a paucity of contrast enhancement.
- Surgery:
  - Tissue diagnosis required: Maximal safe resection recommended. Best available evidence shows aggressive resection associated with improved functional status and possible prolonged survival.
  - If biopsy only, stereotaxic localization should attempt to sample any regions suspicious for high grade on imaging (i.e., enhancement) to limit sampling error in grading.

Treatment Overview

- GBM:
  - Surgery: Maximal safe resection
  - Chemo-RT:
    - Stupp Regimen: RT (see technique below) with concomitant Temozolomide 75 g/m^2 followed by 1 month wash-out, then adjuvant TMZ (150–200 mg/m^2) × up to12 cycles.
- Anaplastic astrocytoma:
  - Surgery: Maximal safe resection
  - Chemo-RT:
    - Extrapolated from GBM data. RT (see Technique section following) with concomitant Temozolomide 75 g/m^2 followed by 1 month wash-out then adjuvant TMZ (150–200 mg/m^2) × up to12 cycles.
    - RT followed by either PCV or TMZ at recurrence is equivalent to PCV or TMZ followed by RT after failure of both drugs *NOA-04*. Chemotherapy as a single agent for first-line adjuvant therapy may be appropriate mostly for patients with favorable molecular markers.
- Anaplastic oligodendroglioma/oligoastrocytoma:
  - Surgery: Maximal safe resection
  - Chemo-RT:
    - Consider Stupp regimen for 1p/19q intact lesions.

- Sequential chemotherapy with PCV and radiotherapy. Order does not matter *EORTC 26951/RTOG 9402.*
  - Subgroup analysis of 1p/19q deletion status demonstrated superiority of sequential therapy in tumors with codeleted tumors but not in nondeleted tumors.
- RT followed by either PCV or TMZ at recurrence is equivalent to PCV or TMZ, followed by RT after failure of both drugs *NOA-04.* Chemotherapy as a single agent for first-line adjuvant therapy may be appropriate mostly for patients with favorable molecular markers.

- *CATNON Intergroup trial randomized non-1p/19/q deleted anaplastic glioma to RT versus RT + concurrent TMZ, versus RT + adjuvant TMZ, versus Stupp regimen. Results pending.*

Radiation Therapy Technique

- Simulation:
  - CT simulation with thermoplastic mask for immobilization in supine position, neck in neutral position
  - Fusion with T1 with pre- and postoperative T2/flair and T1 + C sequences
- Target delineation:
  - Radiation therapy
    - First Course
      - 45 Gy to 46 Gy in 1.8 to 2 Gy fractions
      - GTV: T2/Flair signal intensity including surgical bed
      - CTV: GTV + 1 to 2 cm; may reduce where natural anatomic boundaries exist (such as bone); not lesion may cross corpus callosum
      - PTV: CTV + 0.5 cm (or machine set-up tolerance)
    - Cone down
      - Boost to bring total dose to 59.4 to 60 Gy 1.8 to 2 Gy fractions
      - GTV: Tumor bed + contrast enhancing mass on T1 weighted images
      - CTV: GTV + 1.5 to 2 cm; may reduce where natural anatomic boundaries exist (such as bone); not lesion may cross corpus callosum
      - PTV: CTV + 0.5 cm (or machine set-up tolerance)
- Chemotherapy:
  - Concomitant Temozolomide 75 g/m^2 with RT
  - Adjuvant TMZ (150–200 mg/m^2) × up to12 cycles
  - PCV: 6 cycles

Disease-Specific Management

	Management
Seizure	Levetiracetam 500 mg po bid
Symptomatic edema	Dexamethasone 4 mg po qid and with taper as tolerated GI prophylaxis while on steroid
PJP prophylaxis	Double-strength sulfamethoxazole and trimethoprim or atovaquone: 1,500 mg po QD or pentamidine 300 mg by inhalation q4 wks
Lower extremity swelling	Lower extremity ultrasound to rule out DVT
Respiratory symptoms	Consider pulmonary embolus Other common respiratory and cardiovascular morbidities

Dose constraints based on TD 5/5 (Emami et al., 1991) and QUANTEC (Mayo et al., 2010)

Organ-at-risk (OAR)	Dose constraint (1.8–2 Gy/fx)
Optic nerves and chiasm	less than 54 Gy
Retina	45–50 Gy
Brainstem	54 Gy (Whole brainstem) 59 Gy (1–10 mL)
Cochlea	≤45 Gy, mean dose

Recurrence

- Consider putting patient on protocol; bevacizumab, CCNU, alternating electric field therapy
- Reirradiation with hypo fractionation + bevacizumab; radiosurgery in selected cases

Outcomes

- GBM
  - Median survival 14.6 months with Chemo-RT versus 12.1 with RT alone
  - 2-year survival 26.5 with chemo-RT versus 10.4 with RT alone
  - MGMT-methylated
    - OS 21.7 months with chemo-RT versus 15.3 months with RT alone
    - 2-year survival 46% with chemo-RT versus 22.7% with RT alone
  - MGMT-unmethlyated
    - OS 11.8 months with chemo-RT versus 12.7 months with RT alone
    - 2-year survival 13.8% with chemo-RT versus less than 2% with RT alone
- Anaplastic astrocytoma
  - Median OS: approximately 3 years
- Anaplastic oligodendroglioma/oligoastrocytoma
  - Median OS: 4 to 15 years
  - Nondeleted: 3 years
  - Codeleted: 15 years

Toxicity

- Fatigue, hair loss, skin irritation/dryness, thrush, and edema with symptoms referable to tumor location such as weakness, numbness, gait disturbance, and aphasia. These may potentially require increase in steroids: headache, nausea, and stuffiness in ear. Seizures and bleeding are rare.
- Late complications: Mild to moderate long-term neurocognitive effects are common; severe neurocognitive effects are rare. Optic neuropathy, radiation necrosis and hypopituitarism can occur if gland is in the field. Secondary malignancy is rare but known effect.
- Chemotherapy toxicity:
  - Temozolomide; acute pancytopenia, nausea, vomiting, infertility, and constipation particularly with odansetron GI prophylaxis
  - PCV: Pancytopenia, nausea, vomiting, fatigue, mouth ulcers, GI upset, peripheral neuropathy, liver, and renal dysfunction

Follow-Up

- MRI 4 weeks after RT, then q3 months for 2 to 3 years, then less frequently

10.2   Pituitary

Epidemiology

- This accounts for 10% to 15% of intracranial brain tumors.
- The ratio of female to male is 2–3 to 1.
- 75% of pituitary tumors are secretory.
- Median age of occurrence is 52 years (range 30–60 years).
- Females have more prolactin- or ACTH-secreting tumors and males have more nonsecretory or growth hormone-secreting tumors.
- Etiology is unknown in most cases.
- There is an association with multiple endocrine neoplasia type 1 (MEN-1) in 3% of pituitary adenomas (autosomal dominant).

Pathology

- Most pituitary adenomas arise from the anterior lobe and are benign.
- Prolactin- and growth hormone-secreting tumors account for 30% and 25% of pituitary adenomas, more common than ACTH- secreting tumors.
- TSH-secreting tumors are rare.
- Nelson's Syndrome: Rapid enlargement of ACTH-secreting pituitary adenoma after bilateral adrenalectomy.
- Immunohistochemistry is performed to determine subtype.
- Malignant pituitary neoplasms occur in 1% of all pituitary tumors (diagnosed based on intracranial or extracranial metastasis).

Presentation

- Headaches, visual field deficit (bitemporal hemianopsia), and deficits of functions of III, IV, V1 + 2, and VI nerves

Disease-Specific Feature Related to Hypersecretion

Disease	Clinical Manifestation
Nonsecretory tumor	Symptoms caused by mass effect such as headache and visual field deficits, and hypopituitarism (hypogonadism, hypothyroidism, hypoadrenalism, or panhypopituitarism)
Prolactinoma	Symptoms caused by mass effect such as headache and visual field deficits, and hypopituitarism
	Amenorrhea, galactorrhea, decreased
	libido, impotence, and infertility
Acromegaly	Symptoms caused by mass effect such as headache and visual field deficits, and hypopituitarism
	Gigantism in childhood
	Acromegaly in adult—Enlargement of hands and feet, coarse facial features, macrognathia/ malocclusion, weight gain, arthritis, organomegaly, heat intolerance, glucose intolerance, oily skin, skin tags, and colon polyps
Cushing's disease	Symptoms caused by hypersecretion of ACTH including central obesity, hypertension, psychologic changes, purple skin striae, diabetes, hirsutism, and Nelson's syndrome

Diagnosis and Workup

- History and physical examination: Visual field deficits (tumor compression of optic apparatus), cranial nerve deficits (cavernous sinus involvement), change in sleep, appetite, and behavior (tumor compression of hypothalamus), galactorrhea, amenorrhea, hypogonadism, acromegaly, and Cushingoid features
- Imaging: Thin slice volumetric MRI with contrast, thin slice MRI with small field of view and dynamic contrast acquisition for pituitary microadenoma, CT, and skeletal survey as needed
- Laboratory tests (see following Table):

Laboratory Tests for Pituitary Adenoma

Disease/Target Endocrine Function	Tests
Prolactinoma	Prolactin
Acromegaly	Baseline growth hormone, somatomedin-C, or IGF-1, glucose suppression and insulin tolerance, and thyrotropin-releasing hormone stimulation
Cushing's disease	Serum ACTH, urine 17-hydroxy-corticosteroids, free cortisol, and response to dexamethasone suppression
	Selective bilateral simultaneous venous sampling of ACTH from inferior petrosal sinuses in patients with Cushing's disease with negative neuroimaging
Thyroid function	TSH, T3, and T4
Gonadal function	FSH, LH, estradiol, and testosterone
Adrenal function	Basal plasma or urinary steroids, cortisol response to insulin-induced hypoglycemia, and plasma ACTH response to metyrapone administration

Staging

- Pituitary adenomas can be categorized into microadenomas (<1 cm) or macroadenomas (≥1 cm).
- Hardy's classification (see Table):

Hardy's Radiographic Classification for Pituitary Adenomas and Grading Schema for Suprasellar Extension

Stage (0–IV)/ Grade (A–D)	Diagnostic Criteria
0	Normal pituitary appearance
I	Enclosed within the sella turcica, microadenoma, smaller than 10 mm
II	Enclosed within the sella turcica, macroadenoma, 10 mm or larger
III	Invasive, locally, into the sella turcica
IV	Invasive, diffusely, into the sella turcica
A	0–10 mm suprasellar extension occupying the suprasellar cistern
B	10–20 mm extension and elevation of the third ventricle
C	20–30 mm extension occupying the anterior of the third ventricle
D	A larger than 30 mm extension, beyond the foramen of Monroe, or Grade C with lateral extension

Treatment Overview

- Surgery:
  - Usually the mainstay of treatment.
  - Rapid decompression of optic apparatus and rapid relief of hormonal hypersecretion.
  - Widening the gap between the pituitary tumor and optic apparatus to facilitate stereotactic radiosurgery.
  - Transphenoidal approach is usually preferred.
- RT:
  - Usually offered for medically inoperable disease, persistent hormonal hypersecretion after subtotal resection, or extensive extrasellar disease.
  - External beam RT (EBRT) or stereotactic radiosurgery (SRS), optic apparatus dose permitting for the latter (the goal is to limit the optic apparatus dose to 8–12 Gy in 1 fraction based on data from Harvard University and Mayo Clinic).
- Medical therapy:
  - Bromocriptine—Prolactinoma
  - Somatostatin analogs or pegvisomant (growth hormone receptor Antagonist)—Acromegaly
  - Ketoconazole, metapyone, or mitotane—Cushing's disease

Disease-Specific Management

Disease	Management
Nonsecretory pituitary adenoma	Surgery → Observation or postoperative RT
	Definitive RT
	Postoperative or definitive SRS if adequate gap between tumor and optic apparatus
Prolactinoma	If symptomatic or asymptomatic but macroadenoma→ Medical therapy (bromocriptine, pergolide, or cabergoline)
	If medical therapy poorly tolerated or hypersecretion poorly controlled → Surgery ± RT (depending on endocrine control) or SRS (if adequate gap between tumor and optic apparatus)
	If asymptomatic and microadenoma → Close surveillance → Medical therapy if there is progression
Acromegaly	Surgery → Observation → RT or SRS (if adequate gap between tumor and optic apparatus) for recurrent or progressive elevation of growth hormone or IGF-1
	Definitive RT or SRS (if adequate gap between tumor and optic apparatus) for medically inoperable patients
Cushing's disease	Surgery → Observation → RT or SRS (if adequate gap between tumor and optic apparatus) for recurrent or progressive elevation of ACTH
	Definitive RT or SRS (if adequate gap between tumor and optic apparatus) for medically inoperable patients
TSH-secreting pituitary adenoma	Postoperative RT or SRS (if adequate gap between tumor and optic apparatus) is always needed given the aggressive nature of the disease

Radiation Therapy Technique

- Simulation:
  - o CT simulation with thermoplastic mask for immobilization in supine position Fusion with T1 with gadolinium sequence
- Target delineation:
  - o GTV: Contrast enhanced gross tumor on MRI (axial T1 with gadolinium sequence)
  - o CTV: GTV + 0 to 0.5 cm (none for SRS)
  - o PTV: CTV plus 0.2 to 0.5 cm margin (0 margin if rigid frame placement for SRS, cm for Gill-Thomas-Cosman headframe, and 0.3 to 0.5 cm for 3D-CRT or IMRT)
- External beam radiation therapy (EBRT):
  - o 3D-CRT—Multiple nonopposing with some noncoplanar and vertex beams—6 MV beams ± higher energy beams
  - o IMRT or VMAT—Inverse planning
  - o Doses—45 to 50.4 Gy in 25 to 28 fractions for nonsecretory tumors; 50.4 to 54 Gy in 28 to 30 fractions for secretory tumors
- Stereotactic radiosurgery (SRS):
  - o Nonsecretory tumors—15 to 20 Gy in 1 fraction
  - o Secretory tumors—20 to 30 Gy in 1 fraction
- Dose constraints (see Table):
  - o Dose constraints based on TD 5/5 (Emami et al., 1991) and QUANTEC (Mayo et al., 2010).

Organ-at-Risk (OAR)	TD 5/5	QUANTEC
Optic nerves and chiasm	50 Gy	<55 Gy (<2 Gy/fraction)
		≤8–12 Gy (maximum point dose) in 1 fraction
Retina	45 Gy	Not available
Brainstem	50 Gy	54 Gy (whole brainstem)
		59 Gy (<2 Gy/fraction)
		(1–10 mL)
		12.5 Gy (maximum point dose) in 1 fraction

Outcomes

- Nonsecretory pituitary tumors: Local control rates range from 92% to 100% with EBRT or SRS.
- Acromegaly: Endocrine cure rates range from 52% to 63% with EBRT at 10 years.
- Endocrine cure (IGF-1 normalization) rates range from 42% to 62.2% with SRS.
- Prolactinoma: Endocrine cure rates range from 29% to 50% with EBRT and18% to 52% with SRS.
- Cushing's disease: Endocrine cure rates range from 46% to 84% with EBRT.
- Endocrine cure rates range from 35% to 83% with SRS.

Toxicity

- There are general acute and late side effects, including fatigue, hair loss (variable, depending on RT technique), and skin reaction similar to those observed in patients undergoing RT for other intracranial tumors undergoing RT.
- Serious complications such as optic neuropathy, radiation necrosis, and neurocognitive deficits are uncommon with modern RT techniques.
- Hypopituitarism, especially growth hormone deficiency, can occur.
- Secondary tumor or malignancy is rare.

Follow-Up

- First 2 years: Every 4 to 6 months
- 2 to 5 years: Every 6 to 12 months
- After 5 years: Every year
- History and physical examination: Features of hypopituitarism or hypersecretion, cranial nerve function, and visual field test
- Imaging: MRI every 6 months in the first 2 years, then annually
- Laboratory tests: Growth hormone, TSH, T3, T4, gonadal function, adrenal function, and hypersecreted hormone before treatment every 4 to 6 months

10.3   Spinal Cord

Epidemiology

- Primary spinal cord tumors account for 4% of all CNS tumors.
- 85% to 90% of intramedullary tumors are astrocytoma or ependymoma.
- In adults, 60% to 70% of all spinal cord tumors are ependymomas while, in children, 55% to 65% of intramedullary spinal cord tumors are astrocytomas.
- Extramedullary to intramedullary ratio is 2:1.
- Ependymoma: Mean age is 43 years.
  - Slight female predominance
- Astrocytoma: Male = Female.

Pathology

- Astrocytoma occurs more commonly in cervical and thoracic spinal cord with associated cyst formation.
- Ependymoma occurs more commonly in the lumbar region.
- Extramedullary tumors include meningioma, ependymoma, and schwannoma.
- Intramedullary spinal cord tumors are most commonly astrocytomas and less commonly ependymomas and oligodendrogliomas.
- Astrocytomas and ependymomas are more common in patients with neurofibromatosis type 2 (abnormality on chromosome 22).
- Spinal hemangioblastomas can occur in 30% of patients with von Hippel–Lindau syndrome (abnormality on chromosome 3).

Presentation

- Clinical manifestation is function of local anatomy.
- Symptoms and signs may be distant if long tracts are involved.
- The site of involvement can be localized based on symptoms and signs.

Diagnosis and Workup

- History and physical examination: Weakness or numbness of the extremities, hyperreflexia, sensory level, pain, incontinence, and Brown-Sequard Syndrome;
- slow progression of symptoms for low-grade tumors; rapid progression of symptoms in malignant astrocytomas
- Imaging: MRI spine—Enhancement with gadolinium even in low-grade glioma
- Laboratory tests: CSF cytology—Increased protein

Treatment Overview

- Goal: Maximal safe resection
- Meningioma: Gross total resection → Observation
  - Subtotal resection → Observation or postoperative RT
  - Postoperative RT for grade III regardless of extent of resection
- Low-grade glioma: Gross total resection → Observation
  - Subtotal resection → Postoperative RT
- High-grade glioma: Regardless of extent of resection → Postoperative RT
- Ependymoma: Gross total resection → Observation
  - Subtotal resection → Postoperative RT

Radiation Therapy Technique

- Simulation:
  - CT simulation with thermoplastic mask for immobilization in supine position for cervical spine
  - Fusion with T1 with gadolinium and T2 sequences of MRI of the spine
- Target delineation:
  - Meningioma
    - GTV: T1 with gadolinium
    - CTV: No margin for Grade I, 1 cm for Grade II, and 2 cm for Grade III with volume not extending beyond the spinal canal
    - PTV: 0.5 cm
  - Grade I Glioma
    - GTV: T1 with gadolinium (preoperative and postoperative MRI) including tumor cyst but not syrinx
    - CTV: 1 cm expansion with volume not extending beyond the spinal canal
    - PTV: 0.5 cm
  - Grade II Glioma
    - GTV: T1 with gadolinium and T2 (preoperative and postoperative MRI) including tumor cyst but not syrinx for initial GTV/ T1 with gadolinium (preoperative and postoperative MRI) for boost GTV
    - CTV: 1 cm expansion with volume not extending beyond the spinal canal
    - PTV: 0.5 cm
  - Grade III/IV Glioma
    - GTV: T1 with gadolinium and T2 (preoperative and postoperative MRI) including tumor cyst but not syrinx for initial GTV/ T1 with gadolinium (preoperative and postoperative MRI) for boost GTV
    - CTV: 1 cm expansion with volume not extending beyond the spinal canal
    - PTV: 0.5 cm
- External beam radiation therapy (EBRT):
  - 3D-CRT—A single posterior field, opposed lateral fields, a posterior field with opposed lateral fields, or oblique wedge-pair fields, depending on the tumor location —6 MV beams ± higher energy beams
  - IMRT or VMAT—Inverse planning
- Doses:
  - Meningioma—50.4 to 54 Gy in 28 to 30 fractions/ 54 to 59.4 Gy in 30 to 33 fractions for Grade III
  - Grade I Glioma—45 to 50.4 Gy in 25 to 28 fractions
  - Grade II Glioma—45 Gy in 25 fractions + 5.4 to 9 Gy in 3 to 5 fractions for boost (Total 50.4–54 Gy)
  - Grade III or IV Glioma: 45 to 50.4 Gy in 25 to 28 fractions + 9 to 14.4 Gy in 5 to 8 fractions for boost (Total 54–59.4 Gy in 30–33 fractions)
  - Ependymoma: 45 Gy in 25 fractions + 5.4 to 9 Gy in 3 to 5 fractions for boost (Total 50.4–54 Gy)

Outcomes

- Meningioma—Local control (LC) 94% to 99%; 10-year disease free survival (DFS) 80% after gross total resection or subtotal resection + postoperative RT
- Low-grade glioma: LC 31% to 100%; 5 and 10 DFS 38% to 44% and 10% to 26%, respectively
- High-grade glioma: Median overall survival of 4 to 10 months
- Ependymoma: LC 95% to 100% after surgery alone and 88% to 100% after surgery + RT; 5- and 10-year DFS both 59% after surgery + RT

Toxicity

- Lhermitt's sign:
  - Typically occurs 3 to 4 months after RT
  - Electrical shock-like paresthesia or numbness from the neck to the extremities upon neck flexion
  - Transient demyelination
- Radiation myelopathy (RM):
  - Occurs at least 6 to 12 months
  - 1/2 and 3/4 patients who develop RM in the cervical and thoracic regions will do so within 20 and 30 months, respectively, after irreversible diagnosis by exclusion.

10.4 Brain Metastasis

Epidemiology

- Most common brain tumor
- Incidence 175,000/yr
- Increasing with improving systemic therapies

Pathology

- 50%: Lung
- Other common:
  - Breast
  - Melanoma
  - Renal
  - Unknown primary
- Pathologies with highest incidence of hemorrhage:
  - Renal, melanoma, choriocarcinoma, thyroid
- Pathology most commonly seen with bleeding:
  - Lung due to its prevalence

Presentation

- Referable to area of involvement. Headache, nausea, vomiting, and focal neurologic deficit. Posterior fossa tumors: increased intracranial pressure: headache, nausea, vomiting, ataxia, vertigo, and papilledema. Seizures for supratentorial lesions. Cranial nerve involvement should raise question of leptomeningeal disease.

Diagnosis and Workup

- Full history and physical examination: complete neurological exam and mental status check
- Imaging:
  - If known history of cancer: MRI brain; T1 ± contrast T2/flair. If planning radiosurgery; thin slice with 3D reconstruction

- o If no known history of cancer, in addition to MRI of brain,
  - Chest x-ray
  - Mammogram
  - CT of chest, abdomen, and pelvis
  - Consider FDG-PET
- CSF:
  - o If concerns for leptomeningeal disease and is not detectable on MR. However, due to poor sensitivity, CSF can be determined only diagnostically negative after 3 successive negative samples.
- Surgery:
  - o Resection or biopsy may be used as diagnostic modality if no known primary is detected, no other site of metastasis is detected.
  - o In a randomized controlled study, 11% of patients with a single brain met regardless of extracranial status were found to have pathology different from known cancer.

Treatment Overview

- One lesion:
  - o Surgery followed by whole brain radiation therapy or SRS to cavity.
  - o SRS to lesion ± WBRT.
  - o No comparative trial of efficacy of SRS versus surgery but best available evidence suggests they are comparable.
- Two to three lesions:
  - o SRS ± WBRT; three randomized controlled trials demonstrate that WBRT offers better local and regional brain control, but no survival benefit. May be saved for salvage.
  - o WBRT is associated in some patients with neurocognitive decline, mild to moderate. In some patients may be severe (elderly, uncontrolled diabetics, and uncontrolled hypertensives).
  - o For multiple mets surgery only to relieve symptoms of mass effect not relieved with steroid.
- Four or more metastases:
  - o WBRT.
  - o There is one randomized controlled study that demonstrated that SRS alone for this population was reasonable.
  - o No randomized controlled trials demonstrating SRS alone for less than 4 mets.

Radiation Therapy Technique

- WBRT:
  - o Simulation: CT simulation with thermoplastic mask in supine position.
  - o Dose: 300 cGy × 10 fractions. For patients with more favorable prognosis or who will be receiving SRS, consider 250 cGy × 15 to 3,750 cGy.
  - o Typically interval of approximately 4–6 weeks prior to radiosurgery to allow for maximal tumor response.
  - o Some prefer SRS prior to WBRT.
- Radiosurgery:
  - o Simulation: depends upon treatment platform
    - Frame based Linac
    - Frameless Linac
    - Gamma-knife
    - Cyberknife
      - Frame-based: local anesthetic to pin contact points. Neurosurgical placement of frame. Either CT-based simulation with frame and fusion to diagnostic MRI T1 + C or MR-based simulation.
      - Frameless: aquaplast mask with head in neutral position. ***IV contrast used for intact lesion. Fused with T1 + C MRI.

- o Dose:
  - Lesions ≤2 cm: 20 to 24 Gy
  - Lesions 2.1 to 3 cm: 18 Gy
  - Lesions 3.1 to 4 cm: 15 Gy
  - Various hypo-fractionated schedules used in selected centers.

Outcomes

- Graded Prognostic Assessment (GPA)

	0	0.5	1	Total GPA	OS (Months)
Age	<60	50–59	<50	3.5–4	11
KPS	≥70	70–80	90–100	3	7
Number of CNS mets	≥3	2–4	1	1.5–2.5	4
Extracranial mets	Present		None	0–1	3

- Site-specific GPA:
  - o Breast: KPS, luminal subtype, age (median OS: 3.4–25 months)
  - o Lung: age, KPS, number of lesions
  - o Melanoma/renal: KPS + number of lesions
  - o GI: KPS
- 2-year treatment-specific control:
  - o Surgery alone (not recommended):
    - Treated site: 41%
    - Distant/regional brain: 58%
  - o Surgery + WBRT:
    - Treated site: 75%
    - Distant/regional brain: 77%
  - o SRS + WBRT:
    - Treated site: 80%
    - Distant/regional brain: 67%
  - o SRS alone:
    - Treated site: 70%
    - Distant/regional brain: 52%

Toxicity

- WBRT:
  - o Acute: Fatigue, hair loss, skin irritation/dryness, headaches, nausea, and edema resulting in worsening of presenting symptoms, such as weakness, numbness, gait disturbance, and aphasia. Treated with steroids + GI prophylaxis. Parotid swelling, seizure ear stuffiness, hemorrhage are less common.
  - o Late effects include persistent alopecia. Mild to moderate long-term neurocognitive effects are common; severe neurocognitive effects less common. Likely elderly, patients with other neurocognitive risk factors such as uncontrolled hypertension or diabetes, are at higher risk. Optic neuropathy, radiation necrosis, hypopituitarism, and secondary malignancy are rare.

- SRS:
  - o Acute: Fatigue, hair loss, and skin irritation; less commonly headache or nausea.
  - o Late: Inflammation with focal symptoms referable to location of treatment. May present as flare of initial symptoms. Treated with dexamethasone taper if symptomatic with GI prophylaxis. Rare risk of hemorrhage. Radionecrosis may be imaging finding and asymptomatic. Symptomatic radionecrosis will reflect locality in brain. May be treated with steroid as above. If unable to taper may consider definitive surgery or bevacizumab 7.5 mg/kg at 3 week intervals × 4. Hemorrhage contraindication.
- Work up for radionecrosis:
  - o Trial of steroids and serial MRI for resolution
  - o Dual phase pet scan
  - o Perfusion MRI

Follow-Up

- S/p WBRT: q3 month MRI
- If SRS intended S/p WBRT, MRI 1 to 3 months
  - o If "radioresistant" tumor such as melanoma or renal, consider sooner
- S/p SRS alone: initially 6 to 8 week scan; if no new lesions q3 months
  - o If "radioresistant" tumor such as melanoma or renal, consider sooner
- History and physical examination: Full neurologic history with mini-mental status and physical

10.5   Meningioma

Epidemiology

- This is the most common primary brain tumor in younger adults.
- It accounts for approximately 1/3 of all brain tumors.
- There are 18,000 cases annually.
- 2:1 female/male is the ratio of incidence.
- Risk factors:
  - o Prior ionizing RT
    - Scalp tx with RT for tinea capitis
    - Acne treatment
    - Atom bomb data
    - Dental x-rays?
  - o NF2
  - o Hormonal relationship
    - Female more than male
    - Peak during reproductive years then declines
    - Exogenous hormone use?
    - Association with breast cancer
    - Increased risk with increased BMI?
  - o Cell phone use?

Pathology

- Grade I: 65% to 70%
- Grade II: 23% to 35%
- Grade III: approximately 5%

Grade

I	Don't meet criteria below		
II	Atypical	≥4 mit/10 HPF *or*	Increased cellularity
	Clear Cell	≥3 of the following	*Small cells with high N:C*
	Chordoid		Prominent nucleoli
			Patternless or sheetlike growth
			Foci necrosis
			Brain Invasion
III	Rhabdoid	≥20 mit/10 hpf	Resemble carcinoma, sarcoma, melanoma
	Papillary	and/or	*Loss of usual patterns*
	Anaplastic		Abundant mitoses with atypical forms
			Multifocal foci necrosis

Presentation

- Referable to area of involvement. Seizure-presenting symptom 25% to 40%. Headache, nausea, vomiting, and focal neurologic deficit. Posterior fossa tumors: increased intracranial pressure: headache, nausea, vomiting, ataxia, vertigo, and papilledema. May be asymptomatic and found incidentally.

Diagnosis and Workup

- Full history and physical examination: complete neurological exam
- Imaging:
  - CT: evaluate hyperostosis
  - MRI brain: T1 ± contrast with thin slice with 3D reconstruction, T2/flair
    - Dural tail sign suggestive but not pathognomonic
- Surgery:
  - If surgery definitive therapy also gives definitive diagnosis.
  - If RT definitive therapy, biopsy is controversial.
  - If history of malignancy with likelihood of metastasis, consider surgery.
- If no surgery (active surveillance or RT):
  - Make sure that patient was up-to-date with age-appropriate screening:
    - Mammograms
    - Colonoscopy
    - PSA/Prostate exams
    - Consider SPEP/UPEP

Treatment Overview

- Active surveillance:
  - Age-appropriate screening as mentioned earlier.
  - Recommend repeat MRI in 3 months and, if stable q6 months for 2 years, then yearly, if remains stable. Make sure to compare all prior exams. Consider scanning more frequently if subtle growth noted.

- Surgery:
  - Extent of surgery assessed by Simpson grading criteria:

Grade	Definition	Recurrence (%)
0	Gross total resection (GTR) of tumor, dural attachment, and abnormal bone with stripping of 2 cm of dura	0 (at 5 years)
I	GTR of tumor, dural attachment, and abnormal bone	9
II	GTR of tumor, coagulation of dural attachment	19
III	GTR without resection or coagulation of dural attachment Anaplastic	29
IV	Partial resection of tumor	44
V	Decompression ± biopsy	–

  - Series with 25-year follow-up of all patients demonstrate that even with GTR (Simpson ≤3), there is 10%–15% relapse at 10 years, and ~35%–40% at 25 years with CSS of 50% at 10 and 25 years.
  - Some evidence suggests over-aggressive surgery is associated with worse long-term overall survival.
- Radiation:
  - Adjuvant RT:
    - No role for routine use after total resection of Grade I lesion.
    - Improves PFS after subtotal resection of Grade I lesion, however, routine use somewhat controversial.
    - Controversial after total resection of Grade II lesion.
      - Progression-free survival benefit questionably translates into cause-specific survival benefit.
    - Recommended after subtotal resection of Grade II lesion.
    - Recommended after gross-total and subtotal resection of Grade III lesion.
  - Definitive RT:
    - Control may be comparable to surgery.
    - Possible it is superior to surgery followed by adjuvant RT.
    - Possible there is less toxicity with primary versus adjuvant therapy.
    - Conventional fractionation or SRS is used for Grade I.
    - For higher Grade, conventional fractionation is recommended.

Radiation Therapy Technique

- Simulation:
  - For conventional fractionation, CT simulation with thermoplastic mask in supine position. IV contrast used for intact lesion. Fuse with T1 weighted MRI + Contrast with thin slices and 3D reconstruction. IV contrast used for intact lesion.
  - For SRS, see above sections on radiosurgical sim platform technique.
- Dose:
  - Grade I:
    - GTV is gross lesion + concerning hyperostosis.
    - CTV is GTV + 2 mm to 1 cm along dura only.
    - PTV: CTV + 5 mm (or machine-specific setup tolerance).
    - Dose: 5,400 cGy in 180 cGy fractions to PTV.

- o Grade II:
  - GTV is gross lesion + concerning hyperostosis + surgical bed.
  - CTV is GTV + 5 mm to 2 cm along dura alone unless brain invasion.
  - PTV: CTV + 5 mm (or machine-specific setup tolerance).
  - Dose: 5,400 cGy in 180 cGy fractions to PTV and CD to CTV in 180 Gy fractions to sum of 5,940 to 6,120 cGy respecting critical structures.
- o Grade III:
  - GTV is gross lesion + concerning hyperostosis + tumor bed.
  - CTV is GTV + 1 to 2.5 cm margin (may be smaller into parenchyma than along dura if no evidence of invasion into brain).
  - PTV: CTV + 5 mm (or machine-specific setup tolerance).
  - Dose 5,400 cGy in 180 cGy fractions to PTV and CD to CTV in 180 Gy fractions to sum of 5,940 to 6,120 cGy respecting critical structures. If intact lesion, consider boost of GTV to 6,300 cGy.
- o SRS Dose: 12 to 14 Gy
  - SRS is not recommended around parasagittal/midline para-sinus lesions. Symptomatic toxicity requiring steroids reaches 35% to 45%.

Outcomes

- Grade I: 5-year PFS greater than 95% for surgery, radiation therapy, and radiosurgery.
  - o Long-term control slowly declines with all therapies.
  - o Cause-specific mortality at 10 and 25 years may be as high as 50%.
- Grade II:
  - o 2- and 5-year OS: 93% and 73%.
- Grade III:
  - o 2- and 5-year OS: 57% and 42%.

Toxicity

- Conventional RT:
  - o Fatigue, hair loss, skin irritation/dryness, thrush, and edema with symptoms referable to tumor location such as weakness, numbness, gait disturbance, and aphasia; these may potentially require steroids. Seizure is less common.
  - o Late complications: Mild to moderate long-term neurocognitive effects are less common in modern era. Radionecrosis is low risk for Grade I lesions treated with ≤5,400; however, symptoms referable to region are treated. Treatment around the parasagittal sinus may increase likelihood of symptomatic edema requiring steroids.
- SRS:
  - o Acute: Fatigue, focal hair loss, and skin irritation; less commonly headache or nausea.
  - o Late: Inflammation with focal symptoms referable to location of treatment; may present as flare of initial symptoms. Treated with dexamethasone taper; if symptomatic with GI prophylaxis. Radionecrosis may be imaging finding and asymptomatic. Symptoms from radionecrosis will reflect brain location and may be treated with steroid as above. There is high risk of symptomatic edema requiring steroids if SRS is near parasagittal/midline para-sinus (35%–45%).

Follow-Up

- Active surveillance (see Treatment Overview section)
- Post-therapy
  - o Grade I: MRI T1 ± C and T2/flair with H&P with detailed neurologic exam: q6 months × 2 year, then yearly

- Grade II: MRI T1 ± C and T2/flair with H&P with detailed neurologic exam: at 3 months, then q6 months 2 to 5 years, then annually
- Grade III: MRI T1 ± C and T2/flair with H&P with detailed neurologic exam: at 1 month, then q3 months first year, then q6 months 2 to 5 years, then annually

General Radiosurgery Constraints

Organ-at-Risk (OAR)	QUANTEC
Optic nerves and chiasm	≤8–10 Gy (maximum point dose) in 1 fraction
Retina	Not available
Brainstem	12.5 Gy (maximum point dose) in 1 fraction

10.6   Acoustic Neuroma

Epidemiology

- Incidence: 1 per 100,000 person-years
- Increasing incidence
- Median age at diagnosis: 50
- 90% unilateral affecting right and left equally
- Bilateral gives diagnosis of neurofibromatosis type 2
- Childhood exposure to low-dose radiation risk factor
- Parathyroid adenoma risk factor
- Cell phone use: controversial: note equal left and right incidence of lesions
- Risk of noise exposure controversial

Pathology

- Schwann cell-derived tumors usually arise from vestibular portion of the CN VIII; may arise at other sites.
- NF2 gene encodes merlin.
- They have zones of alternately dense and sparse cellularity called "Antoni A" and "Antoni B" areas respectively.
- Spontaneous malignant degeneration can occur.

Presentation

- Hearing loss, tinnitus: May be of insidious or sudden onset and does not correlate with tumor size. Vestibular and cerebellar symptoms: unsteadiness with walking, matching in place; listing to ipsilateral side objectively or subjectively. True vertigo is uncommon. CN V involvement presents facial numbness or hypesthesia, rarely pain. Facial nerve may present with taste disturbance.

Diagnosis and Workup

- History and physical examination: Full neurologic exam. Detailed documentation of hearing (e.g., Can patients hear out of the affected side on phone? Can they hear alarm clock if contralateral side is against pillow?). Facial sensation changes: taste changes, changes in sensation at the lateral aspect of tongue, facial droop/chewing one side of mouth or biting cheek; food pooling one side of mouth. Changes in balance or coordination: difficulty with vertigo, especially when navigating in dark (e.g., going to bathroom at night). Evaluate subtle signs of CN VII dysfunction by asking patient to mimic risus sardonicus. Flattening of platysma is earliest sign.

- Imaging: MRI with T1 ± C, T2 and flair, thin slice volumetric MRI ± C with 3D reconstruction. FIESTA (fast-imaging employing steady state acquisition) sequencing MRI through auditory canals and cranial nerves. Isointense on T1 weighted images, enhancing brightly with contrast; may be cystic; often extends to cerebellopontine angle. CT bony windows are useful to determine extend of expansion of IAC.
- Audiometry: must be obtained prior to therapy. It is often done as part of making diagnosis. Only 5% have normal test.
  - Pure tone Average (PTA): Average dB score at 500, 1,000, and 2,000 Hz.
  - Speech reception threshold (SRT): dB level at which patients can correctly hear 50% of speech (lower indicates more acute hearing).
  - Speech discrimination (SD): Percentage of words patient can repeat at given dB level. Localizes sidedness of hearing loss and determines if hearing aid is likely to help. Thus may be out of proportion to objective hearing loss.
  - Result will generally demonstrate asymmetric sensorineural hearing loss in the higher frequencies. It does not necessarily correlate with tumor size. On the Gardner–Robertson Hearing Scale, Grades I and II indicate useful hearing.

Gardner–Robertson Hearing Scale

Grade	PTA (dB)	SD (%)
I: Good	0–30	70–100
II: Serviceable	31–50	50–69
III: Nonserviceable	51–90	5–49
IV: Poor	90–100	1–4
V: Deaf	0	0

House–Brackmann Scale

Grade	Description	Features
I	Normal	Normal
II	Mild dysfunction	Slight weakness; slight synkinesis. Noticeable on close inspection
III	Moderate dysfunction	Obvious, not disfiguring
IV	Moderately Severe dysfunction	Obvious; disfiguring asymmetry. Normal symmetry tone at rest. Incomplete eye closure
V	Severe dysfunction	Asymmetry at rest. Brely perceptible motion
VI	Total paralysis	No movement

- Surgery:
  - Typically only when surgery will be used as definitive therapy.

Treatment Overview

- Active surveillance:
  - 40% of patients have growth less than 1 mm/yr; 10% growth rate of ≥3 mm/yr.
  - Approximately 5% regress spontaneously.
  - Hearing loss in 50% followed longitudinally.
  - Reasonable with small tumor size, lack of symptoms or mild symptoms not rapidly progressing, other competing comorbidities.
  - Growth rate may be associated with risk of hearing loss.
  - Rapid tumor growth ≥2.5 mm/yr is indication for tx.
- Surgery—associated with approximately 45% incidence of headaches, often severe. 50% of these resolve; most common in retro sigmoid. Mortality 0.2% to 1%. CSF leak approximately 10% to 15%. Infections 5%, majority meningitis.
  - Retro sigmoid/subscipital: Any tumor size with approximately 30% to 50% hearing preservation. Often, postoperative headache and nausea. Longer healing. More common in women than men.
  - Translabyrinthine: Tumors less than 3 cm or when hearing preservation not consideration. More common CSF leak.
  - Middle fossa: For lesions greater than 1.5 cm with hearing preservation attempted. Higher incidence of seventh nerve palsy.
- Radiation:
  - Conventional fractionation versus SRS

Radiation Therapy Technique

- Simulation:
  - For conventional fractionation: CT simulation with thermoplastic mask for immobilization in supine position, neck in neutral position. Fusion with T1 with T1 + C sequence MRI with thin slicing through the IAC. Fuse with FIESTA sequencing.
  - For SRS: See prior discussion on platform-specific simulation.
- Target delineation:
  - Conventional fractionation:
    - 4,680 cGy to 5,400 cGy in 180 cGy fractions, single course
    - GTV: enhancing lesion on thin slice T1 + C
    - CTV: None
    - PTV: GTV + 0.2 cm (or system-dependent set-up tolerance)
  - Radiosurgery:
    - Restrict to tumors greater than 3 cm; less favorable for cystic lesions
    - 12 to 13 Gy in a single fraction
    - GTV: enhancing lesion on thin slice T1 + C
    - No CTV
    - PTV = GTV. No margin

Outcomes

- Surgery:
  - 5- and 10-year control with GTR: approximately 95%
  - Normal facial movement: 95% small tumors; 50% large tumors
  - Hearing preserved 40% to 80% with preoperative intact hearing and small tumors
  - 10% nonaudio/facial complications
  - 5% infection rate, mostly meningitis
  - 1% hemorrhage/other vascular complication
  - 50% daily headaches, F less than M, resolving in 50% of these

- Conventional fractionated radiation therapy:
  - 5- and 10-year local control less than 95%
  - In patients with serviceable hearing, 5-year hearing preservation 75% to 80% @ 5 years
  - Temporary or permanent trigeminal nerve toxicity; approximately 3%
  - Temporary or permanent facial nerve toxicity; approximately 1%
- Radiosurgery:
  - 5- and 10-year local control less than 95%
  - In patients with serviceable hearing, 5-year hearing preservation 60% to 70% (Worse with fraction sizes less than 13 Gy; likely will continue to decrease to about 25% at 10 years even with current doses)
  - Temporary or permanent trigeminal nerve toxicity; approximately 3%
  - Temporary or permanent facial nerve toxicity; approximately 1%.

Toxicity

- Acute toxicity: Fatigue, regional hair loss with larger volumes; occasional increase in tinnitus or imbalance.
- Late complications:
  - Increase in tinnitus
  - ~3% risk of temporary or permanent trigeminal dysfunction
  - ~1% incidence of facial nerve dysfunction
  - Patients with serviceable hearing: There may be slightly better durable serviceable hearing with fractionation however, this is controversial
  - ~60–80% preservation of serviceable hearing at about 5 years but likely declines over time
  - Less commonly, cystic degeneration potentially requiring surgery
  - RT-induced transformation is rare. There is documentation of spontaneous malignant degeneration in absence of RT
  - Secondary malignancy such as GBM

Follow-Up

- History and physical examination; complete neurologic history and physical exam
- Audiometry yearly
- MRI T1 – Contrast with thin slicing and 3D reconstruction; FIEST sequencing and T2/flair; initially q6 months × 2 years, then 6 months for 5 years, then annually thereafter
- *Tumor enlargement 6 to 18 months after RT common; typically associated with decreased uptake centrally and eventually returning to homogenous enhancement and radiographic stability*
- History and physical examination: mini-mental status with neurologic history and physical

Chapter 10: Practice Questions

1. Rapid enlargement of ACTH-secreting pituitary adenoma after bilateral adrenalectomy is otherwise known as

   A. Nelson's Syndrome
   B. Virchow's Syndrome
   C. Salazar's Syndrome
   D. Rodger's Syndrome

2. Bilateral acoustic neuroma is associated with

   A. NT syndrome
   B. neurofibromatosis type 1A
   C. neurofibromatosis type 1B
   D. neurofibromatosis type 2

3. The 5-year survival rate of a RTOG 98-02 high-risk astrocytoma with postoperative RT is

    A. 82%
    B. 72%
    C. 62%
    D. 52%

4. What is the estimated 5-year disease-free survival rate after surgery and radiation for adult ependymoma?

    A. 40%
    B. 50%
    C. 60%
    D. 70%

5. All of the following cranial nerves can be usually affected by pituitary tumors EXCEPT

    A. III
    B. IV
    C. V1
    D. V3

6. High-risk astrocytomas as defined by RTOG 98-02 is

    A. Age ≥40 years AND/OR less than gross total resection
    B. Both age ≥40 years AND less than gross total resection
    C. Age less than 40 years AND/OR less than gross total resection
    D. Both age less than 40 years AND less than gross total resection

7. The long-term risk of local relapse of a totally resected meningioma is approximately

    A. <5%
    B. 5%–10%
    C. 10%–15%
    D. 15%–20%

8. A 9-mm pituitary tumor that is locally invasive into the sella turcica is Hardy classified as

    A. IIA
    B. IIB
    C. IIIA
    D. IIIB

9. The 2-year local control with surgery for oligometastatic brain mets treated by surgery alone is approximately

    A. 40%
    B. 50%
    C. 60%
    D. 70%

10. Spinal cord ependymomas are most likely located in which region?

    A. Cervical
    B. Thoracic
    C. Lumbar
    D. Sacral

11. A partial resection of a meningioma is categorized as a Simpson grade

    A. 1
    B. 2
    C. 3
    D. 4

12. The clinicopathological hallmark of glioblastoma multiforme is

A. Atypia
B. Mitotic activity
C. Large tumor size
D. Necrosis

13. von Hippel–Lindau Syndrome is associated with which spinal cord tumor?

A. Astrocytoma
B. Ependymoma
C. Oligodendroglioma
D. Hemangioblastoma

14. The most common source of brain metastases is

A. Renal
B. Lung
C. Breast
D. Melanoma

15. Risk factors for Grade II astrocytomas include the following EXCEPT

A. Primary tumor ≥6cm
B. Age less than 40 years
C. Presence of neurological deficits
D. Tumors that cross midline

16. The 5-year survival of a RTOG 98-02 low risk astrocytoma with no postoperative RT is

A. 99%
B. 97%
C. 95%
D. 93%

17. A partial resection of a meningioma is associated with the following approximate recurrence risk:

A. 5%
B. 25%
C. 45%
D. 65%

18. Most adult intramedullary spinal cord tumors are

A. Astrocytomas
B. Ependymomas
C. Germ cell tumors
D. Metastases

19. Typical doses for secretory pituitary tumors are

A. Usually higher than with nonsecretory tumors
B. The same as nonsecretory tumors
C. Lower than nonsecretory tumors
D. Completely different dose per fraction hindering a direct comparison

20. Meningiomas are what proportion of all adult brain tumors?

A. 25%
B. 33%
C. 50%
D. 67%

Chapter 10: Answers

1. A
Nelson's Syndrome: Rapid enlargement of ACTH-secreting pituitary adenoma after bilateral adrenalectomy

2. D
90% of cases are unilateral affecting right and left equally. Bilateral presentation associated with neurofibromatosis type 2.

3. B
High-risk patients with postoperative adjuvant PCV-RT (RTOG 98-02):
    5-year PFS: 61%
    5-year OS: 72%
    10-year PFS: 50%
    10-year OS: 60%

4. C
Ependymoma:
    LC 95%–100% after surgery alone and 88%–100% after surgery + RT; 5- and 10-year DFS both 59% after surgery + RT

5. D
Deficits of functions of III, IV, V1 + 2, and VI nerves can occur in pituitary tumors.

6. A
RTOG 98-02 high-risk definition: age ≥40 and/or less than gross total resection.

7. C
Series with 25-year follow-up of all patients demonstrate that even with GTR (Simpson ≤3) have 10%–15% relapse at 10 years, and approximately 35%–40% at 25 years with CSS 50% at 10 and 25 years.

8. B
Stage III: Invasive, locally, into the sella turcica
Grade A: 0 to 10 mm suprasellar extension occupying the suprasellar cistern.

9. A
2-year treatment-specific control with surgery alone:
    Treated site: 41%
    Distant/regional brain: 58%

10. C
Ependymoma occurs more commonly in the lumbar region.

11. D
Partial resection of tumor is considered a grade IV tumor.

12. D
Necrosis is a clinicopathological hallmark of GBM.

13. D
Spinal hemangioblastomas can occur in 30% of patients with von Hippel–Lindau syndrome (abnormality on chromosome 3).

14. B
50% of brain metastases are associated with primary lung cancer.
Other common primary sites:
  Breast
  Melanoma
  Renal
  Unknown primary

15. B
High-risk features for grade II astrocytoma include ≥3: tumor ≥6 cm, tumor crossing midline, age ≥40, astrocytoma histology, and presence of neurologic deficits.

16. D
Low-risk patients with no postoperative adjuvant tx (RTOG 98-02):
  2-year PFS: 82%
  2-year OS: 99%
  5-year PFS: 48%
  5-year OS: 93%

17. C
A partially resected meningioma is associated with a 44% recurrence risk.

18. A
85%–90% of adult intramedullary tumors are astrocytoma or ependymoma. Intramedullary spinal cord tumors are most commonly astrocytomas and less commonly ependymomas and oligodendrogliomas.

19. A
Conventional radiation:
  45 to 50.4 Gy in 25 to 28 fractions for nonsecretory tumors
  50.4 to 54 Gy in 28 to 30 fractions for secretory tumors
Stereotactic radiosurgery (SRS):
  Nonsecretory tumors: 15 to 20 Gy in 1 fraction
  Secretory tumors: 20 to 30 Gy in 1 fraction

20. B
Most common primary brain tumor in younger adults which is approximately 1/3 of all brain tumors.

Recommended Reading

Andrews DW, Suarez O, Goldman HW, et al. Stereotactic radiosurgery and fractionated stereotactic radiotherapy for the treatment of acoustic schwannomas: comparative observations of 125 patients treated at one institution. *Int J Radiat Oncol Biol Phys.* 2001;50(5):1265-1278.

Andrews DW, Scott CB, Sperduto PW, et al. Whole brain radiation therapy with or without stereotactic radiosurgery boost for patients with one to three brain metastases: phase III results of the RTOG 9508 randomised trial. Lancet. May 22, 2004;363(9422):1665-1672.

Brennan C, Yang TJ, Hilden P, et al. A phase 2 trial of stereotactic radiosurgery boost after surgical resection for brain metastases. *Int J Radiat Oncol Biol Phys.* January 1, 2014;88(1):130-136.

Cairncross G, Wang M, Shaw E, et al. Phase III trial of chemoradiotherapy for anaplastic oligodendroglioma: long-term results of RTOG 9402. *J Clin Oncol.* 2013;31(3):337-343.

Chopra R, Kondziolka D, Niranjan A, et al. Long-term follow-up of acoustic schwannoma radiosurgery with marginal tumor doses of 12 to 13 Gy. *Int J Radiat Oncol Biol Phys.* 2007;68(3):845-851.

Combs SE, Schulz-Ertner D, Debus J, et al. Improved correlation of the neuropathologic classification according to adapted World Health Organization classification and outcome after radiotherapy in patients with atypical and anaplastic meningiomas. *Int J Radiat Oncol Biol Phys.* 2011;81(5):1415-1421.

Combs SE, Welzel T, Schulz-Ertner D, et al. Differences in clinical results after LINAC-based single-dose radiosurgery versus fractionated stereotactic radiotherapy for patients with vestibular schwannomas. *Int J Radiat Oncol Biol Phys.* 2010;76(1):193-200.

Elia AEH, Shih HA, Loeffler JS. Stereotactic radiation treatment for benign meningiomas. *Neurosurgical FOCUS.* 2007;23(4):E5.

Emami B, Lyman J, Brown A, et al. Tolerance of normal tissue to therapeutic radiation. *Int J Radiat Oncol Biol Phys.* 1991;21:109-122.

Fisher BJ, Jeff Lui, David R. Macdonald, et al. A phase II study of a temozolomide-based chemoradiotherapy regimen for high-risk low-grade gliomas: preliminary results of RTOG 0424. *ASCO Meeting Abstracts.* 2013;31(15 suppl):2008.

Goldsmith BJ, Wara WM, Wilson CB, Larson DA. Postoperative irradiation for subtotally resected meningiomas. A retrospective analysis of 140 patients treated from 1967 to 1990. *J Neurosurg.* 1994;80(2):195-201.

Huang D, Halberg FE. Pituitary tumors. In: Leibel SA, Phillips TL, eds. *Textbook of Radiation Oncology*. 2nd ed. Philadelphia, PA: Saunders; 2004:533-548.

Karim AB, Maat B, Hatlevoll R, et al. A randomized trial on dose-response in radiation therapy of low-grade cerebral glioma: European Organization for Research and Treatment of Cancer (EORTC) Study 22844. *Int J Radiat Oncol BiolPhys*. 1996;36(3):549-556.

Lim K, Simon SL. Pituitary adenoma. In: Lu J, Brady L, eds. *Decision Making in Radiation Oncology*. Berlin: Springer;2011:923-940.

Kocher M, Soffietti R, Abacioglu U, et al. Adjuvant whole-brain radiotherapy versus observation after radiosurgery or surgical resection of one to three cerebral metastases: results of the EORTC 22952-26001 study. *J Clin Oncol*. 2011;29(2):134-141.

Kubicky CD, Chan LW, Tsuji SI, et al. Central nervous system. In: Hansen EK, Roach III M, eds. *Handbook of Evidence-Based Radiation Oncology*. 2nd ed. Heidelberg: Springer; 2010:29-71.

Mayo C, Martel MK, Marks LB, et al. Radiation dose–volume effects of optic nerves and chiasm. *Int J Radiat Oncol Biol Phys*. 2010;76:S28-S35.

McLaughlin MP, Marcus RB Jr, Buatti JM, et al. Ependymoma: results, prognostic factors and treatment recommendations. *Int J Radiat Oncol BiolPhys*. 1998;40(4):845-850.

Nabors LB, Portnow J, Ammirati M, et al. NCCN Guidelines Version 1.2015. *J Natl Compr Canc Netw*. 2015;13(10):1191-1202.

Patchell RA, Tibbs PA, Regine WF, et al. Postoperative radiotherapy in the treatment of single metastases to the brain: a randomized trial. *JAMA*. November 4, 1998;280(17):1485-1489.

Patchell RA, Tibbs PA, Walsh JW, et al. A randomized trial of surgery in the treatment of single metastases to the brain. *N Engl J Med*. February 22, 1990;322(8):494-500.

Pettersson-Segerlind J, Orrego A, Lönn S, Mathiesen T. Long-term 25-year follow-up of surgically treated parasagittal meningiomas. *World Neurosurg*. 2011;76(6):564-571.

Rogers L, Pueschel J, Spetzler R, et al. Is gross-total resection sufficient treatment for posterior fossa ependymomas? *J Neurosurg*. 2005;102(4):629-636.

Rogers, L, Shrieve, D, Perry, A. Intracranial meningioma: fractionated radiation therapy perspective. *Principles and Practice of Stereotactic Radiosurgery*. 2008;257-270.

Shaw EG, Berkey B, Coons SW, et al. Recurrence following neurosurgeon-determined gross-total resection of adult supratentorial low-grade glioma: results of a prospective clinical trial. *J Neurosurg*. 2008;109(5):835-841.

Shaw EG, Wang M, Coons SW, et al. Randomized trial of radiation therapy plus procarbazine, lomustine, and vincristine chemotherapy for supratentorial adult low-grade glioma: initial results of RTOG 9802. *J Clin Oncol*. 2012;30(25):3065-3070.

Sheehan JP, Niranjan A, Sheehan JM, et al. Stereotactic radiosurgery for pituitary adenomas: an intermediate review of its safety, efficacy, and role in the neurosurgical treatment armamentarium. *J Neurosurg*. 2005;102:678-691.

Sperduto PW, Berkey B, Gaspar LE, Mehta M, Curran W. A new prognostic index and comparison to three other indices for patients with brain metastases: an analysis of 1,960 patients in the RTOG database. *Int J Radiat Oncol Biol Phys*. February 1, 2008;70(2):510-514.

Sperduto PW, Chao ST, Sneed PK, et al. Diagnosis-specific prognostic factors, indexes, and treatment outcomes for patients with newly diagnosed brain metastases: a multi-institutional analysis of 4,259 patients. *Int J Radiat Oncol Biol Phys*. 2010;77(3):655-661.

Stafford SL, Pollock BE, Leavitt JA, et al. A study on the radiation tolerance of the optic nerves and chiasm after SRS. *Int J Radiat Oncol Biol Phys*. 2003;55:1177-1781.

Stieber VW, SikerML. Spinal cord tumors. In: Gunderson LL, Tepper JE, eds. *Clinical Radiation Oncology*. 3rd ed. Philadelphia, PA: Elsevier Saunders;2012:511-528.

Stupp R, Mason WP, van den Bent MJ, et al. Radiotherapy plus concomitant and adjuvant temozolomide for glioblastoma. *N Engl J Med*. 2005;352(10):987-996.

Tsao MN, Rades D, Wirth A, et al. Radiotherapeutic and surgical management for newly diagnosed brain metastasis(es): an American Society for Radiation Oncology evidence-based guideline. *Pract Radiat Oncol*. July 2012;2(3):210-225.

van den Bent MJ, Brandes AA, Taphoorn MJ, et al. Adjuvant procarbazine, lomustine, and vincristine chemotherapy in newly diagnosed anaplastic oligodendroglioma: long-term follow-up of EORTC brain tumor group study 26951. *J Clin Oncol*. 2013;31(3):344-350.

Wick W, Hartmann C, Engel C, et al. NOA-04 randomized phase III trial of sequential readiochemotherapy of anaplastic glioma with procarbazine, lomustine, and vincristine or temozolomide. *J Clin Oncol*. 2009;27(35):5874-5880.

Witt TC. Stereotactic radiosurgery for pituitary tumors. *Neurosurg Focus*. 2003;14(5):e10.

PART II

Practice Test 1: Basic Science Questions

Practice Questions

Q1. According to the Clark level system, a melanoma that invades into the reticular dermis is classified as

A. Stage I
B. Stage II
C. Stage III
D. Stage IV

Q2. In an area of electronic equilibrium, absorbed dose is

A. Equal to KERMA at all treatment depths
B. Higher than KERMA at all treatment depths
C. Lower than KERMA at all treatment depths
D. Both higher and lower than KERMA depending on treatment depth

Q3. Photon energy is

A. Proportional to both wave frequency and wavelength
B. Proportional to wave frequency and inversely proportional to wavelength
C. Inversely proportional to wave frequency and proportional to wavelength
D. Inversely proportional to both wave frequency and wavelength

Q4. The sensitivity of a test is defined as

A. (True positives) divided by (true positives plus false negatives)
B. (True negatives) divided by (false positives plus true negatives)
C. (True positives) divided by (true and false positives)
D. (True negatives) divided by (true and false negatives)

Q5. Prophylactic bilateral mastectomy for individuals with a BRCA1/BRCA2 mutation is associated with what reduction in breast cancer risk?

A. 75%
B. 90%
C. 99%
D. 100%

Q6. The QUANTEC recommendation of mean esophageal dose to reduce Grade III or greater acute esophagitis to 5% to 20% is

A. <24 Gy
B. <30 Gy
C. <36 Gy
D. <42 Gy

Q7. The sample size for this type of study is usually largest compared to other trial designs:

A. Superiority design
B. Equivalence design
C. Phase II design
D. Noninferiority design

Q8. Tumor hypoxia best relates to oxygen concentrations of approximately

A. <50 mmHg
B. <10 mmHg
C. <5 mmHg
D. <1 mmHg

Q9. The QUANTEC laryngeal maximum dose should be kept less than what dose to keep vocal dysfunction to less than 20%?

A. 50 Gy
B. 60 Gy
C. 66 Gy
D. 70 Gy

Q10. Two atoms with different atomic numbers but the same mass number are referred to as

A. Isotopes
B. Isotones
C. Isobars
D. Isomers

Q11. The number needed to treat is defined by

A. The number inversely related to the number needed to harm
B. The odds ratio between the number of patients who have a positive outcome versus a negative outcome
C. The number of patients who have to be exposed to an intervention to benefit one patient
D. All patients divided the number of patients who did not experience the outcome of interest

Q12. According to the TNM staging system, a macroscopic positive margin is coded as

A. R1
B. R2
C. R+
D. R

Q13. A decreased tissue/organ mass prior to cell maturity is best known as

A. Aplasia
B. Hypoplasia
C. Atrophy
D. Hypertrophy

Q14. Postradiation therapy vasculitis is usually associated with

A. Small vessel injury
B. Medium vessel injury
C. Large vessel injury
D. Fibrosis

Q15. The following are all modes of nucleon emission EXCEPT

A. Electron capture
B. Alpha decay
C. Proton emission
D. Neutron emission

Q16. Tissue with highly undifferentiated cells is best known as

A. Metaplasia
B. Dysplasia
C. Neoplasia
D. Anaplasia

Q17. The standard dose for unresectable pancreatic cancer, as used in ECOG E4201, is

A. 45 Gy in 25 fractions
B. 50.4 Gy in 28 fractions
C. 50 Gy in 25 fractions
D. 54 Gy in 30 fractions

Q18. The electron range for a 12-MeV electron beam is approximately

A. 2 cm
B. 4 cm
C. 6 cm
D. 8 cm

Q19. Changes in the maturation and development of a cell within a tissue or organ system is known as

A. Metaplasia
B. Dysplasia
C. Neoplasia
D. Anaplasia

Q20. According to the Radiation Therapy Oncology Group (RTOG) 0615 nasopharynx clinical trial, the macroscopic volume of disease should receive the following dose fractionation system:

A. 70 Gy in 35 fractions
B. 70 Gy in 33 fractions
C. 59.4 Gy in 33 fractions
D. 54 Gy in 33 fractions

Q21. According to the Radiation Therapy Oncology Group (RTOG) 0912 trial, the macroscopic volume for an anaplastic thyroid cancer should be treated to

A. 70 Gy in 35 fractions
B. 66 Gy in 33 fractions
C. 59.4 Gy in 33 fractions
D. 60 Gy in 30 fractions

Q22. According to the Radiation Therapy Oncology Group (RTOG) 0912 trial, the high-risk microscopic volume for an anaplastic thyroid cancer should be treated to

A. 70 Gy in 35 fractions
B. 66 Gy in 33 fractions
C. 59.4 Gy in 33 fractions
D. 60 Gy in 30 fractions

Q23. As linear energy transfer (LET) increases,

    A. Less energy is deposited along the path of radiation
    B. More direct DNA damage occurs
    C. Less free radical damage occurs
    D. Increased dependence on oxygen levels

Q24. Statistical methods specifically associated with the evidence-based medicine approach include the following EXCEPT

    A. Number needed to treat or harm
    B. Likelihood ratio
    C. Central limit theorem
    D. Receiver-operator curves

Q25. The beta energy of iridium-192 is

    A. 120 kV
    B. 240 kV
    C. 380 kV
    D. 760 kV

Q26. The QUANTEC recommended heart volume dose–volume histogram (DVH) parameter to reduce acute pericarditis to less than 15% is

    A. V30 Gy < 40%
    B. V30 Gy < 46%
    C. V30 Gy < 52%
    D. V30 Gy < 58%

Q27. Differences in important co-interventions in a clinical trial is known as

    A. Assessment bias
    B. Ascertainment bias
    C. Performance bias
    D. Allocation bias

Q28. In terms of photon attenuation, photoelectric effect and Compton scattering have equal importance at the following energy:

    A. 0.026 MV
    B. 0.511 MV
    C. 1.022 MV
    D. 2.451 MV

Q29. The QUANTEC spinal cord maximum dose leading to a 6% risk of injury is

    A. 50 Gy
    B. 54 Gy
    C. 60 Gy
    D. 69 Gy

Q30. Gamma radiation has a wavelength of approximately

    A. 10^{-2} m
    B. 10^{-5} m
    C. 10^{-10} m
    D. 10^{-12} m

Q31. According to the modified Astler–Coller classification, a colon cancer with invasion through the bowel wall muscularis propria is classified as

A. A

B. B

C. B1

D. B2

Q32. Hallmarks of the stochastic effects of radiation therapy include the following EXCEPT

A. Severity of effect independent on dose

B. No threshold dose

C. Related to acute effects of radiation therapy

D. Likelihood of event dependent on dose

Q33. The following radiation therapy considerations can potentially overcome radioresistance EXCEPT

A. Fractionation

B. Radiosensitizers

C. Oxygenation

D. Use of low REB radiation therapy

Q34. The TNM suffix "R" refers to the following concept:

A. Restaging

B. Retreatment

C. Resection margin

D. None of the above

Q35. The following are true regarding the linear attenuation coefficient are true EXCEPT

A. Inversely proportional to half-value layer of the material in question

B. Proportional to the half-value layer of the material in question

C. Directly related to the mass attenuation coefficient

D. A less fundamental concept than the mass attenuation coefficient

Q36. The half-life of cesium-137 is

A. 17 days

B. 60 days

C. 74 days

D. 30 years

Q37. Postradiation therapy cellular atypia is best described as

A. Detrimental premature cell death

B. Replacement of one differentiated cell type by another

C. Abnormal cell development and decrease in cell number and increase in immature cells

D. Distortion of the cell cytoplasm and nucleus

Q38. The likelihood ratio is associated with the following characteristics EXCEPT

A. The likelihood ratio can relate pre- to posttest probability

B. The likelihood ratio is independent to test accuracy

C. The likelihood ratio is related to Bayes' theorem

D. The likelihood ratio is related to sensitivity and specificity

Q39. Which of the following forms of simulation can potentially address organ motion?

A. Conventional simulation
B. Virtual simulation
C. CT simulation
D. Two of the above are correct

Q40. An acquired change of one mature cell type to another mature cell type is known as

A. Metaplasia
B. Dysplasia
C. Neoplasia
D. Anaplasia

Q41. The QUANTEC maximum brain dose related with 5% injury is

A. 50 Gy
B. 60 Gy
C. 72 Gy
D. 90 Gy

Q42. The QUANTEC recommendation to reduce the risk of Grade III late injury to the bladder to less than 6% in the context of bladder cancer radiation therapy is

A. 60-Gy maximum dose
B. 65-Gy maximum dose
C. 70-Gy maximum dose
D. None of the above

Q43. The half-life of iodine-125 is

A. 17 days
B. 60 days
C. 74 days
D. 30 years

Q44. The half-life of palladium-103 is

A. 17 days
B. 60 days
C. 74 days
D. 30 years

Q45. Familial adenomatous polyposis (FAP) is associated with the following lifetime risk of colorectal cancer:

A. 25%
B. 50%
C. 75%
D. 100%

Q46. The QUANTEC recommendation for whole kidney mean dose to keep injury risk less than 5% is

A. 15 to 18 Gy
B. 18 to 21 Gy
C. 21 to 24 Gy
D. 24 to 27 Gy

Q47. A decreased number of cells and absence of tissue is known as

A. Aplasia
B. Hypoplasia
C. Atrophy
D. Hypertrophy

Q48. Lynch syndrome is associated with the following lifetime risk of colorectal cancer:

A. 40%
B. 60%
C. 80%
D. 100%

Q49. The SI unit for radioactive decay is the

A. Curie (Ci)
B. Gray (Gy)
C. Rad (R)
D. Becquerel (Bq)

Q50. The inverse of the decay constant is

A. The half-life
B. Mean lifetime
C. Specific activity
D. Total activity

Q51. The standard dose for locally advanced non-small cell chemoradiation therapy, as confirmed by the Radiation Therapy Oncology Group (RTOG) 0617 clinical trial, is

A. 60 Gy in 30 fractions
B. 66 Gy in 33 fractions
C. 70 Gy in 35 fractions
D. 74 Gy in 37 fractions

Q52. The identification of causality needs to consider all of the following EXCEPT

A. Strength of association
B. Consistency of association
C. Confounding association
D. Temporality of association

Q53. Photon speed is

A. Proportional to both wave frequency and wavelength
B. Proportional to wave frequency and inversely proportional to wavelength
C. Inversely proportional to wave frequency and proportional to wavelength
D. Inversely proportional to both wave frequency and wavelength

Q54. Postradiation therapy vessel thrombi is usually associated with

A. Small vessel injury
B. Medium vessel injury
C. Large vessel injury
D. Fibrosis

Q55. Cancer related to the smooth muscle tissue of origin is known as

    A. Leiomyosarcoma
    B. Rhabdomyosarcoma
    C. Fibromyosarcoma
    D. Dermatofibrosarcoma

Q56. The standard dose for preoperative rectal cancer, as used in Radiation Therapy Oncology Group (RTOG) 0822, is

    A. 45 Gy in 25 fractions
    B. 50.4 Gy in 28 fractions
    C. 50 Gy in 25 fractions
    D. 54 Gy in 30 fractions

Q57. In the context of the high-risk prostate cancer Radiation Therapy Oncology Group (RTOG) 0521 clinical trial, the standard dose for the pelvic radiation therapy component was

    A. 40 Gy in 20 fractions
    B. 44 Gy in 22 fractions
    C. 45 Gy in 25 fractions
    D. 46.8 Gy in 26 fractions

Q58. The negative predictive value of a test is defined as

    A. (True positives) divided by (true positives plus false negatives)
    B. (True negatives) divided by (false positives plus true negatives)
    C. (True positives) divided by (true and false positives)
    D. (True negatives) divided by (true and false negatives)

Q59. X-ray radiation has a wavelength of approximately

    A. 10^{-2} m
    B. 10^{-5} m
    C. 10^{-10} m
    D. 10^{-12} m

Q60. The TNM staging prefix "c" best refers to

    A. Clinical staging prior to treatment within 4 months of diagnosis
    B. Clinical staging prior to treatment within any time from diagnosis
    C. Clinical staging at any time
    D. Clinical staging based on history, physical examination, and investigations except diagnostic scopes and biopsies

Q61. Smoking is related to what percentage of cancers worldwide?

    A. 5%
    B. 10%
    C. 15%
    D. 20%

Q62. The standard dose of low-risk prostate cancer, as used in the Radiation Therapy Oncology Group (RTOG) 0415 clinical trial, is

    A. 70 Gy in 35 fractions
    B. 74 Gy in 37 fractions
    C. 73.8 Gy in 41 fractions
    D. 79.2 Gy in 44 fractions

Q63. Examples of alkaloids include the following EXCEPT

    A. Vincristine

    B. Taxol

    C. Vinorelbine

    D. Topotecan

Q64. A phase IV clinical trial is otherwise known as

    A. A safety and dose finding study

    B. A postmarketing safety study

    C. A confirmatory randomized controlled trial

    D. A crossover randomized controlled trial

Q65. The inverse of the mean lifetime is the

    A. Decay constant

    B. Mean lifetime

    C. Specific activity

    D. Total activity

Q66. According to the Radiation Therapy Oncology Group (RTOG) 0615 nasopharynx clinical trial, the high-risk microscopic volume of disease should receive the following dose fractionation system:

    A. 70 Gy in 35 fractions

    B. 70 Gy in 33 fractions

    C. 59.4 Gy in 33 fractions

    D. 54 Gy in 33 fractions

Q67. The following entities are involved with the production of directly ionizing radiation EXCEPT

    A. Gamma rays

    B. Electrons

    C. Alpha particles

    D. Protons

Q68. The hallmarks of high-quality randomized controlled trials should contain all of the following EXCEPT

    A. Randomization

    B. Placebo control (if feasible)

    C. Blinding

    D. Superiority trial design

Q69. 1 Curie (Ci) of radioactive decay is equivalent to

    A. 3.7×10^{10} Bq

    B. The rate of decay of 1 g of Radium-226

    C. A and B

    D. The rate of decay of 1 g of Radium-222

Q70. Examples of topoisomerase inhibitors include

    A. Topotecan

    B. Etoposide

    C. A and B

    D. Neither A nor B

Q71. The QUANTEC radiosurgery maximum dose to the brainstem to have less than 5% risk of injury is

A. 8.5 Gy
B. 10 Gy
C. 12.5 Gy
D. 15 Gy

Q72. Abnormal cellular proliferation resulting in a new growth is known as

A. Metaplasia
B. Dysplasia
C. Neoplasia
D. Anaplasia

Q73. Important checkpoints in the cell cycle include the following EXCEPT

A. G1–G0 transition
B. G1–S
C. G2–M
D. Metaphase–anaphase

Q74. According to the Radiation Therapy Oncology Group (RTOG) 0615 nasopharynx clinical trial, the low-risk volume of disease should receive the following dose fractionation system:

A. 70 Gy in 35 fractions
B. 70 Gy in 33 fractions
C. 59.4 Gy in 33 fractions
D. 54 Gy in 33 fractions

Q75. The QUANTEC maximum optic nerve/chiasm dose related with 5% injury is

A. <50 Gy
B. <55 Gy
C. 55 to 60 Gy
D. >60 Gy

Q76. Differences in important baseline prognostic factors between control and intervention groups in a clinical trial is known as

A. Assessment bias
B. Ascertainment bias
C. Performance bias
D. Allocation bias

Q77. The model of the atom whereby electrons travel around a positive nucleus in harmonic orbitals explained by the Schrodinger equations is known as the

A. Thompson model
B. Rutherford model
C. Bohr model
D. Quantum model

Q78. An acquired decrease in tissue or organ mass after full cellular maturity due to a decrease in cellular components is best known as

A. Aplasia
B. Hypoplasia
C. Atrophy
D. Hypertrophy

Q79. According to the Dukes classification, a colon cancer with invasion through the bowel wall is classified as

A. A

B. B

C. B1

D. B2

Q80. This class of chemotherapy is chemically similar to DNA bases (purines and pyrimidines):

A. Alkylating agents

B. Tomoisomerase inhibitors

C. Antimetabolites

D. Alkaloids

Q81. According to the QUANTEC report, if cochlea dose is reduced to less than 45-Gy mean dose, the risk of injury should be less than

A. 5%

B. 10%

C. 20%

D. 30%

Q82. The following viruses have been shown to be related to the development of human cancer EXCEPT

A. EBV

B. SV40

C. HPV

D. HTLV-1

Q83. The standards for reporting of a randomized controlled trials are called the

A. Strengthening the Reporting of Observational Studies in Epidemiology (STROBE) statement

B. Consolidated Standards of Reporting Trials (CONSORT) statement

C. Preferred Reporting Items for Systematic Reviews and Meta-Analyses (PRISMA) statement

D. None of the above

Q84. The radius of an electron cloud is approximately

A. 10^{-2} m

B. 10^{-5} m

C. 10^{-10} m

D. 10^{-14} m

Q85. The CT Hounsfield unit (HU) of water is approximately

A. −1,000

B. 0

C. +400

D. +1,000

Q86. The 80% isodose line for a 12-MeV electron beam is approximately at

A. 1 cm

B. 2 cm

C. 3 cm

D. 4 cm

Q87. The standard dose of intermediate-risk prostate cancer, as used in the Radiation Therapy Oncology Group (RTOG) 0815 clinical trial, is

A. 70 Gy in 35 fractions
B. 74 Gy in 37 fractions
C. 73.8 Gy in 41 fractions
D. 79.2 Gy in 44 fractions

Q88. Postradiation therapy metaplasia is best described as

A. Detrimental premature cell death
B. Replacement of one differentiated cell type by another
C. Abnormal cell development and decrease in cell number and increase in immature cells
D. Distortion of the cell cytoplasm and nucleus

Q89. The QUANTEC recommendation of penile bulb mean dose to reduce erectile dysfunction injury is

A. <40 Gy
B. <50 Gy
C. <55 Gy
D. <60 Gy

Q90. The half-life of iridium-192 is

A. 17 days
B. 60 days
C. 74 days
D. 30 years

Q91. According to the U.S. Preventative Services Task Force meta-analysis, women between 40 and 49 years of age have the following reduction in breast cancer mortality associated with screening mammograms:

A. 0%
B. 5%
C. 10%
D. 15%

Q92. The average energy of a cobalt-60 beam is

A. 1.17 MV
B. 1.25 MV
C. 1.33 MV
D. 4 MV

Q93. An acquired increase in tissue or organ mass after full cellular maturity due to a decrease in cellular components is best known as

A. Aplasia
B. Hyperplasia
C. Atrophy
D. Hypertrophy

Q94. The commonly accepted format for the exchange of medical images is known as

A. PACS
B. National Electrical Manufacturers Association (NEMA)
C. DICOM
D. DICOM-RT

Q95. Radiation exposure is consistent with the following EXCEPT

    A. Directly related to total charge
    B. SI unit is the Roentgen (R)
    C. Inversely related to the mass of air
    D. Defined as one Coulomb unit of charge per cubic meter at STP

Q96. Cancer related to the skeletal muscle tissue of origin is known as

    A. Leiomyosarcoma
    B. Rhabdomyosarcoma
    C. Fibromyosarcoma
    D. Dermatofibrosarcoma

Q97. This class of chemotherapy interferes with microtubule formation:

    A. Alkylating agents
    B. Tomoisomerase inhibitors
    C. Antimetabolites
    D. Alkaloids

Q98. A brachytherapy system that delivers radiation at 20 Gy per hour is classified as

    A. A low-dose rate (LDR) system
    B. A medium-dose rate (MDR) system
    C. A high-dose rate (HDR) system
    D. A pulsed-dose rate system

Q99. Characteristic radiation and Auger electrons are created due to

    A. A collision interaction of an electron with the nucleus
    B. A collision interaction of an electron with another electron
    C. Deflection of an electron due to the nucleus
    D. Deflection of an electron due to another electron

Q100. The QUANTEC radiosurgery optic nerve/chiasm maximum dose parameter leading to less than 10% risk of injury is

    A. <8 Gy
    B. <12 Gy
    C. <16 Gy
    D. <20 Gy

Q101. The standard dose for T3–4 or node positive anal canal cancer, as used in Radiation Therapy Oncology Group (RTOG) 0529, is

    A. 45 Gy in 25 fractions
    B. 50.4 Gy in 28 fractions
    C. 50 Gy in 25 fractions
    D. 54 Gy in 30 fractions

Q102. According to the Radiation Therapy Oncology Group (RTOG) 0920 study, the dose fractionation that should be used for high-risk postoperative head and neck radiation therapy is

    A. 63 Gy in 33 fractions
    B. 60 Gy in 30 fractions
    C. 54 Gy in 30 fractions
    D. 50 Gy in 25 fractions

Q103. The standard dose for T2N0 anal canal cancer, as used in Radiation Therapy Oncology Group (RTOG) 0529, is

A. 45 Gy in 25 fractions
B. 50.4 Gy in 28 fractions
C. 50 Gy in 25 fractions
D. 54 Gy in 30 fractions

Q104. In general, a single large dose of radiation therapy versus the same dose given over multiple fractions will lead to

A. Improved cell killing with similar normal tissue effects
B. Improved cell killing with detrimental normal tissue effects
C. Decreased cell killing with similar normal tissue effects
D. Decreased cell killing with detrimental normal tissue effects

Q105. The QUANTEC recommended volume dose parameter for mesothelioma radiation therapy to ensure minimal fatal toxicities is

A. V5 Gy < 60%
B. V5 Gy < 80%
C. V20 Gy < 20%
D. V20 Gy < 30%

Q106. All of the following cancers have been associated with human papillomavirus (HPV) EXCEPT

A. Oropharyngeal cancer
B. Anal cancer
C. Bladder cancer
D. Cervical cancer

Q107. Volumetric arc therapy differs from traditional arc therapy with the inclusion of the following EXCEPT

A. Variable dose rate
B. Variable gantry rotation speed
C. Variable multileaf collimator (MLC) orientation
D. Variance of the MLC aperture shape

Q108. The number of radioactive decays per second per amount of a radioactive material is known as its

A. Decay constant
B. Mean lifetime
C. Specific activity (SA)
D. Total activity

Q109. The MRI technique assumes which of the following statements?

A. Magnetic poles associated with atomic nuclei prior to MRI imaging are not randomly distributed
B. Only magnetic fields are used to align magnetic poles of the atomic nuclei
C. Radio waves are detected by the MRI to create a medical image
D. All of the above

Q110. Two atoms with the same atomic and mass numbers but different energy states are referred to as

A. Isotopes
B. Isotones
C. Isobars
D. Isomers

Q111. Prophylactic bilateral salpingo-oophorectomy for individuals with a BRCA1/BRCA2 mutation is associated with what reduction in breast cancer risk?

A. 50%
B. 75%
C. 95%
D. 100%

Q112. The prevalence of a disease is dependent on the following EXCEPT

A. The incidence of disease
B. The mortality rate of the disease
C. Survival time with the disease
D. The relative prevalence of associated diseases

Q113. The V20 DVH parameter commonly used for lung cancer assessment is known as a

A. Relative dose DVH parameter
B. Absolute dose DVH parameter
C. Relative volume DVH parameter
D. Absolute volume DVH parameter

Q114. A quadruple-blinded study is consistent with a triple-blinded trial and with blinding of

A. Patients
B. Physicians
C. Endpoint assessors
D. Statisticians

Q115. The commonly accepted format for the exchange of radiation oncology contours associated with medical images is known as

A. PACS
B. NEMA
C. DICOM
D. DICOM-RT

Q116. Knowledge of patient assignment in a clinical trial is known as

A. Assessment bias
B. Ascertainment bias
C. Performance bias
D. Allocation bias

Q117. The sample size for a randomized trial is dependent on the following EXCEPT

A. Alpha error
B. Effect size
C. The endpoint selected
D. The expected variance of the endpoint selected

Q118. The gamma energy of iodine-125 is approximately

A. 3 to 7 kV
B. 13 to 17 kV
C. 23 to 27 kV
D. 27 to 36 kV

Q119. The QUANTEC recommended lung volume DVH parameter to keep injury to less than 20% is

A. V20 Gy < 30% to 35%
B. V20 Gy < 20% to 25%
C. V20 Gy < 40%
D. V20 Gy < 25% to 30%

Q120. Examples of aromatase inhibitors include the following EXCEPT

A. Exemestane
B. Letrozole
C. Anastrozole
D. Raloxifene

Q121. The unit of the alpha–beta ratio is

A. Unitless
B. Gy
C. Gy^{-1}
D. Gy^2

Q122. The use of neoadjuvant treatment is denoted by the TNM prefix

A. n
B. na
C. y
D. z

Q123. Radiation fibrosis after radiation therapy is best categorized as

A. Acute injury
B. Consequential late injury
C. Serial late injury
D. Parallel late injury

Q124. Relative biological effectiveness (RBE) and sensitization enhancement ratio (SER) both

A. Compare survival curves to calculate parameters for the linear quadratic model
B. Compare survival curves in terms of dose to have equivalent cell survival
C. Compare survival curves in terms of cell survival percentage to an equivalent dose
D. Compare survival curves to calculate normal tissue complication probabilities

Q125. A brachytherapy system that delivers radiation at 1 Gy per hour is classified as

A. A low-dose rate (LDR) system
B. A medium-dose rate (MDR) system
C. A high-dose rate (HDR) system
D. A pulsed-dose rate system

Q126. The standard dose for adjuvant gastric cancer, as used in Radiation Therapy Oncology Group (RTOG) 0571, is

A. 45 Gy in 25 fractions
B. 50.4 Gy in 28 fractions
C. 50 Gy in 25 fractions
D. 54 Gy in 30 fractions

Q127. A typical Co-60 source for teletherapy contains approximately the following level of activity:

A. 10Ci
B. 100Ci
C. 1,000Ci
D. 10,000Ci

Q128. The QUANTEC recommended mean heart dose to reduce acute pericarditis to less than 15% is

A. <10 Gy
B. <15 Gy
C. <20 Gy
D. <26 Gy

Q129. The QUANTEC radiosurgery volume parameter to keep radionecrosis to less than 20% is

A. V12 Gy < 5 to 10 mL
B. V12 Gy < 20 mL
C. V18 Gy <5 to 10 mL
D. V18 Gy < 20 mL

Q130. According to the European Randomized Study of Screening for Prostate Cancer, one cancer death is prevented for how many PSA screened individuals between the ages of 55 to 69 years?

A. 50
B. 100
C. 1,000
D. 5,000

Q131. Two atoms with the same atomic number but different mass number are referred to as

A. Isotopes
B. Isotones
C. Isobars
D. Isomers

Q132. Examples of cancer oncogenes include the following EXCEPT

A. ras
B. p53
C. HER2/neu
D. EGFR

Q133. The number of radioactive decays per second of a radioactive material is known as its

A. Decay constant
B. Mean lifetime
C. Specific activity
D. Total activity

Q134. The model of the atom whereby electrons travel around a positive nucleus in discrete "planetary" orbits of defined energy states was known as the

A. Thompson model
B. Rutherford model
C. Bohr model
D. Quantum model

Q135. A full body dose of 5 Gy would lead to a

A. Cerebrovascular syndrome
B. Gastrointestinal syndrome
C. Hematopoeitic syndrome
D. Neurological syndrome

Q136. Which radioisotope has been shown to improve survival in metastatic prostate cancer with bone metastases?

A. Radium-223
B. Radium-226
C. Samarium-153
D. Strontium-89

Q137. Improper assessment of primary or secondary outcomes in a clinical trial is known as

A. Assessment bias
B. Ascertainment bias
C. Performance bias
D. Allocation bias

Q138. The standard dose for high-risk meningioma in Radiation Therapy Oncology Group (RTOG) 0539 is

A. 54 Gy in 30 fractions
B. 59.4 Gy in 33 fractions
C. 60 Gy in 30 fractions
D. 66 Gy in 33 fractions

Q139. In terms of photon attenuation, Compton scattering and pair production have equal importance at the following energy:

A. 4 MV
B. 6 MV
C. 18 MV
D. 24 MV

Q140. According to the U.S. Preventative Services Task Force meta-analysis, women between 60 to 69 years of age have the following reduction in breast cancer mortality associated with screening mammograms:

A. 0%
B. 10%
C. 20%
D. 30%

Q141. The maximum spinal cord dose DVH parameter commonly used for treatment assessment is known as a

A. Relative dose DVH parameter
B. Absolute dose DVH parameter
C. Relative volume DVH parameter
D. Absolute volume DVH parameter

Q142. The frequency range for medical ultrasound is

A. 2 to 18 MHz
B. 2 to 18 kHz
C. 20 to 180 MHz
D. 20 to 180 kHz

Q143. The standard dose for postoperative pancreatic cancer, as used in Radiation Therapy Oncology Group (RTOG) 0848, is

A. 45 Gy in 25 fractions
B. 50.4 Gy in 28 fractions
C. 50 Gy in 25 fractions
D. 54 Gy in 30 fractions

Q144. Examples of cytotoxic antibiotics include the following EXCEPT

A. Mitoxantrone
B. Etoposide
C. Epirubicin
D. Bleomycin

Q145. According to the Durie–Salmon system for multiple myeloma, a patient with a hemoglobin level of 7.5 g/dL and creatinine of 3.0 mg/dL is coded as

A. IIIA
B. IIIB
C. IIA
D. IIB

Q146. The half-life of 18 F used for PET imaging is approximately

A. 110 minutes
B. 60 minutes
C. 40 minutes
D. 33 minutes

Q147. Traditional dose–volume histograms (DVHs) routinely used in clinical care and in clinical trials are otherwise known as

A. A differential DVH
B. An inferential DVH
C. A cumulative absolute DVH
D. A cumulative relative DVH

Q148. Alcohol intake is linked to what percentage of worldwide cancer cases?

A. 1%
B. 2%
C. 5%
D. 10%

Q149. According to the Ann Arbor staging system, a patient with lymph node involvement above and below the diaphragm, with extranodal disease, and with fever and drenching night sweats is coded as

A. IIIBE
B. IIBE
C. III
D. IV

Q150. The standard dose for intermediate-risk meningioma in Radiation Therapy Oncology Group (RTOG) 0539 is

A. 54 Gy in 30 fractions
B. 59.4 Gy in 33 fractions
C. 60 Gy in 30 fractions
D. 66 Gy in 33 fractions

Q151. The QUANTEC recommendation for mean radiation therapy dose to both parotid glands to keep injury to less than 20% is

A. 10 Gy
B. 15 Gy
C. 20 Gy
D. 30 Gy

Q152. According to the American Society for Radiation Oncology (ASTRO) bone metastases guideline, the retreatment rate for 30 Gy in 10 fractions is

A. 4%
B. 8%
C. 20%
D. 40%

Q153. According to the U.S. Preventative Services Task Force, the level of evidence associated with expert opinion alone is known as

A. Level III
B. Level I
C. Level A
D. Level D

Q154. The QUANTEC recommended mean lung dose to keep injury to less than 20% is

A. 10 to 13 Gy
B. 15 to 18 Gy
C. 20 to 23 Gy
D. 27 to 30 Gy

Q155. Biologically equivalent dose (BED) is related to the following EXCEPT

A. Related to the dose per fraction
B. Directly related to total dose
C. Inversely proportional to the alpha–beta ratio
D. Directly related to fraction number

Q156. According to the U.S. Preventative Services Task Force meta-analysis, women between 50 and 59 years of age have the following reduction in breast cancer mortality associated with screening mammograms:

A. 0%
B. 5%
C. 10%
D. 15%

Q157. Successful strategies to improve the therapeutic ratio between tumor control and normal tissue complications include:

A. Altered fractionation
B. Radiation therapy planning and image-guidance
C. Tumor radiosensitization
D. All of the above

Q158. According the ICRU 62, the internal target volume is equivalent to

A. The planning target volume (PTV)
B. The clinical target volume (CTV)
C. The CTV and internal margin (IM)
D. The CTV and set-up margin

Q159. The following treatments are generally considered to be "particle" therapy EXCEPT

    A. Proton

    B. Photon

    C. Neutron

    D. Carbon ion

Q160. The photon–atomic interaction that absorbs and releases a photon of the same energy but with different direction is known as

    A. Coherent scattering

    B. Photoelectric effect

    C. Compton scattering

    D. Photodisintegration

Q161. The standard dose for resectable and unresectable esophageal cancer, as used in Radiation Therapy Oncology Group (RTOG) 1010 and RTOG 0436, is

    A. 45 Gy in 25 fractions

    B. 50.4 Gy in 28 fractions

    C. 50 Gy in 25 fractions

    D. 54 Gy in 30 fractions

Q162. Examples of alkylating agents include the following EXCEPT

    A. Chlorambucil

    B. Cyclophosphamide

    C. Carboplatin

    D. Epirubicin

Q163. In general for all screening maneuvers for colorectal cancers, screening is associated with the following decrease in mortality:

    A. 0%

    B. 15%

    C. 30%

    D. 45%

Q164. The photon–atomic interaction that absorbs a photon and releases a separate photon and electron each with less energy is known as

    A. Coherent scattering

    B. Photoelectric effect

    C. Compton scattering

    D. Photodisintegration

Q165. Ionizing radiation generally has wavelengths of

    A. 10^{-2} m or larger

    B. 10^{-2} m or smaller

    C. 10^{-8} m or larger

    D. 10^{-8} m or smaller

Q166. The computed tomography (CT) Hounsfield unit of cortical bone is approximately

    A. −1,000

    B. 0

    C. +400

    D. +1,000

Q167. A hot spot according to ICRU 50 is defined as

    A. The maximum point dose within the planning target volume (PTV)
    B. The maximum point dose outside the PTV
    C. The dose to a small volume of interest within the PTV
    D. The dose to a small volume of interest outside the PTV

Q168. All of the following are examples of functional imaging EXCEPT

    A. Positron emission tomography
    B. Single-photon emission tomography
    C. Functional MRI
    D. T1 weighted MRI

Q169. Heritable DNA repair syndromes related to the development of lymphoma include the following EXCEPT

    A. Ataxia telangiectasia
    B. Nijmegen breakage syndrome
    C. Xeroderma pigmentosum
    D. Bloom syndrome

Q170. The number of photons within a cross-sectional area in space at an instant in time is known as

    A. Energy fluence
    B. Fluence
    C. Linear attenuation coefficient
    D. Mass attenuation coefficient

Q171. Two atoms with the different atomic numbers and mass numbers but the same number of neutrons are referred to as

    A. Isotopes
    B. Isotones
    C. Isobars
    D. Isomers

Q172. The TNM staging prefix "p" best refers to

    A. Pathology staging prior to treatment within 4 months of diagnosis
    B. Pathological staging prior to treatment within any time from diagnosis
    C. Pathological staging at the time of surgical resection
    D. Pathological staging based on history, physical examination, and investigations except diagnostic scopes and biopsies

Q173. Prophylactic bilateral salpingo-oophorectomy for individuals with a BRCA1/BRCA2 mutation is associated with what reduction in ovarian cancer risk?

    A. 50%
    B. 75%
    C. 95%
    D. 100%

Q174. The sum of energy of all photons within a cross-sectional area in space at an instant in time is known as

    A. Energy fluence
    B. Fluence
    C. Linear attenuation coefficient
    D. Mass attenuation coefficient

Q175. Examples of antimetabolites include the following EXCEPT

A. Chlorambucil
B. Pemetrexed
C. 5-fluorouracil
D. Fludarabine

Q176. Which of the following cancers can usually be treated with low-dose rate (LDR), high-dose rate (HDR), and pulsed-dose rate (PDR) brachytherapy?

A. Prostate cancer
B. Gynecological cancer
C. Lung cancer
D. Breast cancer

Q177. The following statements regarding randomization are correct EXCEPT

A. Stratification can be used to better ensure similar groups for comparison
B. Randomization is performed to ensure that similar groups will always occur
C. If 1:1 randomization is not used, sample size will increase
D. Block randomization can be used for small trials

Q178. Examples of gonadotropin-releasing hormone (GnRH) agonists include the following EXCEPT

A. Degarelix
B. Leuprolide
C. Goserelin
D. Buserelin

Q179. The signal intensity for each voxel in traditional hydrogen-based MRI is

A. Electron density
B. Proton density
C. Hounsfield unit
D. Flow rate

Q180. Hallmarks of apoptosis include the following EXCEPT

A. Lack of inflammation
B. Antigenic release
C. Programmed cell death
D. Cell remnant phagocytosis

Q181. A full body dose of 50 Gy would lead to a

A. Cerebrovascular syndrome
B. Gastrointestinal syndrome
C. Hematopoeitic syndrome
D. Neurological syndrome

Q182. Stereotactic radiosurgery and stereotactic body radiation therapy are generally similar except for the following considerations:

A. Fraction number
B. Treatment location
C. A and B
D. Use of IMRT

Q183. According to the Radiation Therapy Oncology Group (RTOG) 0413/NSABP B-39 study, the following dose fractionation schedule should be used for partial breast irradiation:

A. 40 Gy in 10 fractions BID
B. 38.5 Gy in 10 fractions BID
C. 40 Gy in 10 fractions
D. 38.5 Gy in 10 fractions

Q184. According the TNM staging system for testicular cancer, the S subclassification for a patient with a lactate dehydrogenase (LDH) of 11 times the upper normal limit is

A. S
B. S1
C. S2
D. S3

Q185. Poor dietary intake of fruits and vegetables is associated to what percentage of worldwide cancer cases?

A. 1%
B. 2%
C. 5%
D. 10%

Q186. The half-life and mean lifetime are

A. Directly proportional to each other
B. Quadratically proportional to each other
C. Inversely proportional to each other
D. Not related to each other

Q187. Single-photon emission computed tomography (SPECT) has routine clinical applications in all of the following EXCEPT

A. Thyroid
B. Lung
C. Prostate
D. Glioblastoma

Q188. Nonhealing mucosal injury after radiation therapy is best categorized as

A. Acute injury
B. Consequential late injury
C. Serial late injury
D. Parallel late injury

Q189. Bremsstrahlung radiation is created due to

A. A collision interaction of an electron with the nucleus
B. A collision interaction of an electron with another electron
C. Deflection of an electron due to the nucleus
D. Deflection of an electron due to another electron

Q190. With respect to the invasion to metastasis cascade pathway, the step prior to micrometastatic lesion formation is

A. Extravasation
B. Cell arrest
C. Intravasation
D. Detachment

Q191. Obesity is linked to what percentage of worldwide cancer cases?

    A. 1%

    B. 2%

    C. 5%

    D. 10%

Q192. Postradiation therapy vessel fibrosis and cell necrosis are usually associated with

    A. Small vessel injury

    B. Medium vessel injury

    C. Large vessel injury

    D. Fibrosis

Q193. Radiation spinal cord myelopathy after radiation therapy is best categorized as

    A. Acute injury

    B. Consequential late injury

    C. Serial late injury

    D. Parallel late injury

Q194. Postradiation therapy necrosis is best described as

    A. Detrimental premature cell death

    B. Replacement of one differentiated cell type by another

    C. Abnormal cell development and decrease in cell number and increase in immature cells

    D. Distortion of the cell cytoplasm and nucleus

Q195. The area under a receiver operator curve that is associated with a test that is no better than random chance is

    A. −1

    B. 0

    C. 0.5

    D. 1

Q196. Comparison of two survival curves can be performed by

    A. Cox proportional hazards test

    B. Nonparametric log-rank test

    C. A and B

    D. Neither A nor B

Q197. Systemic therapy for bone metastases can utilize which of the following radionuclides?

    A. Sr-89

    B. Sa-153

    C. Ra-223

    D. All of the above

Q198. According to the American Society for Radiation Oncology (ASTRO) palliative thoracic guideline, a modest improvement in survival and symptom score for good prognosis patients is associated with the following dose fractionation system:

    A. 20 Gy in 5 fractions or higher

    B. 30 Gy in 10 fractions or higher

    C. 39 Gy in 13 fractions or higher

    D. 60 Gy in 30 fractions or higher

Q199. Single-strand breaks are usually corrected by

A. Homologous repair
B. Nonhomologous repair
C. Base excision, repair, and sealing
D. All of the above

Q200. The QUANTEC recommendation to reduce rectal injury to less than 10% to 15% is

A. V75 Gy less than 15%
B. V70 Gy less than 20%
C. V60 Gy less than35%
D. All of the above

Q201. The QUANTEC recommendation liver mean dose to reduce injury to less than 5% in patients with no preexisting liver dysfunction is

A. 30 to 32 Gy
B. 34 to 36 Gy
C. 38 to 40 Gy
D. No recommendation was made

Q202. Alkylating agents alkylate which base of DNA?

A. Guanine
B. Cytosine
C. Adenine
D. Thymine

Q203. The surface dose for a 6-MeV electron beam is approximately

A. 25%
B. 50%
C. 75%
D. 100%

Q204. The beta energy of palladium-103 is

A. 7 kV
B. 14 kV
C. 21 kV
D. 28 kV

Q205. The following are all modes of beta decay EXCEPT

A. Electron capture
B. Beta decay
C. Positron emission
D. Proton emission

Q206. The standard dose for anaplastic glioma in Radiation Therapy Oncology Group (RTOG) 1071 and RTOG 0834 is

A. 50.4 Gy in 28 fractions
B. 59.4 Gy in 33 fractions
C. 60 Gy in 30 fractions
D. 66 Gy in 33 fractions

Q207. The specificity of a test is defined as

A. (True positives) divided by (true positives plus false negatives)
B. (True negatives) divided by (false positives plus true negatives)
C. (True positives) divided by (true and false positives)
D. (True negatives) divided by (true and false negatives)

Q208. The computed tomography (CT) Hounsfield unit (HU) of air is approximately

A. −1,000
B. 0
C. +400
D. +1,000

Q209. Hallmarks of cancer include the following EXCEPT

A. Tissue invasion and metastasis
B. Limitless replication potential
C. Dependency to external growth signals
D. Sustained angiogenesis

Q210. The minimum threshold energy for pair production is

A. 0.511 MeV
B. 0.745 MeV
C. 1.000 MeV
D. 1.022 MeV

Q211. According the ICRU 62, the conformity index for perfect coverage of a planning target volume (PTV) is

A. 0
B. 1
C. 10
D. Infinitely large

Q212. A full body dose of 150 Gy would lead to a

A. Cerebrovascular syndrome
B. Gastrointestinal syndrome
C. Hematopoeitic syndrome
D. Neurological syndrome

Q213. The model of the atom whereby electrons travel around a positive nucleus in "planetary" orbits was known as the

A. Thompson model
B. Rutherford model
C. Bohr model
D. Quantum model

Q214. According to the American Society for Radiation Oncology (ASTRO) bone metastases guideline, the retreatment rate for 8 Gy in 1 fraction is

A. 4%
B. 8%
C. 20%
D. 40%

Q215. All of the following cancers have been associated with Epstein–Barr virus (EBV) EXCEPT

    A. Nasopharyngeal cancer
    B. Burkitt lymphoma
    C. Hodgkin's lymphoma
    D. Hepatocellular carcinoma

Q216. In the context of an x-ray tube, a cathode is

    A. A positive electrode used to attract an electron beam
    B. A positive electrode used to generate and repel an electron beam
    C. A negative electrode used to attract an electron beam
    D. A negative electrode used to generate and repel an electron beam

Q217. The standard dose for glioblastoma in Radiation Therapy Oncology Group (RTOG) 0825 is

    A. 50.4 Gy in 28 fractions
    B. 59.4 Gy in 33 fractions
    C. 60 Gy in 30 fractions
    D. 66 Gy in 33 fractions

Q218. The gamma energy of cesium-137 is

    A. 0.33 MeV
    B. 0.66 MeV
    C. 1.01 MeV
    D. 3.3 MeV

Q219. According the linear quadratic model, the cell survival fraction is related to the following EXCEPT

    A. Dose
    B. Alpha component of the alpha/beta ratio
    C. Beta component of the alpha/beta ratio
    D. Directly to the alpha/beta ratio

Q220. The photon–atomic interaction that absorbs a photon and releases protons or neutrons is known as

    A. Coherent scattering
    B. Photoelectric effect
    C. Compton scattering
    D. Photodisintegration

Q221. The QUANTEC recommendation volume DVH parameter for small bowel (contoured as a peritoneal space) is

    A. V15 Gy < 195 mL
    B. V30 Gy < 195 mL
    C. V45 Gy < 195 mL
    D. V60 Gy < 195 mL

Q222. The SI unit for effective dose is the

    A. Becquerel (Bq)
    B. Sievert (Sv)
    C. Gray (Gy)
    D. Roentgen (R)

Q223. The standard dose for central nervous system (CNS) lymphoma used in Radiation Therapy Oncology Group (RTOG) 1114 is

    A. 30 Gy in 15 fractions
    B. 30 Gy in 10 fractions
    C. 23.4 Gy in 13 fractions
    D. 27 Gy in 15 fractions

Q224. In the context of an x-ray tube, an anode is

    A. A positive electrode used to attract an electron beam
    B. A positive electrode used to generate and repel an electron beam
    C. A negative electrode used to attract an electron beam
    D. A negative electrode used to generate and repel an electron beam

Q225. Examples of antiandrogens include the following EXCEPT

    A. Bicalutamide
    B. Flutamide
    C. Goserelide
    D. Finasteride

Q226. According to the Breslow stage system, a melanoma with depth of 1 mm is categorized as

    A. Stage I
    B. Stage II
    C. Stage III
    D. Stage IV

Q227. The reduction in cervical cancer incidence and mortality likely associated with the introduction of the Pap smear is approximately

    A. 20%
    B. 40%
    C. 60%
    D. 80%

Q228. Transient bone marrow suppression after radiation therapy is best categorized as

    A. Acute injury
    B. Consequential late injury
    C. Serial late injury
    D. Parallel late injury

Q229. The QUANTEC maximum dose to less than 1 mL of brainstem volume leading to less than a 5% risk of injury is

    A. 54 Gy
    B. 57 Gy
    C. 60 Gy
    D. 64 Gy

Q230. The 90% isodose line for a 12-MeV electron beam is approximately at

    A. 1 cm
    B. 2 cm
    C. 3 cm
    D. 4 cm

Q231. Examples of cancer tumor suppressor genes include the following EXCEPT

    A. BRCA-1/2
    B. p53
    C. HER2/neu
    D. RB

Q232. The impact of dose rate on cell survival based on experimental evidence can be best described as

    A. Continuous improvement in cell killing with increasing dose rate
    B. Continuous reduction in cell killing with increasing dose rate
    C. No relationship between cell killing with increasing dose rate
    D. A complex relationship of improvements and reduction of cell killing depending on dose rate and cell redistribution

Q233. The positive predictive value of a test is defined as

    A. (True positives) divided by (true positives plus false negatives)
    B. (True negatives) divided by (false positives plus true negatives)
    C. (True positives) divided by (true and false positives)
    D. (True negatives) divided by (true and false negatives)

Q234. Depth dose distribution profiles depend on the following EXCEPT

    A. Beam energy
    B. Tissue density
    C. Field size and shape
    D. Beam dose rate

Q235. The following statements regarding linear energy transfer (LET) are true EXCEPT

    A. Energy is deposited evenly through the medium
    B. Low LET radiation is sparsely ionizing
    C. LET is defined as the change in kinetic energy per unit length
    D. Is dependent of particle charge and medium density

Q236. The model of the atom whereby electrons were free to travel within an area of positive charge was known as the

    A. Thompson model
    B. Rutherford model
    C. Bohr model
    D. Quantum model

Q237. CT simulation provides the following important information for the treatment-planning process:

    A. Anatomical cancer delineation
    B. Electron densities for treatment planning
    C. External contours for treatment planning
    D. All of the above

Q238. According to the U.S. Preventative Services Task Force, the level of evidence associated with multiple well-conducted randomized controlled trials is known as

    A. Level III
    B. Level I
    C. Level A
    D. Level D

Q239. Properties of electromagnetic radiation include the following EXCEPT

A. Superposition
B. Refraction
C. Dispersion
D. Interposition

Q240. H_2O hydrolysis creates the following free radicals EXCEPT

A. H_3O^+
B. OH^-
C. e^-
D. O_3^-

Q241. The TNM prefix "r" refers to the following concept:

A. Restaging
B. Retreatment
C. Resection margin
D. None of the above

Q242. The following two statistical concepts are directly related to each other:

A. Alpha error and beta error
B. Alpha error and statistical power
C. Alpha error and effect size
D. Beta error and statistical power

Q243. The following are generally considered to be prerequisites for brain stereotactic radiosurgery EXCEPT

A. Cranial immobilization
B. Advanced treatment conformality
C. Image-guided radiation therapy
D. Single fraction delivery

Q244. The following radionuclides can be utilized for brachytherapy EXCEPT

A. I-131
B. Ir-192
C. I-125
D. Pd-103

Q245. The signal intensity for each voxel in computed tomography is

A. Electron density
B. Proton density
C. Hounsfield unit (HU)
D. Flow rate

Q246. Unsafe sexual practices are associated with what percentage of worldwide cancer cases?

A. 1%
B. 2%
C. 3%
D. 5%

Q247. The role of combined chemoradiation has been shown to be important in the following localized cancers EXCEPT

A. Bladder cancer
B. Cervical cancer
C. Intermediate-risk prostate cancer
D. Anal canal cancer

Q248. According to the Radiation Therapy Oncology Group (RTOG) brain metastases recursive partitioning analysis (RPA), a patient with Karnofsky performance scores (KPS) of 70, 70 years of age with no extracranial metastases or active primary, would be classified as

A. Class I
B. Class II
C. Class III
D. There is insufficient information to classify this patient

Q249. For radioresistant tumors, the tumor control curve is where in comparison to a normal tissue complication curve?

A. Overlapping
B. To the right
C. To the left
D. They cross over each other

Q250. Which of the following concepts are NOT considered to be purely an anatomical concept in ICRU 50?

A. Gross tumor volume (GTV)
B. Clinical target volume (CTV)
C. Planning target volume (PTV)
D. Organ at risk

Q251. The dominant forms of DNA damage due to ionizing radiation therapy include the following EXCEPT

A. Base damage
B. Single-strand break (SSB)
C. Double-strand break (DSB)
D. Epigenetic instability

Q252. Tumor response to therapy is usually assessed by

A. The NCI-CTCAE criteria
B. The Response Evaluation Criteria in Solid Tumor (RECIST) criteria
C. The LENT-SOMA criteria
D. None of the above

Q253. A brachytherapy system that delivers radiation at 8 Gy per hour is classified as

A. A low-dose rate (LDR) system
B. A medium-dose rate (MDR) system
C. A high-dose rate (HDR) system
D. A pulsed-dose rate system

Q254. The main difference between a projectional radiograph and fluoroscopy is that

A. Fluoroscopy utilizes a digital cine display
B. Fluoroscopy utilizes different energy of radiation
C. Fluoroscopy can be used only in radiation oncology procedures
D. Fluoroscopy requires contrast procedures as a prerequisite for imaging

Q255. According to the Radiation Therapy Oncology Group (RTOG) 1005 local breast cancer trial, the following dose fractionations are acceptable for the whole breast component of treatment

A. 50 Gy in 25 fractions
B. 42.5 Gy in 16 fractions
C. A and B
D. 40 Gy in 15 fractions

Q256. According to the Radiation Therapy Oncology Group (RTOG) 0618 early stage lung cancer SBRT trial, the following dose fractionation is acceptable

A. 60 Gy in 3 fractions over 1.5 to 2 weeks (with heterogeneity correction)
B. 60 Gy in 3 fractions over 1.5 to 2 weeks (without heterogeneity correction)
C. 54 Gy in 3 fractions over 1 week (with heterogeneity correction)
D. 54 Gy in 3 fractions over 1 week (without heterogeneity correction)

Q257. According to the ICRU 62, the planning organ at risk volume (PRV) is equivalent to

A. The organ at risk (OAR) volume
B. The OAR volume plus internal margin
C. The OAR volume plus set-up margin
D. The OAR volume plus both internal and set-up margins

Q258. All of the following are noncontinuous endpoints EXCEPT

A. Survival
B. Mortality
C. Tumor response
D. Treatment toxicity

Q259. The four R's of radiation therapy:

A. All improve cell death with no impact on cell survival
B. All improve cell survival with no impact on cell death
C. All improve cell survival and cell death
D. Two of them improve cell survival and two improve cell death

Q260. The photon–atomic interaction that absorbs a photon and releases an electron with less energy is known as

A. Coherent scattering
B. Photoelectric effect
C. Compton scattering
D. Photodisintegration

Q261. A linear accelerator-based conebeam CT is otherwise known as a

    A. 2D-kV scan

    B. 2D-MV scan

    C. 3D-kV scan

    D. 3D-MV scan

Q262. The following radionuclides can be utilized for cancer diagnostics EXCEPT

    A. Tc-99 m

    B. F-18

    C. Ga-67

    D. Sa-153

Q263. The radius of an atomic nucleus is approximately

    A. 10^{-2} m

    B. 10^{-5} m

    C. 10^{-10} m

    D. 10^{-14} m

Practice Test 2: Clinical Questions

Practice Questions

Q1. Denys–Drash syndrome (associated with Wilms' tumor) have the following disorders EXCEPT

A. Developmental delay
B. Intersex disorders
C. Renal failure
D. Mesangial sclerosis

Q2. A patient with Hodgkin's lymphoma on both sides of the diaphragm, splenic involvement, and unexplained fevers greater than 38°C is best staged as

A. IIIES
B. IIIBS
C. IVBS
D. IIBS

Q3. The most common histological subtype of kidney cancer is

A. Chromophilic
B. Chromophobic
C. Collecting duct
D. Clear cell

Q4. The NSABP B32 was a clinical trial assessing

A. Chemotherapy
B. Hormonal therapy
C. Sentinel node biopsy and node dissection
D. Radiation therapy

Q5. Retroperitoneal sarcomas make up what percentage of all soft tissue sarcomas?

A. 1%
B. 5%
C. 15%
D. 25%

Q6. The risk of pelvic lymph node involvement with inguinal node positivity in the context of vulvar cancer is

A. 10%
B. 15%
C. 20%
D. 30%

Q7. A breast cancer patient with metastases in ipsilateral internal mammary nodes and level 1/2 axillary nodes is best N staged as

    A. N3

    B. N3a

    C. N3b

    D. N3c

Q8. The most frequent mutation in non-squamous lung cancer is

    A. KRAS

    B. EGFR

    C. FGFR1

    D. EML4-ALK

Q9. The most frequent cause of pancreatic cancer is

    A. Smoking

    B. Diet

    C. Hereditary

    D. Sporadic

Q10. Lung cancer patients with T4N2 and T1N3 diseases are considered to be best described as having

    A. Stage III disease

    B. Stage IIIA disease

    C. Stage IIIB disease

    D. Stage IVA disease

Q11. The following percentage of clinically node negative penile cancer will have positive nodes at surgery:

    A. 20%

    B. 40%

    C. 60%

    D. 80%

Q12. Metastatic disease at the diagnosis of pediatric neuroblastoma is confirmed in what percentage of patients?

    A. 5%

    B. 20%

    C. 50%

    D. 70%

Q13. Pediatric endocrinopathies occur more commonly when doses to the pituitary/hypothalamus exceed this level:

    A. 10–15 Gy

    B. 20–25 Gy

    C. 30–35 Gy

    D. 40–45 Gy

Q14. All of the following are contraindications for brachytherapy in extremity soft tissue sarcoma (STS) EXCEPT

    A. Positive margin

    B. Skin involvement

    C. Inadequate CTV coverage

    D. Primary tumor size

Q15. The following are all subtypes of cutaneous B-cell lymphomas EXCEPT

    A. Follicle center
    B. Large cell
    C. Plasmablastic
    D. Marginal zone

Q16. All of the following are hallmarks of high-risk prostate cancer EXCEPT

    A. PSA >20 ng/mL
    B. T1 with PSA >10 ng/ml
    C. T3/T4 disease
    D. Gleason score ≥8

Q17. The 5-year disease-free survival rate with resection and radiation therapy for osteosarcoma is approximately

    A. 70%
    B. 50%
    C. 40%
    D. 25%

Q18. Invasion/encasement of the following structures are all considered to be absolute contraindications to pancreatic surgery EXCEPT

    A. >50% superior mesenteric artery
    B. Portal vein
    C. >50% celiac artery
    D. >50% hepatic artery

Q19. The WAGR syndrome is associated with the following lifetime risk of the development of Wilms' tumor:

    A. 10%
    B. 30%
    C. 50%
    D. 70%

Q20. Hepatocellular carcinoma is ranked as which following leading cause of cancer death worldwide?

    A. 3rd
    B. 5th
    C. 7th
    D. 9th

Q21. Three randomized trials in postprostatectomy radiation have consistently demonstrated

    A. Survival benefit
    B. Metastases free survival benefit
    C. Biochemical control/disease specific control benefits
    D. No benefits

Q22. The clinical complete response rate after 45 Gy of chemoradiation in a bladder preservation approach is approximately

    A. 45%
    B. 55%
    C. 70%
    D. 90%

Q23. All of the following are considered potential indications for postoperative prostate radiation therapy EXCEPT

A. Perineural invasion
B. Extracapsular extension (T3a)
C. Seminal vesicle invasion (T3b)
D. Positive margin

Q24. The risk of nodal metastases from basal cell carcinoma of the skin is approximately

A. 1/100
B. 1/1,000
C. 1/10,000
D. 1/1,000,000

Q25. The NSABP B17 DCIS trial assessing lumpectomy alone versus lumpectomy with radiation demonstrated an absolute reduction of 15-year in-breast recurrence of

A. 15%
B. 25%
C. 35%
D. 5%

Q26. What percentage of all anterior mediastinal masses are thymomas?

A. 30%
B. 40%
C. 50%
D. 60%

Q27. The most common subtype of astrocytomas are

A. Fibrillary
B. Genistocytic
C. Genistoblastic
D. Protoplasmic

Q28. The local control of limb-sparing surgery with adjuvant radiation therapy is approximately

A. 40%
B. 60%
C. 75%
D. 90%

Q29. The 5-year overall survival rate with resection and radiation therapy for osteosarcoma is approximately

A. 70%
B. 50%
C. 40%
D. 25%

Q30. The expected 5-year survival rate of Stage III esophageal cancer is

A. 15%
B. 30%
C. 40%
D. 80%

Q31. The majority of vulvar cancer arise from the

    A. Labia majora/minora
    B. Clitoris
    C. Perineum
    D. Bartholin's gland

Q32. The lymphedema risk after sentinel lymph node biopsy (SNLB) alone is

    A. 0%
    B. 5%
    C. 10%
    D. 20%

Q33. The following subtype of meningioma is considered to be a Grade II tumor:

    A. Clear cell
    B. Rhabdoid
    C. Papillary
    D. Anaplastic

Q34. Lifetime risk of developing a colon cancer in the United States is estimated at

    A. 3%
    B. 6%
    C. 9%
    D. 12%

Q35. Common risk factors for the development of hepatocellular are the following EXCEPT

    A. Alcoholic cirrhosis
    B. Hepatitis A
    C. Hepatitis B
    D. Hepatitis C

Q36. An 0.5-cm anaplastic thyroid cancer that is confined to the thyroid gland without extracapsular extension is T staged as

    A. T1
    B. T1a
    C. T1b
    D. T4

Q37. Osseous involvement of a primary orbital cancer is T staged as

    A. T4a
    B. T4b
    C. T4c
    D. T4d

Q38. Which of the following histologies is least likely to seed the cerebrospinal fluid (CSF) in pediatric malignancies?

    A. Astrocytomas
    B. Embryonal tumors
    C. Germ cell tumors
    D. Ependymal tumors

Q39. All of the following are factors associated with the graded prognostic assessment EXCEPT

    A. Performance status
    B. Number of mets
    C. Control of primary disease
    D. Age

Q40. Mesotheliomas generally express the following markers EXCEPT

    A. TTF-1
    B. WT-1
    C. D2-40
    D. Calretinin

Q41. Screening with low-dose CT for lung cancer is best targeted to the following patient criteria EXCEPT

    A. Current/former smokers
    B. Age 55–80 years
    C. >30 pack years smoking
    D. Presence of COPD

Q42. The use of higher doses of radiation therapy (range of 45–55 Gy) in the context of diffuse large B-cell lymphoma is usually reserved for

    A. Consolidation RT
    B. Complimentary RT
    C. Primary RT prior to chemotherapy
    D. Primary RT for refractory postchemotherapy patients

Q43. A typical dose fractionation schedule used for partial breast external beam irradiation is

    A. 38.5 Gy in 10 fractions BID
    B. 34 Gy in 10 fractions
    C. 30 Gy in 10 fractions
    D. 36 Gy in 24 fractions TID

Q44. The pathological complete response rate with the use of neoadjuvant docetaxel and AC chemotherapy in locally advanced breast cancer is approximately

    A. 15%
    B. 25%
    C. 35%
    D. 45%

Q45. Five-year survival rate for Stage III vulvar cancer is approximately

    A. 90%
    B. 75%
    C. 50%
    D. 20%

Q46. All of the following are known toxicities of temozolomide EXCEPT

    A. Infertility
    B. Pancytopenia
    C. Diarrhea
    D. Nausea and vomiting

Q47. Retroperitoneal sarcoma grade is based on all of the following EXCEPT

A. Abnormal cell density
B. Differentiation
C. Mitotic rate
D. Necrosis

Q48. Acoustic neuromas are associated with which cranial nerve?

A. VI
B. VII
C. VIII
D. IX

Q49. The following subtype of mesothelioma has the best outcomes:

A. Epitheloid
B. Sarcomatoid
C. Biphasic
D. Mixed

Q50. Which World Health Organization (WHO) class of nasopharyngeal cancer is least frequently diagnosed?

A. Type 1
B. Type 2a
C. Type 2b
D. Type 3

Q51. All of the following factors are common between the non-Hodgkin's lymphoma International Prognostic Index (IPI) and follicular lymphoma IPI EXCEPT

A. Performance status
B. Age
C. Tumor stage
D. LDH level

Q52. All of the following syndromes are associated with the development of kidney cancer EXCEPT

A. Von Hippel–Lindau disease
B. Dirt–Hogg–Dubé syndrome
C. Tuberous sclerosis
D. Lynch syndrome

Q53. In a case of adult ependymoma with evidence of metastases in the CNS neuraxis, craniospinal RT should be given with the following dose:

A. 25 Gy
B. 30 Gy
C. 36 Gy
D. 45 Gy

Q54. A typical dose fractionation schedule used for pediatric HIGH grade astrocytoma is

A. 45 Gy in 25 fractions
B. 50.4 Gy in 28 fractions
C. 59.4 Gy in 33 fractions
D. 66 Gy in 33 fractions

Q55. A cutaneous palpable 1.5 cm tumor of cutaneous lymphoma is T staged as

A. T1
B. T2
C. T3
D. T4

Q56. The median survival for all pancreatic cancer patients is

A. 2–3 months
B. 4–6 months
C. 8–10 months
D. 10–12 months

Q57. A 2-year-old Stage IV patient with N-myc nonamplified neuroblastoma would be considered to have this risk stratification assignment:

A. Low
B. Intermediate
C. High
D. Cannot determine risk stratification based on the available information

Q58. The following hereditary syndromes are associated with gallbladder cancer EXCEPT

A. Gardner syndrome
B. Hereditary nonpolyposis colon cancer
C. Lynch syndrome
D. Neurofibromatosis type I

Q59. Myasthesia gravis is seen in what percentage of thymoma patients?

A. 5%
B. 15%
C. 40%
D. 65%

Q60. All of the following are important factors for local control of Ewing's sarcoma EXCEPT

A. Tumor grade
B. Primary tumor volume
C. Response post chemotherapy
D. Tumor diameter

Q61. Risk factors of the development of squamous cell cervix cancer include the following EXCEPT

A. Prenatal exposure to DES
B. HPV infection
C. Immunosuppression
D. Early first intercourse

Q62. The current rate of clinically significant radiation pneumonitis associated with radical radiation planning is on the order of

A. Rare <1%
B. Uncommon <5%
C. Common 15%
D. Unknown

Q63. Various studies have shown that doses above the following have been associated with improved local control:

  A. 45 Gy
  B. 50.4 Gy
  C. 55.8 Gy
  D. 59 Gy

Q64. The lifetime risk of developing ovarian cancer with BRCA1 syndrome is

  A. 5%–10%
  B. 15%–25%
  C. 35%–45%
  D. 55%–60%

Q65. According to the American Society for Radiation Oncology (ASTRO) bone mets guideline, the retreatment rate of single fraction radiation therapy is

  A. 4%
  B. 8%
  C. 15%
  D. 20%

Q66. Which of the following prostate brachytherapy isotopes have the longest half-life?

  A. 103-Pd
  B. 125-I
  C. 192-Ir
  D. 128-I

Q67. The following are relative contraindications to prostate brachytherapy EXCEPT

  A. AUA score >5
  B. Seminal vesicle invasion
  C. Gland size >60 mL
  D. Pubic arch interference

Q68. In terms of site-specific graded prognostic assessment for brain metastases, gastrointestinal (GI) tumors have how many factors making the index?

  A. 1
  B. 2
  C. 3
  D. 4

Q69. Local control of radiation versus surgery for the definitive treatment of Ewing's sarcoma is

  A. Radiation is superior
  B. Radiation and surgery are equivalent
  C. Surgery is superior
  D. Radiation and surgery can both be superior depending on patient selection

Q70. In the definitive radiation (or chemoradiation) treatment of cervix cancer, adequate radiation dose at point A is considered to be

  A. 65 Gy
  B. 75 Gy
  C. 85 Gy
  D. 95 Gy

Q71. The expected 5-year survival outcome with a Stage IVA cervix cancer is

A. 40%
B. 30%
C. 20%
D. 10%

Q72. The NSABP B24 DCIS trial assessing 5 years of Tamoxifen with surgery/radiation demonstrated what absolute reduction in ipsilateral breast recurrence?

A. No reduction
B. 2%–3%
C. 5%–10%
D. 15%–20%

Q73. Which of the following is common to typical cases of both classical and nodular lymphocyte predominant Hodgkin's lymphoma?

A. CD15+
B. CD30+
C. CD20–
D. CD3–

Q74. Stage I–IIB non-bulky Hodgkin's disease is usually treated with the following radiation dose:

A. 20 Gy
B. 30 Gy
C. 36 Gy
D. 40 Gy

Q75. An en-bloc resection of involved pleura, lung, ipsilateral diaphragm, and pericardium in mesothelioma is called

A. Pleurectomy/decortication
B. Extrapleural pneumonectomy
C. Radical pneumonectomy
D. Extended pneumonectomy

Q76. The most frequent form of cutaneous lymphoma is

A. Mycosis fungoides
B. Sezary syndrome
C. Cutaneous B-cell lymphoma
D. Natural killer cutaneous lymphoma

Q77. The most common paraneoplastic syndrome associated with small cell lung cancer is

A. Cushing's syndrome
B. Eaton-Lambert
C. Cerebellar degeneration
D. Syndrome of Inappropriate Anti-diuretic Hormone production (SIADH)

Q78. All of the following tumors are associated with the development of hemorrhagic brain metastases EXCEPT

A. Lung
B. Renal
C. Melanoma
D. Choriocarcinoma

Q79. A pediatric anaplastic oligodendroglioma cancer is graded as

   A. Grade I
   B. Grade II
   C. Grade III
   D. Grade IV

Q80. Multiagent chemotherapy for osteosarcoma utilizes all the following drugs EXCEPT

   A. Cisplatin
   B. Methotrexate
   C. Doxorubicin
   D. Gemcitabine

Q81. Which of the following is the least frequently diagnosed endometrial cancer histology?

   A. Papillary serous
   B. Sarcoma
   C. Clear cell
   D. Adenocarcinoma

Q82. A MALT lymphoma is

   A. Indolent B-cell lymphoma
   B. Aggressive B-cell lymphoma
   C. Indolent T-cell lymphoma
   D. Aggressive T-cell lymphoma

Q83. The NSABP B18 trial assessed

   A. Chemotherapy dosage
   B. Number of chemotherapy cycles
   C. Sequencing of chemotherapy with surgery
   D. Various chemotherapy regimens

Q84. The typical dose for gross disease for a thymoma is approximately

   A. 40 Gy
   B. 50 Gy
   C. 60 Gy
   D. 70 Gy

Q85. The age distribution related with Hodgkin's lymphoma is best described as

   A. Increasing with age
   B. Decreasing with age
   C. Bimodal age distribution
   D. Normal age distribution

Q86. All of the following are manifestations of Cushing's disease EXCEPT

   A. Central obesity
   B. Heat intolerance
   C. Hypertension
   D. Diabetes

Q87. The following has been shown to statistically significantly improve survival in high-risk prostate cancer treated with radiation therapy:

A. Androgen therapy
B. Brachytherapy
C. Chemotherapy
D. Pelvic nodal irradiation

Q88. Relative contraindications for bladder preservation include the following EXCEPT

A. Multifocal disease
B. In situ disease
C. Hydronephrosis
D. T2 disease

Q89. Bulky Hodgkin's lymphoma is usually described as tumors that are larger than

A. 5 cm
B. 10 cm
C. 15 cm
D. 20 cm

Q90. The most frequent primary head and neck cancer site in the context of a level 5 node is

A. Nasopharynx
B. Thyroid
C. Oropharynx
D. Oral cavity

Q91. The expected 5-year survival rate of Stage III vaginal cancer is

A. 50%
B. 40%
C. 30%
D. 20%

Q92. The expected 5-year survival outcome with a stage IIA cervix cancer is

A. 70%
B. 60%
C. 50%
D. 40%

Q93. The use of D2 surgical resections in gastric cancer has

A. Been shown to be potentially associated with overall survival benefits in all patient populations
B. Been shown to be potentially associated with overall survival benefits in T1–T2 tumors
C. Been shown to be potentially associated with overall survival benefits in T3 tumors
D. Been shown to be potentially associated with overall survival benefits in N positive tumors

Q94. A typical dose fractionation range for plasmacytoma in terms of primary (non-palliative) treatment is

A. 20–26 Gy
B. 30–36Gy
C. 45–50Gy
D. 60–66 Gy

Q95. In terms of colorectal cancer, tumors that invade into but not through the muscularis propria are considered what T stage?

A. T1
B. T2
C. T3
D. T4

Q96. The most common anatomical subtype of hypopharynx cancer is

A. Pyriform sinus
B. Posterior pharyngeal wall
C. Lateral pharyngeal wall
D. Postcricoid

Q97. High-risk features in terms of the GOG99 endometrial cancer trial include all of the following EXCEPT

A. Grade
B. Age >60 years
C. Lymphovascular invasion
D. Outer 1/3 myometrial invasion

Q98. Acceptable dose fractionation schedules for thoracic treatment for limited small cell lung cancer include the following EXCEPT

A. 45 Gy in 30 fractions BID
B. 45 Gy in 25 fractions
C. 60 Gy in 30 fractions
D. 45 Gy in 15 fractions

Q99. An osteosarcoma patient that has 75% tumor necrosis with chemotherapy has what overall grade of response?

A. Grade I
B. Grade II
C. Grade III
D. Grade IV

Q100. All of the following are important prognostic factors for Ewing's sarcoma EXCEPT

A. Age
B. Grade
C. Site of metastases
D. Primary local control

Q101. The 5-year distant metastases rate with resection and radiation therapy for osteosarcoma is approximately

A. 70%
B. 50%
C. 40%
D. 25%

Q102. The addition of pemetrexed to cisplatin for mesothelioma has been shown to improve median survival by

A. Less than 1 month
B. 3 months
C. 6 months
D. 12 months

Q103. A low-risk oropharynx cancer will have what 3-year overall survival rate according to RTOG 0129?

  A. 50%
  B. 60%
  C. 80%
  D. 95%

Q104. In the context of intermediate-risk prostate cancer treated with nondose escalated radiation therapy the use of short-term androgen therapy has been associated with

  A. No improvement in biochemical control or survival
  B. Improvement in biochemical control only
  C. Improvement in survival only
  D. Improvement in biochemical control and survival

Q105. A T1N1 oral cavity cancer is overall stage

  A. II
  B. III
  C. IVa
  D. IVb

Q106. A patient with a single extralymphatic presentation of non-Hodgkin's lymphoma is best staged as

  A. Stage I
  B. Stage IE
  C. Stage IV
  D. Stage IVE

Q107. The most favorable histology of gallbladder cancer is

  A. Small cell
  B. Sclerosing
  C. Sodular
  D. Papillary

Q108. The usual dose of temozolomide used adjuvantly after RT for glioblastoma multiforme is

  A. 50 g/m^2
  B. 75 g/m^2
  C. 100 g/m^2
  D. 150 g/m^2

Q109. The 5-year overall survival rate for localized Ewing's sarcoma is

  A. 70%
  B. 50%
  C. 30%
  D. 10%

Q110. Which of the following is NOT associated with neurofibromatosis in childhood CNS tumors?

  A. Tumors are more indolent
  B. Increased RT complications
  C. Increased tumor response
  D. Increased second malignancies

Q111. The following are B symptoms EXCEPT

    A. Unexplained fatigue
    B. Unexplained loss of more than 10% of body weight in the 6 months before diagnosis
    C. Unexplained fever with temperatures above 38°C
    D. Drenching night sweats

Q112. What percentage of patients with skin melanomas present with localized disease?

    A. 50%
    B. 85%
    C. 95%
    D. 99%

Q113. Spinal cord compression leading to complete paralysis is classified as a Frankel grade

    A. A
    B. B
    C. C
    D. D

Q114. The difference in median survival for anaplastic oligodendroglioma/oligoastrocytoma in terms of 1p/19q deletion status is

    A. 1 month
    B. 1 year
    C. 2 years
    D. 10 years

Q115. What proportion of acoustic neuroma patients have a normal audiometry test?

    A. 0%
    B. 5%
    C. 15%
    D. 50%

Q116. Nonseminomas are associated with the following histologies EXCEPT

    A. Embroyal
    B. Choriocarcinoma
    C. Sertoli cell
    D. Teratoma

Q117. The risk of metastatic disease at diagnosis of Ewing's sarcoma is

    A. 5%
    B. 25%
    C. 50%
    D. 75%

Q118. Regional nodal irradiation for breast cancer is generally indicated for

    A. Any node positivity
    B. 2 or more nodes
    C. 2 or more nodes with extracapsular extension
    D. 4 or more nodes

Q119. The usual dose of temozolomide used concomitantly with radiation therapy (RT) for glioblastoma multiforme is

A. 50 g/m^2
B. 75 g/m^2
C. 100 g/m^2
D. 150 g/m^2

Q120. A typical total dose range for a Grade II astrocytoma is typically considered to be

A. 40–45 Gy
B. 45–50 Gy
C. 50–54 Gy
D. 55–60 Gy

Q121. The risk of positive lymph nodes in early-stage hypopharynx cancer is

A. 20%
B. 40%
C. 60%
D. 80%

Q122. The outermost layer of the stomach wall is called the

A. Submucosa
B. Serosa
C. Subserosa
D. Muscularis

Q123. Which of the following presenting symptoms are considered to be a favorable prognostic factor?

A. Headache
B. Seizure
C. Nausea
D. Altered mental status

Q124. For children over the age of 10 years, the progression-free survival rate to be expected after a course of radiation therapy is in the order of

A. 20%–30%
B. 40%–50%
C. 70%–80%
D. over 90%

Q125. The absolute benefit in survival (at 3 years) with the use of prophylactic cranial irradiation in limited stage small cell lung cancer is

A. 5%
B. 20%
C. 30%
D. 50%

Q126. The lifetime risk of developing ovarian cancer with BRCA2 syndrome is

A. 5–10%
B. 15–25%
C. 35–45%
D. 55–60%

Q127. The international prognostic index for non-Hodgkin's lymphoma consists of the following EXCEPT

   A. Age
   B. Tumor stage
   C. Number of nodal sites
   D. LDH level

Q128. What proportion of ependymoma occur in the brain?

   A. 5%
   B. 15%
   C. 25%
   D. 35%

Q129. The median survival of glioblastoma multiforme treated with chemoradiation is estimated at

   A. 6 months
   B. 9 months
   C. 12 months
   D. 15 months

Q130. A typical dose fractionation schedule used for partial breast intracavitary irradiation is

   A. 34 Gy in 10 fractions BID
   B. 34 Gy in 10 fractions
   C. 30 Gy in 10 fractions
   D. 36 Gy in 24 fractions TID

Q131. Paraneoplastic syndromes associated with kidney cancer usually have the following findings EXCEPT

   A. Elevated calcium
   B. Elevated white count
   C. Hypertension
   D. Transaminitis

Q132. The 5-year local control with resection and radiation therapy for osteosarcoma is approximately

   A. 70%
   B. 50%
   C. 40%
   D. 25%

Q133. In terms of vulvar cancer, the risk of primary recurrence is increased by the following EXCEPT

   A. Margin status
   B. Tumor size
   C. Grade
   D. Depth of invasion >1 mm

Q134. A high-risk international prognostic index non-Hodgkin's lymphoma patient has an estimated 5-year survival rate of

   A. 50%
   B. 40%
   C. 25%
   D. 5%

Q135. According to the Canadian breast hypofractionation study, 10-year local recurrence for both the standard and hypofractionated arms was approximately

A. 2%

B. 6%

C. 13%

D. 20%

Q136. Radiation dose for neuroblastoma gross residual disease is usually on the order of

A. 10 Gy

B. 15 Gy

C. 20 Gy

D. 35 Gy

Q137. A low-risk international prognostic index non-Hodgkin's lymphoma patient has an estimated 5-year survival rate of

A. 50%

B. 60%

C. 75%

D. 85%

Q138. In the United States, lung cancer is ranked as the following in terms of cancer mortality:

A. First

B. Second

C. Third

D. Fourth

Q139. In which trimesters can chemotherapy be delivered for breast cancer during pregnancy?

A. First

B. Second

C. Third

D. Any trimester

Q140. An unresectable Wilms' tumor is considered to be what stage?

A. I

B. II

C. III

D. IV

Q141. A breast cancer patient with T1N2 disease is best overall Stage grouped as

A. IIB

B. IIIA

C. IIIB

D. IIIC

Q142. In a randomized controlled trial, the use of long-term androgen deprivation in pathologically staged node positive prostate cancer is associated with

A. A 5-year improvement in overall survival (OS)

B. A 2-year improvement in OS

C. A 1-year improvement in OS

D. No improvement in OS

Q143. All of the following factors correlate with risk of nodal metastases with skin melanoma EXCEPT

    A. Anatomical site

    B. Breslow thickness

    C. Mitotic rate

    D. Ulceration

Q144. In standard fractionation radiation therapy for whole breast treatment, an ipsilateral lung should be kept to the following dose-volume constraint:

    A. Ipsilateral lung: V20 ≤1%

    B. Ipsilateral lung: V20 ≤15%

    C. Ipsilateral lung: V20 ≤10%

    D. Ipsilateral lung: V20 ≤20%

Q145. The sensitivity of positron emission tomography (PET) staging for mediastinal nodes is approximately

    A. 80%

    B. 85%

    C. 90%

    D. 95%

Q146. A prostate cancer with seminal vesicle involvement is T staged as

    A. T2c

    B. T3a

    C. T3b

    D. T4

Q147. What percentage of supraglottic cancers are node positive?

    A. 25%

    B. 35%

    C. 45%

    D. 55%

Q148. Postoperative rhabdomyosarcoma (RMS) with positive margins is considered to be what Stage grouping?

    A. IIA

    B. IIB

    C. IIC

    D. IID

Q149. What is the long-term local control acoustic neuroma treated with surgery or radiation?

    A. 80%

    B. 85%

    C. 90%

    D. 95%

Q150. Neuroendocrine markers for small cell cancer include the following EXCEPT

    A. Synaptophysin

    B. Chromogranin

    C. CD56

    D. AE1/AE3

Q151. The most common histological subtype of non-small cell lung cancer is

A. Squamous cell carcinoma
B. Large cell carcinoma
C. Adenocarcinoma
D. Carcinoid

Q152. The difference in median survival for chemoradiation of glioblastoma multiforme in MGMT methylated versus non-methylated cases is approximately

A. No difference
B. 2 months
C. 6 months
D. 10 months

Q153. A luminal-A breast cancer is defined as

A. ER/PR + Her2neu–
B. ER/PR + Her2neu+
C. ER/PR – Her2 neu– (triple negative)
D. ER/PR – Her2 neu+

Q154. In terms of the stereotactic treatment of early-stage non-small cell lung cancer, the best local control results have been demonstrated with a biologically equivalent dose greater than

A. 60 Gy
B. 80 Gy
C. 100 Gy
D. 120 Gy

Q155. The most common salivary gland cancers are

A. Parotid
B. Submandibular
C. Sublingual
D. Minor salivary

Q156. The majority of ocular melanomas arise from

A. Iris
B. Ciliary body
C. Choroid
D. Intraocular

Q157. The 5-year survival rate with 64 Gy with no chemotherapy as reported by the RTOG 85-01 study (Herskovic et al.) is

A. 0%
B. 5%
C. 10%
D. 15%

Q158. The MAGIC protocol assessing perioperative chemotherapy that included distal esophageal adenocarcinoma demonstrated a median survival improvement of what magnitude?

A. No difference in median survival
B. 4 months but not statistically significant
C. 4 months and statistically significant
D. 7 months and statistically significant

Q159. The NSABP B21 trial assessed the following types of breast treatment:

A. Hormonal therapy
B. Radiation therapy
C. Both A and B
D. Surgery

Q160. The maximum heart dose for a regional breast irradiation technique should be limited to the following:

A. V25 <5%
B. V25 <10%
C. V25 <15%
D. V25 <25%

Q161. A T4N1M0 kidney cancer is staged as

A. Stage I
B. Stage II
C. Stage III
D. Stage IV

Q162. The presence of level 6 nodes is consistent with the following primary head and neck sites EXCEPT

A. Anterior cervical skin
B. Larynx
C. Esophagus
D. Thyroid

Q163. Positive ipsilateral nodes in the setting of pediatric neuroblastoma is what stage?

A. 2A
B. 2B
C. 2C
D. 3

Q164. Risk factors for the development of squamous cell vaginal cancer includes the following EXCEPT

A. Smoker
B. Immunosuppression
C. In utero exposure to DES
D. Early age first intercourse

Q165. Overall 5-year survival rate for retroperitoneal sarcoma is approximately

A. 10%
B. 25%
C. 50%
D. 75%

Q166. The majority of cholangiocarcinomas are

A. Adenocarcinomas
B. Squamous cell carcinomas
C. Mixed tumors
D. Small cell carcinomas

Q167. All of the following are risk factors associated with spread of squamous cell carcinoma of the skin EXCEPT

    A. Lesion size

    B. Lymphovascular invasion

    C. Grade

    D. Anatomic site

Q168. The overall 5-year survival rate for multiple myeloma according to Surveillance, Epidemiology and End Results (SEER) data is

    A. 15%

    B. 35%

    C. 55%

    D. 75%

Q169. The most common M-protein involved with multiple myeloma is

    A. IgG

    B. IgM

    C. IgA

    D. IgD

Q170. Bilateral Wilms' tumor confined to the kidney is classified as

    A. Bilateral stage I disease

    B. Stage III

    C. Stage IV

    D. Stage V

Q171. The NSABP B14 trial assessed

    A. Hormonal therapy

    B. Radiation therapy

    C. Chemotherapy

    D. Surgery

Q172. The expected 5-year survival rate after complete pathological response following neoadjuvant chemoradiation for esophageal cancer is approximately

    A. 20%

    B. 50%

    C. 70%

    D. 90%

Q173. Which of the following head and neck primary tumor sites have the highest predilection to retropharngeal and level 5 lymph node spread?

    A. Nasopharynx

    B. Oropharynx

    C. Parotid

    D. Hypopharynx

Q174. All the following are high-risk features for cervix cancer risk stratification EXCEPT

    A. Parametrial involvement

    B. Lymph node positivity

    C. Histology

    D. Lymphovascular invasion

Q175. Progression-free survival for pediatric craniopharyngioma treated with radiation therapy should be on the order of

    A. 20%

    B. 50%

    C. 70%

    D. 90%

Q176. A vulvar cancer with upper urethral involvement is staged as

    A. II

    B. III

    C. IVA

    D. IVB

Q177. A typical craniocaudal CTV margin (on GTV) for extremity soft tissue sarcoma (STS) is on the order of

    A. 1 cm

    B. 2 cm

    C. 3 cm

    D. 4 cm

Q178. An axillary node in the setting of gastric cancer is otherwise known as a

    A. Sister Mary Joseph nodule

    B. Virchow node

    C. Irish node

    D. Kruckenberg tumor

Q179. The following are prognostic for poor survival for anal cancer EXCEPT

    A. Tumor size greater than 5 cm

    B. Node positive

    C. Female sex

    D. Tumor site

Q180. Invasion of the cricoid cartilage in terms of hypopharynx cancer is T staged as

    A. T3

    B. T4

    C. T4a

    D. T4b

Q181. The majority of nasal cavity/sinus cancers arise from which anatomical subtype

    A. Maxillary sinus

    B. Ethmoid sinus

    C. Nasal cavity

    D. Sphenoid sinus

Q182. Expected 5-year survival rate for Stage IIIA endometrial cancer is approximately

    A. 90%

    B. 80%

    C. 70%

    D. 60%

Q183. The least common M-protein involved with multiple myeloma is

A. IgG
B. IgM
C. IgA
D. IgD

Q184. All of the following are common sites of origin for neuroblastoma EXCEPT

A. Adrenal medulla
B. Cauda equina
C. Posterior mediastinum
D. Paraspinal ganglia

Q185. A mesothelioma with direct invasion into the spine is T staged as

A. T3
B. T3a
C. T3s
D. T4

Q186. The risk of vaginal stenosis/fibrosis postradiation therapy (RT) for vaginal cancer is estimated at

A. 5%
B. 15%
C. 50%
D. nearly 100%

Q187. The risk of second malignancies after radiation therapy for Ewing's sarcoma (within 20 years) is

A. 1%
B. 10%
C. 20%
D. 30%

Q188. The lymphedema risk after regional post mastectomy radiation therapy after a sentinel lymph node biopsy (SNLB) is

A. 0%
B. 5%
C. 10%
D. 20%

Q189. Preoperative radiation therapy (RT) is favored over postoperative RT for retroperitoneal sarcoma for the following reasons EXCEPT

A. Randomized phase III evidence
B. Better tumor definition
C. Critical structure displacement
D. Less tumor seeding

Q190. The half-life of bHCG is

A. 1 day
B. 5 days
C. 14 days
D. 28 days

Q191. The categorization between macro- and micro-adenomas is based on which size cutoff?

    A. 1 mm

    B. 5 mm

    C. 10 mm

    D. 20 mm

Q192. A PSA bounce associated with prostate brachytherapy can occur in this percentage of cases:

    A. Rarely happens

    B. 5%

    C. 15%

    D. 35%

Q193. The overall mortality rate of pancreaticoduodenectomy (Whipple procedure) is approximately

    A. 0.5%

    B. 2%

    C. 6.5%

    D. 10%

Q194. Which of the following syndromes are NOT associated with childhood central nervous system (CNS) tumors?

    A. Tuberous sclerosis

    B. Von Hippel Lindau

    C. Gorlin

    D. Neurofibromatosis type 3

Q195. The NSABP B-04 was a clinical trial assessing

    A. Mastectomy

    B. Radiation therapy

    C. Chemotherapy

    D. Hormonal therapy

Q196. The most common malignancy in the orbit is

    A. Metastases

    B. Melanoma

    C. Lymphoma

    D. Carcinoma

Q197. What is the staging of a 3-cm cervical cancer with lower 1/3 vaginal involvement?

    A. 1B1

    B. 1B2

    C. IIB

    D. IIIA

Q198. What proportion of pediatric central nervous system (CNS) tumors occur extracranially?

    A. 1%

    B. 5%

    C. 10%

    D. 15%

Q199. What proportion of bladder tumors are either premalignant or T1 at diagnosis?

    A. 25%

    B. 50%

    C. 75%

    D. 90%

Q200. Which of the following subtypes of HPV is associated with the highest risk of adenocarcinoma?

    A. 6

    B. 11

    C. 16

    D. 18

Practice Test 1: Basic Science Answers

Answers With Rationales

A1. D   RO P + R 2013, Ch 10.

The Clark levels are:
I—in situ disease confined to epidermis
II—invasion into papillary dermis
III—invasion into junction of papillary and reticular dermis
IV—invasion into reticular dermis
V—invasion into subcutaneous fat

A2. B   RO P + R 2013, Ch 1.

KERMA will exceed absorbed dose in the so called "build-up region" due to electronic adisequilibrium (more electrons leaving the volume/mass than entering it). After equilibrium, absorbed dose will be higher than KERMA due to the law of conservation of mass and energy.

A3. B   RO P + R 2013, Ch 1.

Photon energy is directly proportional to frequency by the mathematical relationship of photon energy equals frequency times 6.626×10^{-34} Js. Photon frequency and wavelength are inversely proportional to each other; therefore, wavelength is inversely proportional to photon energy.

A4. A   RO P + R 2013, Ch 7.

Sensitivity = (true positives) divided by (true positives plus false negatives).

A5. B   RO P + R 2013, Ch 9.

Patients at high risk of breast cancer or with known BRCA mutations should have a discussion regarding the use of prophylactic mastectomy, as this surgical approach has been demonstrated to prevent up to 90% of breast cancers, and up to 95% when combined with bilateral salpingo-oophorectomy.

A6. C   RO P + R 2013, Ch 5.

In the context of 1.8 to 2 Gy/day chemoradiation therapy, a mean dose of 34 Gy or less should lead to a severe (Grade III or greater) acute esophagitis risk of 5% to 20%.

A7. B   RO P + R 2013, Ch 7.

Equivalence trials are designed to prove that the intervention and control arms are identical. They generally have larger sample size requirements due to the narrow confidence intervals required for such studies.

Note: RO P + R 2013 refer's to this book's previously published companion volume, *Radiation Oncology Primer and Review: Essential Concepts and Protocols* (Demos Medical Publishing, 2013), which can be used as a reference for further study.

A8. C   RO P + R 2013, Ch 2.

Tumors tend to have regions of hypoxic environments, with oxygen concentration less than 5 mmHg. Normal tissue oxygen concentration typically ranges between 10 and 80 mmHg.

A9. C   RO P + R 2013, Ch 5.

Dose–volume histogram recommendations from the QUANTEC document include maximum dose of less than 66 Gy (1.8–2 Gy/day with chemo) to keep vocal dysfunction to less than 20%. Other parameters include mean dose less than 50 Gy (30% risk of aspiration), mean less than 44 Gy (20% risk of edema, nonchemotherapy), and V50 Gy (20% risk of edema).

A10. C   RO P + R 2013, Ch 1.

Examples of isobars include $^{40}S_{16}$, $^{40}K_{19}$, and $^{40}Ca_{20}$ with all species having identical mass numbers of 40 and different atomic numbers (16, 19, and 20, respectively).

A11. C   RO P + R 2013, Ch 7.

Defined as the number of individuals who have to be exposed to an intervention (compared to standard of care intervention or placebo) to either obtain a desired benefit (NNT: number needed to treat) or an undesired clinically important negative event (e.g., death, NNH: number needed to harm).

A12. B   RO P + R 2013, Ch 10.

The R subclassifications are: R0—no residual primary tumor, R1—microscopic residual tumor, R2—macroscopic residual tumor, and Rx—presence of residual primary tumor not assessed.

A13. B   RO P + R 2013, Ch 4.

Aplasia, hypoplasia, and hyperplasia are all related to changes in cell number.

A14. B   RO P + R 2013, Ch 5.

Medium vessel injury is usually associated with intimal fibrosis, macrophage infiltration, and vasculitis.

A15. A   RO P + R 2013, Ch 1.

Electron capture is not a mode of nucleon emission radioactive decay; it is a form of beta decay where a nucleus captures an orbital electron (functionally equivalent to positron emission) with a daughter nucleus $^{A}X_{Z-1}$.

A16. D   RO P + R 2013, Ch 4.

Metaplasia, dysplasia, neoplasia, and anaplasia are related to change of cell maturity as opposed to change in cell number or size.

A17. D   RO P + R 2013, Ch 18.

The standard dose for unresectable pancreatic cancer, as used in ECOG E4201, is 54 Gy in 30 fractions.

A18. C   RO P + R 2013, Ch 1.

The electron range is estimated by the following equation: electron range (in cm) = electron energy (in MeV)/2.

A19. B   RO P + R 2013, Ch 4.

Metaplasia, dysplasia, neoplasia, and anaplasia are related to change of cell maturity as opposed to change in cell number or size.

A20. B   RO P + R 2013, Ch 15.

According to the RTOG 0615 clinical trial, the macroscopic volume of disease should receive 70 Gy in 33 fractions.

A21. B   RO P + R 2013, Ch 15.

According to the RTOG 0912 trial, the macroscopic volume for an anaplastic thyroid cancer should be treated to 66 Gy in 33 fractions.

A22. C   RO P + R 2013, Ch 15.

According to the RTOG 0912 trial, the high-risk microscopic volume for an anaplastic thyroid cancer should be treated to 59.4 Gy in 33 fractions.

A23. B   RO P + R 2013, Ch 3.

As the LET increases, more energy is deposited along the path of radiation. This results in a significantly increased amount of water hydrolysis and resulting free radical formation. As the density of free radicals increases, there is increased likelihood of these particles recombining and neutralizing themselves prior to mediating DNA damage.

A24. C   RO P + R 2013, Ch 7.

Various statistical concepts exist that are important in the context of evidence-based medicine:
  1. Number needed to treat/harm.
  2. Receiver-operator curves.
  3. Likelihood ratio.

A25. C   RO P + R 2013, Ch 12.

Iridium-192 has an energy of 380 kV.

A26. B   RO P + R 2013, Ch 5.

For acute pericarditis, V30 Gy (in 1.8–2 Gy/day) should be less than 46%.

A27. C   RO P + R 2013, Ch 7.

Performance Bias: Systematic differences in nonprotocol treatment (i.e., co-interventions) between control and intervention groups.

A28. A   RO P + R 2013, Ch 1.

At 0.026 MV, an equal contribution to total attenuation between photoelectric effect (50%) and Compton scattering (50%) exists.

A29. C   RO P+R 2013, Ch 5.

In the context of traditional 3DCRT planning at 1.8 to 2 Gy/day, the following maximum cord doses for full cord irradiation are related to associated estimates of spinal cord injury risk: 50 Gy (0.2%), 54 Gy (1%), 60 Gy (6%), 61 Gy (10%), and 69 Gy (50%).

A30. D   RO P + R 2013, Ch 1.

Gamma radiation is more energetic than x-ray radiation with higher frequency and lower wavelengths.

A31. D   RO P + R 2013, Ch 10.

The modified Astler–Coller (MAC) classification:
Stage A: mucosa only
Stage B1:   extending into muscularis propria, but not penetrating through
Stage B2:   penetrating through muscularis propria

Stage C1: extending into muscularis propria but not penetrating through, and nodal involvement
Stage C2: penetrating through muscularis propria, nodal involvement
Stage D: distant metastatic spread

A32. C RO P + R 2013, Ch 3.

Stochastic effects are nonguaranteed effects typically associated with lower dose exposures that are variable and are not associated with a threshold dose, but become more likely with increasing dose. The severity of these effects is not proportional to the exposure. Long term and delayed effects of radiation, such as inherited genetic mutations and cancer, are examples of stochastic (random) effects.

A33. D RO P + R 2013, Ch 3.

High REB radiation therapy (e.g., neutrons) can be potentially used for overcoming radioresistance.

A34. C RO P + R 2013, Ch 10.

The R denotation is applied following definitive surgery to comment on the status of surgical margins, and can incorporate both the surgeon's operative observations and the pathological findings.

A35. B RO P + R 2013, Ch 1.

The equation that relates the linear attenuation coefficient and half-value layer is $\ln 2/HVL = 0.693/HVL$.

A36. D RO P + R 2013, Ch 12.

The half-life of cesium-137 is 30 years.

A37. D RO P + R 2013, Ch 5.

Postradiation therapy cellular atypia is a form of parenchymal injury.

A38. B RO P + R 2013, Ch 7.

As a result of Bayes' theorem, a pretest probability of a diagnosis can be modified by the likelihood ratio of either a positive or negative test in order to calculate a posttest probability. This posttest probability, therefore, takes into account both the test result, as well as the prevalence of the disease in the patient population being assessed. The likelihood ratio is mathematically related to other concepts such as sensitivity, specificity, positive/negative predictive value, and accuracy.

A39. D RO P + R 2013, Ch 12.

Virtual simulation is a set of simulation procedures similar to conventional simulation; yet, a CT-based system is used instead of a fluoroscopy unit. Radiation beams can be placed to direct therapy in a manner similar to conventional simulation; however, the radiation oncologist can review and utilize the 3D information available in the CT to help define beam direction, size, and shielding. It is generally not used to address organ motion as opposed to conventional and CT simulation.

A40. A RO P + R 2013, Ch 4.

Metaplasia, dysplasia, neoplasia, and anaplasia are related to change of cell maturity as opposed to change in cell number or size.

A41. C RO P + R 2013, Ch 5.

QUANTEC maximum brain dose (in 1.8–2 Gy/day fractions) parameters for 5% and 10% risk of primary endpoint injury are 72 and 90 Gy, respectively.

A42. B   RO P + R 2013, Ch 5.

Various dose–volume histogram (DVH) parameters are used to assist in defining tolerance doses, in the context of prostate cancer (V65 Gy ≤50%, V70 Gy ≤35%, V75 Gy ≤25%, and V80 Gy ≤15%), bladder cancer (65-Gy maximum dose for <6% grade 3 late toxicity risk), and gynecological (40–50-Gy maximum dose of external beam) 1.8 to 2-Gy/day treatment.

A43. B   RO P + R 2013, Ch 12.

The half-life of iodine-125 is 60 days.

A44. A   RO P + R 2013, Ch 12.

The half-life of palladium-103 is 17 days.

A45. D   RO P + R 2013, Ch 9.

FAP is characterized by numerous adenomas within the colon, and a near 100% risk of developing colorectal cancer by age 40.

A46. A   RO P + R 2013, Ch 5.

In the context of whole kidney radiation therapy in 1.8 to 2 Gy, a mean dose of less than 15 to 18 Gy is related to less than 5% risk of renal dysfunction.

A47. A   RO P + R 2013, Ch 4.

Aplasia, hypoplasia, and hyperplasia are all related to changes in cell number.

A48. C   RO P + R 2013, Ch 9.

Patients with Lynch syndrome have an 80% lifetime risk of colorectal cancer development. For patients with confirmed Lynch syndrome, the use of prophylactic colectomy is more controversial, because frequent colonoscopies at an interval of between 1 and 2 years should identify most cancers and premalignant polyps.

A49. D   RO P + R 2013, Ch 1.

The rate of radioactive decay is known as the activity and is measured in Becquerel (Bq). One Bq is defined as one radioactive decay per second.

A50. B   RO P + R 2013, Ch 1.

The decay constant is the inverse of mean lifetime (average lifetime of a radionuclide prior to decay).

A51. A   RO P + R 2013, Ch 17.

The standard dose for locally advanced non-small cell chemoradiation therapy as confirmed by the RTOG 0617 clinical trial is 60 Gy in 30 fractions.

A52. C   RO P + R 2013, Ch 8.

Causality is highly difficult to prove; yet, the following features are considered to increase the evidence of causation: strength of association, consistency, specificity, temporality, biological gradient, plausibility, coherence, analogy, and experimental evidence.

A53. A   RO P + R 2013, Ch 1.

Photon speed, which is at the speed of light, is equal to frequency × wavelength.

A54. C   RO P + R 2013, Ch 5.

Large vessel injury is associated with myointimal proliferation, vessel thrombi, and vessel dissection/rupture.

A55. A   RO P + R 2013, Ch 4.

Leiomyosarcoma, rhabdomyosarcoma, fibromyosarcoma, and dermatofibrosarcoma are all forms of mesenchymal tumors.

A56. B   RO P + R 2013, Ch 18.

The standard dose for preoperative rectal cancer, as used in RTOG 0822, is 50.4 Gy in 28 fractions.

A57. D   RO P + R 2013, Ch 19.

In the context of the high-risk prostate cancer RTOG 0521 clinical trial, the standard dose for the pelvic radiation therapy component was 46.8 Gy in 26 fractions.

A58. D   RO P + R 2013, Ch 7.

Negative predictive value = (true negatives) divided by (true and false negatives).

A59. C   RO P + R 2013, Ch 1.

X-ray radiation is a high energy and ionizing with very short wavelengths of 10^{-10} m.

A60. A   RO P + R 2013, Ch 10.

Clinical (c)—defined as stage before definitive treatment and within 4 months of diagnosis (pretreatment), based on symptoms, physical examination, imaging, investigations including diagnostic scopes and biopsies.

A61. D   RO P + R 2013, Ch 9.

Use of tobacco is currently considered as the number one avoidable risk factor for cancer development, and is linked to the development of approximately 21% of the world's cancers, and nearly 1.5 million cancer-related deaths annually.

A62. C   RO P + R 2013, Ch 19.

The standard dose of low-risk prostate cancer as used in the RTOG 0415 clinical trial is 73.8 Gy in 41 fractions.

A63. D   RO P + R 2013, Ch 11.

Alkaloids include the vinca alkaloids (vincristine, vinblastine, and vinorelbine), stabilizing microtubules (taxanes, creating anaphase arrest, e.g., taxol, docetaxel) or drugs initiating G1/S cell arrest (podophyllotoxin).

A64. B   RO P + R 2013, Ch 7.

Trials can be classified by: level of intervention (observational vs. interventional), technology to be assessed (prevention vs. screening vs. diagnostic vs. therapy), phase (I—safety and dose finding study, II—preliminary efficacy study, III—definitive randomized controlled trial, and IV—postmarketing safety monitoring for rare side effects), design (parallel group assignment vs. factorial trials vs. crossover study vs. cluster trials), hypothesis (superiority vs. equivalence vs. noninferiority), and trial aim (explanatory vs. pragmatic trials).

A65. A   RO P + R 2013, Ch 1.

Mean lifetime (T) is defined as the average lifetime of a radionuclide prior to decay.

A66. C   RO P + R 2013, Ch 15.

According to the RTOG 0615 clinical trial, the high-risk microscopic volume of disease should receive 59.4 Gy in 33 fractions.

A67. A   RO P + R 2013, Ch 1.

Directly ionizing radiation requires the interaction of a charged particle with an atom or molecule. Gamma rays are uncharged and act by indirect mechanisms.

A68. D   RO P + R 2013, Ch 7.

The most robust evidence for confirming or changing medical practice usually comes from a well-designed and reported randomized controlled trial. These trials can have the following design features to reduce bias:
1. Randomization
2. Blinding
3. Placebo-control

A69. C   RO P + R 2013, Ch 1.

Historically, another unit of radioactivity was the Curie (Ci), which was defined as the rate of decay of 1 g of Radium-226 (equal to $3.7 \times 1,010$ Bq).

A70. C   RO P + R 2013, Ch 11.

This class of chemotherapy drug is DNA topology inhibitors that interfere with both the transcription and replication of DNA by disruption of appropriate DNA coiling. Examples include topotecan and etoposide.

A71. C   RO P + R 2013, Ch 5.

In single-fraction stereotactic radiosurgery, a maximum brainstem dose of 12.5 Gy should lead to less than 5% risk of necrosis and/or cranial neuropathy.

A72. C   RO P + R 2013, Ch 4.

Metaplasia, dysplasia, neoplasia, and anaplasia are related to change of cell maturity as opposed to change in cell number or size.

A73. A   RO P + R 2013, Ch 2.

Important cell cycle checkpoints include the G1–S checkpoint, G2–M checkpoint, and the metaphase–anaphase checkpoint.

A74. D   RO P + R 2013, Ch 15.

According to the RTOG 0615 nasopharynx clinical trial, the low-risk volume of disease should receive 54 Gy in 33 fractions.

A75. C   RO P + R 2013, Ch 5.

QUANTEC (1.8–2 Gy/day) maximum optic nerve/chiasm doses are listed as less than 55 Gy (<3% risk), 55 to 60 Gy (3%–7% risk), more than 60 Gy (7%–20% risk).

A76. D   RO P + R 2013, Ch 7.

Attrition Bias: A difference in length of follow-up between intervention and control groups.

A77. D   RO P + R 2013, Ch 1.

This model of the atom builds upon the existence of the wave particle duality of matter. Electrons have wave-like properties that manifest themselves in statistically based electron probability clouds (also known as electron orbitals) when they are part of an atom.

A78. C   RO P + R 2013, Ch 4.

Atrophy, agenesis, and hypertrophy are all related to changes in cell size.

A79. B   RO P + R 2013, Ch 10.

The Dukes classification system is:
Dukes A—invasion into, but not through the bowel wall
Dukes B—invasion through bowel wall, but no lymph node invasion
Dukes C—lymph node involvement
Dukes D—distant metastases

A80. C   RO P + R 2013, Ch 11.

Antimetabolites: This class of chemotherapy drugs is chemically similar to purines or pyrimidines and interferes with DNA replication and RNA synthesis.

A81. D   RO P + R 2013, Ch 5.

The mean dose to the cochlea should be limited to less than 45 Gy (preferably <35 Gy) to reduce the risk of toxicity to below 30%.

A82. B   RO P + R 2013, Ch 2.

SV40 has been associated with cancer in monkeys.

A83. B   RO P + R 2013, Ch 7.

Different reporting standards do exist; the dominant approach utilized by major medical journals is the CONSORT. The 2010 version of the CONSORT statement consists of a 25-item checklist, listing the technical requirements for the reporting of trial design, patient flow, results, and interpretation.

A84. C   RO P + R 2013, Ch 1.

The radius of an electron cloud is 10^{-10} m.

A85. B   RO P + R 2013, Ch 6.

By definition, water has an HU value of 0.

A86. D   RO P + R 2013, Ch 1.

The depth of a 80% isodose line of an electron beam is estimated by the following equation:

80% isodose line = electron energy (in MeV)/3 (in cm)

A87. D   RO P + R 2013, Ch 19.

The standard dose of intermediate-risk prostate cancer as used in the RTOG 0815 clinical trial is 79.2 Gy in 44 fractions.

A88. B   RO P + R 2013, Ch 5.

Postradiation therapy metaplasia is a form of parenchymal injury.

A89. B   RO P + R 2013, Ch 5.

QUANTEC (1.8–2 Gy/day) constraints to the penile bulb include a mean dose to 95% of the penile bulb of less than 50 Gy, as well as other recommended parameters such as D70% less than 70 Gy and D50% less than 50 Gy.

A90. C   RO P + R 2013, Ch 12.

The half-life of iridium-192 is 74 days.

A91. D   RO P + R 2013, Ch 9.

A recent U.S. Preventative Services Task Force meta-analysis reveals that the relative risk of breast cancer mortality with mammography for women aged 40 to 49 is 0.85 (15% reduction).

A92. B   RO P + R 2013, Ch 12.

Teletherapy radiation treatment machines utilize cobalt-60 to deliver a 1.25-MV photon beam.

A93. D   RO P + R 2013, Ch 4.

Aplasia, hypoplasia, and hyperplasia are all related to changes in cell number.

A94. C   RO P + R 2013, Ch 6.

DICOM is an imaging standard (from the NEMA) for the storage, data exchange, and handling of a variety of forms of medical imaging information.

A95. D   RO P + R 2013, Ch 1.

The definition of radiation exposure in air is defined as: radiation exposure = total charge/mass of air.

The SI unit for exposure is the Roentgen (R), and it is defined as 2.58×10^{-4} C/kg air.

A96. B   RO P + R 2013, Ch 4.

Leiomyosarcoma, rhabdomyosarcoma, fibromyosarcoma, and dermatofibrosarcoma are all forms of mesenchymal tumors.

A97. D   RO P + R 2013, Ch 11.

Alkaloids: Plant-based drugs that interfere with cell division by preventing microtubule formation.

A98. C   RO P + R 2013, Ch 12.

Various systems can deliver different rates of radiation therapy dosage (i.e., dose rate). These include LDR (<2 Gy/h, e.g., prostate seed implant), MDR (2–12 Gy/h), and HDR (>12 Gy/h, e.g., prostate, lung, esophagus, and cervix).

A99. B   RO P + R 2013, Ch 1.

Characteristic x-rays are created by the interaction between a free electron and an orbital electron (as opposed to an atomic nucleus). In this interaction, the free-moving electron imparts energy to the orbital electron, freeing the orbital electron from the atom. Auger electrons can be created in a related process whereby the atom can release energy by ejecting an additional electron from the atom.

A100. B   RO P + R 2013, Ch 5.

In the context of stereotactic radiosurgery, a maximum dose of less than 12 Gy in a single dose will lead to a less than 10% risk of blindness. A maximum dose of 8 Gy or less will lead to rare risk of complications.

A101. D   RO P + R 2013, Ch 18.

The standard dose for T3–4 or node positive anal canal cancer, as used in RTOG 0529, is 54 Gy in 30 fractions.

A102. B   RO P + R 2013, Ch 15.

According to the RTOG 0920 study, the dose fractionation that should be used for high-risk postoperative head and neck radiation therapy is 60 Gy in 30 fractions.

A103. B   RO P + R 2013, Ch 18.

The standard dose for T2N0 anal canal cancer, as used in RTOG 0529, is 50.4 Gy in 28 fractions.

A104. B   RO P + R 2013, Ch 3.

Giving a single fraction of high-dose radiation would have a significant tumor effect, but would also grossly impact surrounding normal tissues. Fractionating the dose allows divergence of the two cell survival curves, as the normal tissue curve continues to re-express the shoulder of the curve sparing more normal tissue.

A105. A   RO P + R 2013, Ch 5.

Mesothelioma or pneumonectomy situations require more stringent dose parameters such as V5 Gy less than 60% and V20 Gy less than 4% to 10% to ensure minimal risk of severe or fatal radiation pneumonitis.

A106. C   RO P + R 2013, Ch 9.

HPV has been associated with oropharyngeal, anal, and cervical cancers.

A107. D   RO P + R 2013, Ch 12.

Hallmarks of volumetric arc therapy include: variable dose rate, variable gantry rotation speed, and variable MLC orientation.

A108. C   RO P + R 2013, Ch 1.

SA is defined as the number of decays per second per amount (can be based on mass or volume).

A109. C   RO P + R 2013, Ch 6.

An MRI uses a very strong magnetic field to change the nuclear polar alignment, which leads to a rotating magnetic field. The MRI scanning coil can detect these rotating magnetic fields as they relax back to a normal equilibrium (nonaligned) state. A mathematical algorithm is used to construct a 3D imaging dataset that can be visualized for anatomic and pathological diagnostic purposes.

A110. D   RO P + R 2013, Ch 1.

Examples of isomers include the stable and metastable forms of $^{99}\text{Tc}_{43}$.

A111. A   RO P + R 2013, Ch 9.

Studies have suggested a decreased breast cancer risk of 50% in patients of this population undergoing the procedure.

A112. D   RO P + R 2013, Ch 8.

Also known as "point" prevalence, cancer prevalence is defined as the number of cases of cancer present in a population at a specific point in time, divided by the number of individuals in the population.

A113. C   RO P + R 2013, Ch 5.

The V20 Gy is a parameter expressing a relative volume between 0% and 100% of lung volume receiving a cumulative dose of 20 Gy or greater.

A114. D   RO P + R 2013, Ch 7.

Various terms are used to describe blinding in the literature and include: single-blind (patient blinded to intervention), double-blind (patients and researchers blinded to intervention assignment), triple-blind (patients, researchers, and endpoint assessors), and quadruple-blind (like triple-blind but with statistical personnel included in the blinding procedures).

A115. D   RO P + R 2013, Ch 6.

In terms of radiation therapy another related standard is the DICOM-RT standard. This standard encodes radiation therapy point-of-interest (i.e., isocenter), volume-of-interest (i.e., contours), and dose (i.e., isodose) information coregistered on the same coordinate system as DICOM information from the associated CT and/or MRI simulation imaging.

A116. B   RO P + R 2013, Ch 7.

Ascertainment Bias: Patient assignment is known within a blinded study (e.g., due to specific side effects of the intervention), which can lead to biased outcome reporting.

A117. C   RO P + R 2013, Ch 7.

Sample size determination (for an RCT) can be calculated by mathematical formulas, tables, and computer calculators depending on the following parameters:
1. Statistical power
2. Type I (alpha) error
3. Type II (beta) error
4. Effect size
5. Baseline endpoint variance

A118. D   RO P + R 2013, Ch 12.

Iodine-125 has an energy of 27 to 36 kV.

A119. A   RO P + R 2013, Ch 5.

In terms of radiation pneumonitis, the V20 Gy parameter should be kept under 30% to 35%.

A120. D   RO P + R 2013, Ch 11.

Aromatase Inhibitors: An inhibitor of the steroid enzyme aromatase that can reduce estrogen levels in postmenopausal women leading to cell arrest and programmed death in hormone responsive cells. Examples include: letrozole, anastrozole, and exemestane.

A121. B   RO P + R 2013, Ch 3.

The alpha–beta ratio is the dose at which the killing effect of single track damage is equal to that caused by dual track damage, and is expressed in Gy.

A122. C   RO P + R 2013, Ch 10.

Post(neoadjuvant) treatment (y)—the y modifier is used to restage a patient to communicate response to a given therapy, and can be done either clinically (denoted as yc) or pathologically (denoted as yp).

A123. D   RO P + R 2013, Ch 3.

Fibrosis is a late injury to tissue usually in parallel organs such as lung or liver.

A124. B   RO P + R 2013, Ch 3.

RBE is the comparison of effects of different radiation types on similar cell populations or conditions. SER is the comparison of the same radiation on variations of cell populations or conditions. Both the RBE and SER are calculated by the ratio of the dose required to population B (Db), to that required to achieve the same surviving cell fraction in population A (Da).

A125. A   RO P + R 2013, Ch 12.

Various systems can deliver different rates of radiation therapy dosage (i.e., dose rate). These include LDR (<2 Gy/h, e.g., prostate seed implant), MDR (2–12 Gy/h), and HDR (>12 Gy/h, e.g., prostate, lung, esophagus, and cervix).

A126. A   RO P + R 2013, Ch 18.

The standard dose for adjuvant gastric cancer, as used in RTOG 0571, is 45 Gy in 25 fractions.

A127. D   RO P + R 2013, Ch 1.

Cobalt-60 pellets, cylinders, and/or discs are stored within a 1- to 2-cm sealed steel container containing approximately 10,000 Ci of activity.

A128. D   RO P + R 2013, Ch 5.

The mean heart dose should be less than 26 Gy to keep toxicity rates under 15%.

A129. A   RO P + R 2013, Ch 5.

In the context of stereotactic radiosurgery, V12 Gy should be kept to less than 5 to 10 mL in order to ensure a less than 20% risk of symptomatic brain necrosis.

A130. C   RO P + R 2013, Ch 9.

Two very large randomized control trials, the U.S. Prostate, Lung, Colorectal, and Ovarian Cancer Screening Trial (PLCO) and European Randomized Study of Screening for Prostate Cancer (ERSPC), have found either nonexistent or very small and minimal mortality benefit of screening, respectively. The European study found that one cancer death is prevented for every thousand men screened between the ages of 55 and 69 years.

A131. A   RO P + R 2013, Ch 1.

Examples of isotopes are $^{12}C_6$ and $^{13}C_6$ with both species having an atomic number of six and different mass numbers (12 and 13, respectively).

A132. B   RO P + R 2013, Ch 2.

p53 is a tumor suppressor gene. Ras, Her2/neu, and EGFR are all examples of oncogenes.

A133. D   RO P + R 2013, Ch 1.

Total activity (A) is defined as the number of decays per second (A_0 = initial activity at time zero, A_t = activity at time t).

A134. C   RO P + R 2013, Ch 1.

For any specific atom, electrons were required to exist in very specific quantum orbits with correspondingly specific energy states. Electrons moving from one quantum energy state to another would either release or absorb a discrete amount of energy.

A135. C   RO P + R 2013, Ch 3.

The hematopoietic syndrome will lead to death within 60 days without remedial treatment (antibiotics and/or bone marrow transplant).

A136. A   RO P + R 2013, Ch 12.

Radium-223 chloride: A new agent for bone metastases treatment demonstrating a survival benefit of 2.8 months in phase III randomized controlled trial testing. Radium-223 has a half-life of 11.4 days and is a beta emitter with a short range equivalent to 10 cell diameters or less.

A137. A   RO P + R 2013, Ch 7.

Assessment Bias: Improper assessment of primary or secondary study outcomes.

A138. C   RO P + R 2013, Ch 14.

The standard dose for high-risk meningioma in RTOG 0539 is 60 Gy in 30 fractions.

A139. D   RO P + R 2013, Ch 1.

At 24 MV an equal proportion of attenuation from Compton (50%) and pair production (50%) exists. At 4 MV, 94% of attenuation is from Compton effect, and at 10 MV, 77% of attenuation is Compton based (with the remainder from pair production).

A140. D   RO P + R 2013, Ch 9.

A recent U.S. Preventative Services Task Force meta-analysis reveals that the relative risk of breast cancer mortality with mammography for women in the 60- to 69-year age group is 0.68 (32% reduction).

A141. B   RO P + R 2013, Ch 5.

The maximum spinal cord dose is a dose parameter expressing a specific absolute dose (i.e., 48 Gy).

A142. A   RO P + R 2013, Ch 6.

Medical ultrasonography (US) refers to an imaging technique that uses high-frequency ultrasound sound waves (between 2- and 18-MHz range).

A143. B   RO P + R 2013, Ch 18.

The standard dose for postoperative pancreatic cancer, as used in RTOG 0848, is 50.4 Gy in 28 fractions.

A144. B   RO P + R 2013, Ch 11.

Examples include epirubicin, doxorubicin, bleomycin, and mitoxantrone.

A145. B   RO P + R 2013, Ch 10.

The Durie–Salmon system is:
Stage I: Requires all of: Hb >10.0 g/dL, serum calcium ≤12 mg/dL, normal bone x-rays or solitary bone lesions, IgG <5 g/dL, IgA <3 g/dL, urine M-protein <4 g/24 h
Stage II: Does not fit stage I or III criteria
Stage III: Requires one of: Hb <8.5 g/dL, serum calcium >12 mg/dL, 3 or more bone lesions, IgG >7 g/dL, IgA >5 g/dL, urine M-protein >12 g/24 h
Subtypes: A or B for serum creatinine < or ≥2.0 mg/dL, respectively

A146. A   RO P + R 2013, Ch 6.

Various positron-emitting radionuclides can be used for PET imaging. These include: ^{11}C (t1/2 20.3 minutes), ^{13}N (t1/2 9.9 minutes), ^{15}O (t1/2 122.2 minutes), and ^{18}F (t1/2 109.7 minutes).

A147. D   RO P + R 2013, Ch 5.

A cumulative DVH; however, y-axis reflects the volume associated with the x-axis bin dose or greater. By definition, the first and lowest dose bin will have 100% relative volume. Similarly, 0% relative volume will occur beyond the last dose bin of the target or organ at risk under consideration. This leads to the traditional DVH which is graphs both cumulative dose and relative volume.

A148. C   RO P + R 2013, Ch 9.

Excess consumption of alcohol is linked as a primary risk factor in 5% of all human cancer cases, and most commonly is linked to head and neck and liver malignancies.

A149. A   RO P + R 2013, Ch 10.

The Ann Arbor staging system is based primarily on anatomical location of lymph node regions of involvement:

Stage I: single nodal region

Stage II: two or more lymph node regions on the same side of diaphragm, or one nodal region associated with spread to one extra-lymphatic site on the same side of diaphragm

Stage III: involvement of lymph node regions above and below diaphragm, which may include involvement of the spleen

Stage IV: diffuse involvement of one or more extra-lymphatic organs or spread to distant organ, including bone marrow

Use of the suffix E denotes the presence of extra-nodal disease in other organs and viscera (i.e., skin, liver, lungs), and includes bone marrow. Waldeyer's ring, thymus, and spleen are considered as part of the nodal regions, but splenic involvement is denoted with the suffix S. Each Roman numeric stage is further subclassified clinically as A or B, with the latter denoting the clinical presence of B-symptoms at the time of diagnosis (fever, drenching night sweats, and weight loss).

A150. A   RO P + R 2013, Ch 14.

The standard dose for intermediate-risk meningioma in RTOG 0539 is 54 Gy in 30 fractions.

A151. C   RO P + R 2013, Ch 5.

Mean radiation therapy dose (at 1.8–2 Gy/day) for one or both parotid glands should be below 20 and 25 Gy, respectively, in order to keep the risk of clinically significant xerostomia less than 20%. If possible, maintaining mean submandibular dose to less than 35 Gy can also assist in preserving salivary function.

A152. B   RO P + R 2013, Ch 13.

30 Gy in 10 fractions is associated with 20% retreatment rate in bone metastases.

A153. A   RO P + R 2013, Ch 7.

The U.S. Preventive Services Task Force consists of the following (Level I: one or more randomized controlled trial, Level II: 1. nonrandomized controlled trial, 2. cohort/case-control, 3. time series, and Level III: expert opinion).

A154. C   RO P + R 2013, Ch 5.

The mean dose should be less than 20 to 23 Gy to keep the primary symptomatic pneumonitis risk to less than 20%.

A155. C   RO P + R 2013, Ch 3.

The following calculation defines the BED: BED = nd (1 + d/(alpha/beta)) [in units Gy(alpha/beta)] where n is number of fractions, and d is the dose per fraction.

A156. D   RO P + R 2013, Ch 9.

A recent U.S. Preventative Services Task Force meta-analysis reveals that the relative risk of breast cancer mortality with mammography for women ages 50 to 59 is 0.86 (14% reduction).

A157. D   RO P + R 2013, Ch 11.

Factors that can improve therapeutic ratio include: altered fractionation, radiation therapy planning and image-guidance (to reduce normal tissue dose), and tumor radiosensitization/normal tissue radioprotection.

A158. C   RO P + R 2013, Ch 12.

Internal Target Volume (ITV): A subcomponent of the PTV that contains the CTV and IM. All components of the ITV are tumor-related and patient-related. Uncertainty due to treatment-related factors is contained within the set-up margin.

A159. B   RO P + R 2013, Ch 12.

Examples of hadron particles include protons, neutrons, and heavy ions (e.g., carbon ions), and all of these particles have been exploited for therapeutic purposes.

A160. A   RO P + R 2013, Ch 1.

This process, which is also known as "Rayleigh scattering," essentially absorbs and releases a photon from an atom with the same energy, although the direction of the photon has changed.

A161. B   RO P + R 2013, Ch 18.

The standard dose for resectable and unresectable esophageal cancer, as used in RTOG 1010 and RTOG 0436, is 50.4 Gy in 28 fractions.

A162. D   RO P + R 2013, Ch 11.

Examples of alkylating agents include: cisplatin, carboplatin, oxaliplatin, chlorambucil, and cyclophosphamide.

A163. B   RO P + R 2013, Ch 9.

Screening for colorectal cancers has been associated with an approximately 16% decrease in mortality. This benefit is derived from identification of premalignant polyps (adenomas), which can be removed endoscopically before they progress to invasive carcinomas, thus significantly reducing colorectal cancer incidence.

A164. C   RO P + R 2013, Ch 1.

In this interaction scenario, an incident photon will lose a portion of its energy, usually to an outer orbital electron, which will result in the release of that electron with some kinetic energy (equal to transferred energy minus binding energy) and the creation of a new photon with reduced energy (and reduced frequency/increased wavelength) and a new direction (up to maximum 180° change in direction from incident direction; the 180° situation is commonly known as "photon backscatter").

A165. D   RO P + R 2013, Ch 1.

High-energy ionizing radiation generally has high frequency (and corresponding low wavelengths). For ionizing radiation, the transition occurs at 10^{-8} m or smaller.

A166. C   RO P + R 2013, Ch 6.

Other structures can have variable values but the following are known representative values: cortical bone (+400), titanium (+1,000), and cranial bone (+2,000).

A167. D   RO P + R 2013, Ch 12.

Hot Spot: This refers to a volume outside the PTV that receives dosage higher than the prescription dose (100% of PTV dose). Usually considered significant for volumes with greater than 1.5-cm diameter (rule not used for small organs, e.g., orbit).

A168. D   RO P + R 2013, Ch 6.

T1 weighted MRI is an example of anatomical imaging.

A169. C   RO P + R 2013, Ch 2.

Xeroderma pigmentosum is associated with UV-induced skin cancer.

A170. B   RO P + R 2013, Ch 1.

The unit for fluence is m^{-2}.

A171. B   RO P + R 2013, Ch 1.

Examples of isotones are $^{12}B_5$ and $^{13}C_6$ with both species having 7 neutrons and different atomic numbers (5 and 6, respectively).

A172. C   RO P + R 2013, Ch 10.

Pathologic (p)—staging based on surgical resection or the primary and/or lymph nodes and examination of the specimen by pathologist, and is generally given preference over clinical stage when it can be assessed, as it is more predictive of prognosis.

A173. C   RO P + R 2013, Ch 9.

Patients with known BRCA mutations should have a discussion regarding prophylactic risk reducing bilateral salpingo-oopherectomy, which has been shown in studies to reduce ovarian cancer risk up to 96%.

A174. A   RO P + R 2013, Ch 1.

The unit for energy fluence is Jm^{-2}.

A175. A   RO P + R 2013, Ch 11.

Examples for agents include: fludarabine (purine), 5-fluorouracil (pyrimidine), and pemetrexed (antifolate).

A176. B   RO P + R 2013, Ch 12.

An intermittent treatment intensity system called PDR (intermittent dose given once per hour, e.g., gynecological) can be used to deliver LDR- or HDR-like treatment.

A177. B   RO P + R 2013, Ch 7.

Randomization procedures will create very similar groups for comparison in terms of both known and unknown risk factors. If any bias between groups occurs after randomization, that bias would have been generated in a random fashion and can be adjusted by various statistical techniques.

A178. A   RO P + R 2013, Ch 11.

GnRH Analogs/Antagonists: A drug that causes chemical castration due to the downregulation of GnRH receptors (analogs) or direct blockage (antagonists) in the pituitary gland. Examples include leuprolide and goserelin (analogs) and degarelix (antagonist).

A179. B   RO P + R 2013, Ch 6.

The primary paramagnetic atomic target for MRI scanning is the proton (1H MRI). In biological tissue, water is a dominant constituent in cells. Additionally, fat has high concentrations of protons within the hydrocarbon structures and provides an important signal in many MRI sequences.

A180. B   RO P + R 2013, Ch 2.

Antigenic release is a hallmark of necrotic death.

A181. B   RO P + R 2013, Ch 3.

The gastrointestinal syndrome will lead to death in 3 to 10 days with no possibility of remediation.

A182. B   RO P + R 2013, Ch 12.

Stereotactic body radiation is similar to stereotactic radiosurgery but is directed to other areas of the body (e.g., small lung tumors).

A183. B   RO P + R 2013, Ch 16.

According to the RTOG 0413/NSABP B-39 study, 38.5 Gy in 10 fractions BID should be used for partial breast irradiation.

A184. D   RO P+R 2013, Ch 10.

The S subclassifications are:
SX: marker studies not available or performed
S0:   marker study levels within normal limits
S1:   LDH <1.5 × upper limit normal, hCG <5,000 mg/mL, and AFP <1,000 ng/mL
S2:   LDH 1.5 to 10 × upper limit normal or hCG 5,000 to 50,000 mg/mL, or AFP 1,000 to 10,000 ng/mL
S3:   LDH >10 × upper limit normal or hCG >50,000 mg/mL, or AFP >10,000 ng/mL

A185. C   RO P + R 2013, Ch 9.

Low fruit and vegetable intake has been associated with approximately 5% of human cancer cases, most commonly those affecting the aerodigestive tract.

A186. A   RO P + R 2013, Ch 1.

The relationship between half-life, mean lifetime, and the decay constant is defined by the following equation:
$t1/2 = \ln 2/\lambda = T \ln 2$ where $\ln 2 = 0.693$.

A187. D   RO P + R 2013, Ch 6.

SPECT scanning is routinely utilized in bone scanning (technetium-99m phosphonate or bisphosphonate) for the staging of many solid tumors including prostate, breast, lung, and colorectal cancers. Thyroid scans with Iodine-123 labeled metaiodobenzylguanidine (MIBG) can be used to investigate and stage several tumor subtypes such as pheochromocytomas and neuroblastomas. Normal tissue functional perfusion and ventilation imaging (e.g., quantitative ventilation/perfusion scan) can also assist the thoracic radiation oncologists and surgeons in the management of lung cancer patients with borderline pulmonary function.

A188. B   RO P + R 2013, Ch 3.

Early/acute effects that lead to permanent dysfunction are termed consequential late effects and are likely due to stem cell depletion or irreversible damage to underlying tissue structure(s).

A189. C   RO P + R 2013, Ch 1.

One method by which electrons can interact with atoms to create x-ray radiation is by travelling near to the atomic nucleus. The positive charge of the nucleus will cause the trajectory of the travelling electron track to detect toward the nucleus. The electron will lose energy (and speed) in the process; however, the total amount of energy will be conserved by the creation of an x-ray photon.

A190. A   RO P + R 2013, Ch 2.

Arrested tumor cells may extravasate into the tissue parenchyma through complex interactions between the tumor cells, endothelial cells of the capillary, and the basement membrane. The tumor cells may extend projections known as invadopodia between the endothelial cell junctions, which facilitates proteolytic penetrance and allows access to the basement membrane.

A191. B   RO P + R 2013, Ch 9.

Being overweight (body mass index [BMI] >25) or obese [BMI >30]) is associated as a prime risk factor in approximately 2% of all cancer cases, most commonly linked to the development of colorectal, postmenopausal breast, endometrial, esophageal, kidney, and pancreatic malignancies.

A192. A   RO P + R 2013, Ch 5.

Small vessel injury is associated with intimal macrophage infiltration, vessel fibrosis, and fibrin deposition with cell necrosis.

A193. C   RO P + R 2013, Ch 3.

A serial organ is one where dysfunction at any given part of the organ would result in downstream dysfunction.

A194. A   RO P + R 2013, Ch 5.

Necrosis is defined as detrimental premature cell death (as opposed to apoptosis which is programmed cell death).

A195. C   RO P + R 2013, Ch 7.

In the context of diagnostic tests where various cut-off points are possible (each with a unique sensitivity and specificity for each cut-off value), a receiver-operator curve graphing sensitivity (i.e., the true positive rate) versus 1-specificity (i.e., the false positive rate) can be performed. The area under the receiver-operator curve is proportional to the general usefulness of the test (with area under curve of 1 being a perfect test and 0.5 being no better that random chance).

A196. C   RO P + R 2013, Ch 7.

The comparison of two survival curves can be performed with the parametric Cox proportional hazards test or a nonparametric-based log-rank test.

A197. D   RO P + R 2013, Ch 1.

All three of these radionuclides have been utilized for the systemic therapy for bone metastases.

A198. B   RO P + R 2013, Ch 13.

30 Gy in 10 fractions or higher is associated with a modest improvement in survival and symptom score, primarily in patients with good performance status (5% at 1 year, 3% at 2 years).

A199. C   RO P + R 2013, Ch 3.

Single-strand breaks are typically repaired by the cell sensing DNA damage and excising the damaged portion. Single base codon damage can be readily repaired through excision of the damaged base. DNA polymerase then acts to replace the excised portion, using the opposite intact strand as a template. DNA ligase then seals the break in the sugar-phosphate backbone.

A200. D   RO P + R 2013, Ch 5.

In the context of 1.8- to 2-Gy/day radiation therapy the following DVH recommendation should be followed to reduce grade two or greater rectal toxicity to less than 10% to 15% (V50 Gy ≤50%, V60 Gy ≤35%, V65 Gy ≤25%, V70 Gy ≤20%, V75 Gy ≤15%).

A201. A   RO P + R 2013, Ch 5.

In the setting of 1.8- to 2-Gy/day therapy, DVH limits depend on the level of preexisting liver disease. In the case of no preexisting disease, mean liver dose of <30 to 32 Gy leads to <5% risk.

A202. A   RO P + R 2013, Ch 11.

Alkylating Agents: The mechanism of action is via the alkylation of the guanine base of DNA.

A203. C   RO P + R 2013, Ch 1.

The surface dose for an electron beam can be estimated by the following equation: surface dose (in percent) = 70 + electron beam energy.

A204. C   RO P + R 2013, Ch 12.

Palladium-103 has an energy of 21 kV.

A205. D   RO P + R 2013, Ch 1.

Proton emission is a form of nucleon emission with a daughter nucleus $^{A-1}X_{Z-1}$.

A206. B   RO P + R 2013, Ch 14.

The standard dose for anaplastic glioma in RTOG 1071 and RTOG 0834 is 59.4 Gy in 33 fractions (1.8 Gy/fraction).

A207. B   RO P + R 2013, Ch 7.

Specificity = (true negatives) divided by (false positives plus true negatives).

A208. A   RO P + R 2013, Ch 6.

Air has an HU value of −1,000.

A209. C   RO P + R 2013, Ch 2.

The hallmarks of cancer include: evading apoptosis, self-sufficiency in growth signals, insensitivity to antigrowth signals, tissue invasion and metastasis, limitless replication potential, and sustained angiogenesis.

A210. D   RO P + R 2013, Ch 1.

A minimum threshold energy applies to this form of interaction, which is equal to the energy equivalent of the electron pair mass that was created (2 × 0.511 MeV = 1.022 MeV).

A211. B   RO P + R 2013, Ch 12.

Conformity Index (CI): The conformity index describes the mathematical ratio between the treated volume to the PTV. For a perfect treatment, the CI is 1. Practically, assuming adequate coverage of the PTV volume, clinical CI usually is greater than 1.

A212. A   RO P + R 2013, Ch 3.

The cerebrovascular syndrome leads to death within 24 to 48 hours with no possibility of remediation.

A213. B   RO P + R 2013, Ch 1.

This model introduced the concept of a central dense positively charged nucleus with electrons orbiting this nucleus in a manner similar to planetary motion.

A214. C   RO P + R 2013, Ch 13.

8 Gy in 1 fraction is associated with 20% retreatment rate in bone metastases.

A215. D   RO P + R 2013, Ch 9.

Hepatitis B virus (HBV) is associated with hepatocellular carcinoma. Nasopharyngeal cancer, Burkitt lymphoma, and Hodgkin's lymphoma are associated with EBV.

A216. D   RO P + R 2013, Ch 1.

A cathode is a negative electrode used to generate and repel an electron beam toward an anode target.

A217. C   RO P + R 2013, Ch 14.

The standard dose for glioblastoma in RTOG 0825 is 60 Gy in 30 fractions.

A218. B   RO P + R 2013, Ch 12.

Cesium-137 has an energy of 0.66 MeV.

A219. D   RO P + R 2013, Ch 3.

The linear quadratic model is expressed by the equation:

$S(D) = e(-alpha \times D - beta \times D2)$ where S is surviving fraction, D is the dose exposed, alpha is the initial slope of the curve at low dose, and represents the susceptibility to single track damage, beta is the slope at larger doses and represents the susceptibility to dual track damage.

A220. D   RO P + R 2013, Ch 1.

This concept relates to the absorption of a high-energy photon by an atomic nucleus with the release of a subatomic particle (e.g., proton or neutron) and potential disruption of the nucleus itself.

A221. C   RO P + R 2013, Ch 5.

Recommended dose limits for small bowel at 2 Gy/day include: V15 Gy <120 mL (small bowel contoured) or V45 Gy <195 mL (peritoneal space contoured as a surrogate to account for small bowel motion).

A222. B   RO P + R 2013, Ch 3.

Effective dose is the product of cumulative dose to each organ or tissue with a weighting factor for that tissue type.

Effective dose = Sum of (DTi × WTi) where DTi is the total dose to each organ, and WTi is the tissue weighting factors.

A223. C   RO P + R 2013, Ch 14.

The standard dose for CNS lymphoma used in RTOG 1114 is 23.4 Gy in 13 fractions.

A224. A   RO P + R 2013, Ch 1.

An anode is a positive electrode to attract an electron beam and dissipate heat generated in the x-ray process.

A225. C   RO P + R 2013, Ch 11.

Antiandrogens: This class of drugs can either bind to androgen receptors (nonsteroidal antiandrogens) or block the peripheral conversion of steroid hormone metabolites into testosterone (5-alpha reductase inhibitors). Examples include bicalutamide/flutamide (nonsteroidal antiandrogen) and dutasteride/finasteride (5-alpha reductase inhibitors).

A226. B   RO P + R 2013, Ch 10.

The original Breslow stages, on the basis of depth of pathologic invasion were I = less or equal to 0.75 mm, II = 0.75 to 1.5 mm, III = 1.51 to 2.25 mm, IV = 2.25 to 3.0 mm, V = <3.0 mm.

A227. D   RO P + R 2013, Ch 9.

A prime example of an effective cancer-screening program is the implementation of the Papanicolaou test, commonly called a "Pap smear," which has resulted in a significant decline in cervical cancer incidence and mortality by approximately 80% since its adoption as a screening tool in the last 60 years.

A228. A   RO P + R 2013, Ch 3.

Early/acute effects manifest within a few days to weeks, caused by the death of a large number of cells. This is typically seen in tissues with rapid rates of turnover, such as the gastrointestinal epithelium, skin epidermis, and hematopoietic system.

A229. D   RO P + R 2013, Ch 5.

The QUANTEC (1.8–2 Gy/day) brainstem tolerance is 54 Gy to the entire organ, 59 Gy to 1 to 10 mL of the brainstem, and 64 Gy to a point dose of less than 1 mL in volume.

A230. C   RO P + R 2013, Ch 1.

The depth of the 90% isodose line of an electron beam is estimated by the following equation:

90% isodose line (in cm) = electron energy (in MeV)/4.

A231. C   RO P + R 2013, Ch 2.

HER2/neu is an example of an oncogene. BRCA1/2, p53, and RB are all examples of tumor suppressor genes.

A232. D   RO P + R 2013, Ch 3.

Within the therapeutic realm of radiation, external beam radiation is delivered at higher dose rates than interstitial and intracavitary brachytherapy. Lower dose rates can be associated with increased DNA repair. At very low doses, the paradoxical inverse dose rate effect is noted, and tumor cell kill can be enhanced.

A233. C   RO P + R 2013, Ch 7.

Positive predictive value = (true positives) divided by (true and false positives).

A234. D   RO P + R 2013, Ch 1.

Depth dose distribution profiles can vary according to various parameters including: radiation type, radiation energy, density (or density changes) in the medium, field size, field shape (shielding), and source-to-skin distance (SSD). Depth dose distributions do not depend on the dose rate of the radiation beam.

A235. A   RO P + R 2013, Ch 3.

LET is not evenly deposited through tissue medium. LET is commonly expressed in units of KeV/μm. The LET depends on the particle charge, energy (speed), absorbed (tissue) type, and its density.

A236. A   RO P + R 2013, Ch 1.

Otherwise known as the "plum and pudding" model of the atom, electrons were considered to be residing within an area of positive charge but free to travel within this positive charge area.

A237. D   RO P + R 2013, Ch 12.

CT simulation not only provides anatomical information regarding targets, normal tissues, and the external patient contour for treatment planning but also provides voxel-based Hounsfield unit information for dose calculation to support isodose generation for planning optimization, review, and acceptance.

A238. B   RO P + R 2013, Ch 7.

The U.S. Preventive Services Task Force consists of the following (Level I: one or more randomized controlled trial; Level II: 1. nonrandomized controlled trial, 2. cohort/case control, 3. time series; and Level III: expert opinion).

A239. D   RO P + R 2013, Ch 1.

Superposition (interference), refraction (alteration of direction), and dispersion (separation into component parts) are all properties of electromagnetic radiation.

A240. D   RO P + R 2013, Ch 3.

Reactive species formed by the radiolysis of water include OH^-, H_3O^+, e^-_{aq}, and H.

A241. B   RO P + R 2013, Ch 10.

Retreatment (r)—used for restaging of a recurrent or progressive tumor following initial therapy.

A242. D   RO P + R 2013, Ch 7.

The type II error rate is the probability that a study will not find a difference when a true difference between the control and intervention arms exists. This is otherwise known as the "false negative rate," which is mathematically related to the power probability by the following equation: power = 1 − beta.

A243. D   RO P + R 2013, Ch 12.

This approach uses highly focused radiation therapy beams guided by pretreatment and on-treatment imaging (image-guided radiation therapy) to treat brain and spine tumors. This approach is usually combined with invasive fixation of the cranium (for brain tumors) to achieve high levels of immobilization to support the high dose of radiation therapy delivered to usually small target volumes. Commonly single fractions of radiation therapy are delivered; however, multiple fractions of radiation therapy can also be used particularly for larger tumors where normal tissue toxicity is a concern.

A244. A   RO P + R 2013, Ch 1.

I-131 is utilized for radioactive iodine thyroid treatment. Ir-192, I-125, and Pd-103 are utilized for various seed-based brachytherapy applications. Ir-192 is also utilized as a high-dose brachytherapy source.

A245. C   RO P + R 2013, Ch 6.

A CT pixel is related to relative x-ray radio density on the HU scale (ranging from low attenuation −1,024 to high attenuation +3,071). By definition, water has an HU value of 0 and air is −1,000. Other structures can have variable values but the following are known representative values: bone (+400), titanium (+1,000), and cranial bone (+2,000).

A246. C   RO P + R 2013, Ch 9.

Unsafe sexual practices contribute to 3% of worldwide cancer cases, but most concerning is the major risk factor for development of cervical cancer, one of the most preventable female malignancies.

A247. C   RO P + R 2013, Ch 11.

Several examples (not exhaustive) of the clinical role of chemoradiation therapy that are established in the medical literature are listed in the following:
1. Central nervous system (CNS) high-grade gliomas
2. Head and neck cancers
3. Lung cancer
4. Esophageal cancer

5. Stomach and rectal cancer
6. Anal canal cancer
7. Bladder cancer
8. Cervical cancer

A248. B   RO P + R 2013, Ch 13.

Recursive Partitioning Analysis System:
Class I: KPS ≥70, <65 years old, controlled primary, no extracranial metastasis
Class II: all others
Class III: KPS <70

A249. B   RO P + R 2013, Ch 11.

The tumor control curve is to the right of the normal tissue curve reflecting the fact that at any particular dose there is a higher rate of toxicity than tumor control.

A250. C   RO P + R 2013, Ch 12.

Planning target volume (PTV): This is a geometrical concept which defines a new volume containing the CTV (and hence the GTV) but also includes a three-dimensional margin to take into account any set-up, organ, patient, or beam inaccuracies. This volume will define the "target" for radiation therapy planning as it is not considered to be a pure anatomical construct.

A251. D   RO P + R 2013, Ch 3.

There are three important types of DNA damage: SSBs, DSBs, and base damage. SSBs are formed by the deposition of energy directly into the sugar-phosphate backbone structure. DSBs are formed when two SSBs occur on opposite strands of DNA at a distance of less than 10 base pairs apart.

A252. B   RO P + R 2013, Ch 7.

A commonly used system for the assessment of solid tumors is the RECIST criteria that have specific rules for measurable and nonmeasurable lesions/disease to classify patients into complete response (CR—complete resolution), partial response (PR—at least 30% cross sectional sum reduction), stable disease (SD—neither PR or PD), and progressive disease (PD—at least 20% cross-sectional sum increase).

A253. B   RO P + R 2013, Ch 12.

Various systems can deliver different rates of radiation therapy dosage (i.e., dose rate). These include LDR (<2 Gy/h, e.g., prostate seed implant), MDR (2–12 Gy/h), and HDR (>12 Gy/h, e.g., prostate, lung, esophagus, and cervix).

A254. A   RO P + R 2013, Ch 6.

The fluoroscopy imaging technique is related to a projectional radiograph, but utilizes a cine display (multiple images over time).

A255. C   RO P + R 2013, Ch 16.

According to the RTOG 1005 local breast cancer trial, 50 Gy in 25 fractions (2 Gy/fraction) or 42.5 Gy in 16 fractions (2.67 Gy/fraction) are acceptable for the whole breast component of treatment.

A256. B   RO P + R 2013, Ch 17.

According to the RTOG 0618 early-stage lung cancer SBRT trial, 60 Gy in 3 fractions over 1.5 to 2 weeks (without heterogeneity correction) is an acceptable dose fractionation schedule.

A257. D   RO P + R 2013, Ch 12.

PRV: This is an extension of the OAR concept, which is similar to the PTV for target specification. The PRV includes physiological (IM) and technical (SM) uncertainty margins around the OAR to provide a final avoidance volume for radiation therapy planning.

A258. A   RO P + R 2013, Ch 7.

Survival is usually calculated from the date of death (or last follow-up) to the date of diagnosis, start of treatment, or end of treatment.

A259. D   RO P + R 2013, Ch 3.

Repair and repopulation result in lower tumor cell kill, but increased normal tissue recovery. Conversely, reassortment and reoxygenation are associated with improved tumor cell kill, but likely more normal tissue effects.

A260. B   RO P + R 2013, Ch 1.

In this photon–atomic interaction, the photon is completely absorbed by the atom with the release of an electron (usually an inner orbital electron) with kinetic energy equal to the photon energy minus the binding electron energy (potential energy to be overcome to release the electron).

A261. C   RO P + R 2013, Ch 12.

Modern image-guided radiation therapy (IGRT) utilizes either kilovoltage (kV) diagnostic quality on-board imaging (e.g., fluoroscopy or kV cone-beam CT) or megavoltage (MV) treatment energy on-board imaging (e.g., two-dimensional kV planar portal image or a three-dimensional MV cone-beam CT).

A262. D   RO P + R 2013, Ch 1.

Sa-153 is utilized for systemic bone metastases treatment. F-18 is utilized for PET scanning. Ga-67 is used for thyroid imaging. Tc-99m is used for bone scanning.

A263. D   RO P + R 2013, Ch 1.

The radium of the atomic nucleus is several orders of magnitude smaller than the radius of an electron cloud at 10^{-14} m.

Practice Test 2: Clinical Answers

Answers With Rationales

A1. A

Denys–Drash syndrome consists of mesangial sclerosis, renal failure, and intersex disorders. Most will develop Wilms' tumor.

A2. B

Stage III disease is described by the involvement of lymph node regions on both sides of the diaphragm (III), which also may be accompanied by extra lymphatic extension in association with adjacent lymph node involvement (IIIE) or by involvement of the spleen (IIIS) or both (IIIE, S).

B symptoms are: unexplained loss of more than 10% of body weight in the 6 months before diagnosis, unexplained fever with temperatures above 38°C, drenching night sweats.

A3. D

Pathologic subtypes of kidney cancers include: clear cell (70% of cases), chromophilic, chromophobic, collecting duct.

A4. C

NSABP B-32: Clinically node negative patients randomized to sentinel lymph node (SLN) biopsy (with ancillary lymph node dissection [ALND] if sentinel node positive) versus SLN biopsy + ALND. No overall survival (OS), progression free survival (PFS), or disease free survival (DFS) difference.

A5. C

10% to 15% of soft tissue sarcomas are retroperitoneal.

A6. D

If inguinal LNs involved, risk of pelvic LN involvement = 30%.

A7. C

N3 breast nodal staging:
    N3a—Metastases in ipsilateral infraclavicular (level III) axillary lymph node(s)
    N3b—Metastases in ipsilateral internal mammary node(s) and level I, II axillary lymph nodes
    N3c—Metastases in ipsilateral supraclavicular lymph node(s)

A8. A

The KRAS mutation is seen in approximately 25% of nonsquamous lung cancer cases.

A9. D

40% of pancreatic cancer cases are sporadic in nature. 30% are related to smoking. 20% may be associated with dietary factors. 5% to 10% are hereditary.

A10. B

Any lung cancer patients with N3 or T4N2 disease are considered to have Stage IIIB cancer.

A11. A

20% of patients with cN0 inguinal lymph nodes will be pN+. 30% to 50% of patients with cN+ inguinal lymph nodes will be pN0.

A12. D

Metastatic disease is very common, occurring in approximately 70% at diagnosis with common metastatic sites including the lymph nodes, bone, bone marrow, liver, orbits, and skin.

A13. C

Endocrinopathies are common when dose to the pituitary/hypothalamus exceeds 30 to 35 Gy. Most common are growth hormone deficits and secondary hypothyroidism.

A14. D

Brachytherapy for extremity STS is contraindicated as primary adjuvant treatment if:
    CTV cannot be adequately covered by implant geometry
    Critical anatomic structures would receive a meaningful dose
    Positive margins
    Skin involvement

A15. C

Primary cutaneous B cell lymphoma (PCBCL) has three main subtypes:
    Primary cutaneous follicle center lymphoma (PCFCL)—most common PCBCL, presentation on head or trunk, indolent course, excellent prognosis.
    Primary cutaneous large B cell lymphoma (PCLBCL), leg type—presentation on legs, older age at diagnosis, most commonly elderly women, aggressive lymphoma, intermediate prognosis.
    Primary cutaneous marginal zone lymphoma (PCMZL)—indolent PCBCL.

A16. B

The three commonly accepted features of high-risk prostate cancer are:
    PSA >20 ng/mL
    Gleason score ≥8
    T3/T4

A17. A

Osteosarcoma outcomes: 5 year Local control—72%, 5-year OS—67%, 5-year DFS—65%, 5-year distant metastases—26%.

A18. B

Invasion or encasement of >50% of the superior mesenteric, celiac, and hepatic arteries are considered contrain- dications to surgery (T4 = unresectable). Invasion or encasement of the superior mesenteric or portal vein is no longer considered an absolute contraindication surgery as they can be partially resected or reconstructed.

A19. C

The WAGR syndrome consists of Wilms' tumor, aniridia, genitourinary abnormalities, and mental retardation. Approximately 50% will develop Wilms' tumor. Other syndromes associated with Wilms' tumor include Denys– Drash, Beckwith–Weidemann, and Simpson–Golabi–Behmel.

A20. A

Third leading cause of cancer deaths worldwide, >500,000 affected. Worldwide, incidence in developing nations >2× incidence in developed countries.

A21. C

Three randomized trials have reported informed on the role of adjuvant radiation therapy in patients with adverse pathologic features (pT3 and/or positive margin).

A22. C

About 70% of patients will have a clinical CR after 45 Gy of chemoradiation (cT0 and negative cytology).

A23. A

Three randomized trials have reported informed on the role of adjuvant radiation therapy in patients with adverse pathologic feature (pT3 and/or positive margin).

A24. C

Basal cell carcinomas are generally slow growing over many years. Spread to lymph nodes or distant organs is rare, <0.01%. Squamous cell carcinomas usually are more aggressive than basal cell carcinoma. Incidence of regional metastasis at diagnosis is 2%; eventually 10% develop regional metastasis.

A25. A

NSABP B17 demonstrated that RT reduced the rate of breast recurrence from 35% to 19.8% at 15 years.

A26. A

Thymic neoplasms are predominantly thymomas (90%) and constitute 30% of all anterior mediastinal masses among adults.

A27. A

Astrocytoma subtypes:
   Fibrillary are the most common.
   Gemistocytic may be more aggressive.
   Protoplasmic have a better prognosis.

A28. D

Limb-sparing surgery alone has a 30% to 50% local control rate; the addition of adjuvant radiation increases this to 90% but with no effect on overall survival.

A29. A

Osteosarcoma outcomes: 5 year Local control—72%, 5-year OS—67%, 5-year DFS—65%, 5-year distant metastases—26%.

A30. A

Survival in patients with esophageal cancer depends on the Stage of the disease.
   AJCC TNM Stage 0—100% 5-year OS
   AJCC TNM Stage I—80% 5-year OS
   AJCC TNM Stage IIA—40% 5-year OS
   AJCC TNM Stage IIB—30% 5-year OS
   AJCC TNM Stage III—15% 5-year OS
   AJCC TNM Stage IV—0% 5-year OS

A31. A

70% of vulvar cancers arise from the labia majora/minora; 10% to 15% from the clitoris; 5% from the perineum and <1% Bartholin's gland/vestibule.

A32. B

Lymphedema risk is approximately 5% after SNLB, 10% with ALND, and up to 20% with ALND and regional nodal radiation.

A33. A

Grade 2:
  Atypical
  Clear Cell
  Chordoid

Grade 3:
  Rhabdoid
  Papillary
  Anaplastic

A34. B

93,090 new cases of colon cancer and 39,610 new cases of rectal cancer were diagnosed in 2015. Lifetime risk of developing a colorectal cancer is approximately 6% in the United States.

A35. B

Risk factors for the development of hepatocellular carcinoma in the United States include:
  Alcoholic cirrhosis
  Hepatitis B (250 times more common with Hep B)
  Hepatitis C
  Hemochromatosis
  Combination of hepatitis and alcohol significantly increases risk of cirrhosis and hepatocellular carcinoma (HCC)
  Obesity with nonalcoholic fatty liver disease (NAFLD) or nonalcoholic steatohepatitis (NASH) can progress to fibrosis, cirrhosis, and HCC

A36. D

All anaplastic carcinomas are considered as T4 tumor:
  T4a: Intrathyroidal anaplastic carcinoma
  T4b: Anaplastic carcinoma with gross extrathyroid extension

A37. B

Locally advanced orbital cancers are T staged as:
  T4a: Involvement of nasopharynx
  T4b: Osseous involvement (including periosteum)
  T4c: Involvement of maxillofacial, ethmoidal, and/or frontal sinuses
  T4d: Intracranial spread

A38. A

Although all four of these histologies (embryonal tumors, germ cell tumors, ependymal tumors, and astrocytomas) can seed the CSF, astrocytomas have the lowest relative propensity of such spread.

A39. C

The graded prognostic assessment consists of age, KPS, number of mets, and extracranial mets.

A40. A

A panel of immunohistochemical markers is used to distinguish MPM from lung adenocarcinoma. MPMs typically express Wilms' tumor protein (WT-1), D2-40, and calretinin and do not express TTF-1 or CEA.

A41. D

Currently, low dose computed tomographic scan (LDCT) is recommended in healthy current or former smokers (≥30 pack years of smoking, quit <15 years ago), age 55 to 80 years.

A42. D

DLBCL dose fractionation schedules:
    Consolidation RT after chemotherapy CR: 30 to 36 Gy
    Complimentary RT after PR: 40 to 50 Gy
    Primary RT for refractory or noncandidates for chemotherapy: 45 to55 Gy

A43. A

Typical prescription for PBI: 38.5 Gy BID in 10 fractions

A44. B

The addition of docetaxel (T) to AC preoperatively increased pathological complete response (pCR) rate (26% vs. 13%). Patients with pCR had improved survival rate compared to those without pCR.

A45. C

5-year OS by stage for vulvar cancer:
    I: 90%
    II: 77%
    III: 51%
    IV: 18%

A46. C

Temozolomide toxicities include: acute pancytopenia, nausea, vomiting, infertility, and constipation particularly with ondansetron GI prophylaxis.

A47. A

Grade is based on differentiation, mitotic rate, and necrosis.

A48. C

Acoustic neuroma is associated with the Schwann cell-derived tumors usually arising from vestibular portion of the CN VIII.

A49. A

Patients with epitheloid histology in mesothelioma have better outcomes than those with either mixed or sarcomatoid histologies.

A50. B

WHO type 2a: nonkeratinizing squamous cell carcinoma is the most uncommon subtype of nasopharyngeal cancer.

A51. A

Age, tumor stage, and LDH level are common between the two IPI risk stratification systems.

A52. D

Several genetic conditions can predispose to the development of renal cell carcinoma (RCC):

von Hippel–Lindau disease (VHL): Autosomal dominant mutation of the VHL gene (3p25.3). Commonly associated with RCC, hemangioblastoma, pheochromocytoma, and pancreatic cysts.

Dirt–Hogg–Dubé syndrome: Associated with RCC, renal and pulmonary cysts, and fibrofolliculoma of the skin.

Tuberous sclerosis: Mutation of TSC1 or TSC2, tumor suppressor genes. Predisposes to various tumors including RCC as well as developmental delay.

A53. C

Craniospinal RT should be given to the whole brain and spine to bottom of thecal sac with a dose fractionation schedule of 36 Gy/1.8 Gy/fractions.

A54. C

The usual dose is 59.4 in 1.8 Gy fractions.

A55. C

T staging of cutaneous lymphoma:

T1   Limited patches, papules, and/or plaques covering <10% of the skin surface

T2   Patches, papules, or plaques covering ≥10% of the skin surface

T3   One or more tumors (≥1 cm diameter)

T4   Confluence of erythema covering ≥80% body surface area.

A56. B

Pancreatic carcinoma is usually fatal with MS for all patients on the order of 4 to 6 months.

1-year OS rate is about 24%

5-year OS rate is about 5%

For the 20% of patients able to undergo a successful curative resection, MS ranges from 12 to 19 months, and the 5-year survival rate is 15% to 20%.

A57. C

High-risk neuroblastoma disease is defined by either:

N-myc amplified (stage II–IVs) disease

or

N-myc nonamplified disease, >1-year old, and stage IV

A58. C

Hereditary syndromes associated with gallbladder cancer include:

Gardner syndrome

Neurofibromatosis type I

Hereditary nonpolyposis colon cancer

A59. C

Myasthenia Gravis (MG) is the most common autoimmune disorder and can be present in 30% to 50% of patients. Younger females and older males are usually affected; the female to male ratio is 2:1.

A60. A

Local disease prognostic factors for Ewing's sarcoma: primary tumor volume >200 mL or 8 cm in diameter, and histologic response seen after chemotherapy in resection patients.

A61. A

Risk factors for cervical cancer includes: HPV infection, smoking, immunosuppression (HIV/AIDS), early first intercourse, multiple sexual partners, history of venereal disease, high parity, and prenatal exposure to DES (for clear cell histology).

A62. C

Radiation pneumonitis is dose and volume dependent. With mean lung dose of <20 Gy, and V20 <30% to 35% the incidence of significant RT pneumonitis is <20%.

A63. C

Conventionally, doses of radiation between 50.4 and 59.4 Gy are appropriate. Two studies suggest that doses in excess of 55.8 Gy result in higher LC than lower doses (Rich, Radiother Oncol, 1993; Fung IJROBP, 1993). But increased radiation dose did not increase LC when given with split-course in a phase II RTOG study, so a maximum dose of 59 Gy is considered standard.

A64. C

Genetic syndromes with increased risk of ovarian cancer:
  BRCA1: 35% to 45% lifetime risk
  BRCA2: 15% to 25% lifetime risk

A65. D

ASTRO recommendations for bone mets:
  8 Gy × 1 noninferior to 3 Gy × 10, 4 Gy × 6, 4 Gy × 5 in providing pain relief
  Higher retreat rate with single fractionation treatment versus fractionated RT 20% versus 8% because of recurrent pain
  No difference in long-term toxicity between 8 Gy × 1 and prolonged RT courses for uncomplicated, painful bone mets

A66. C

Common isotopes for prostate brachytherapy:
  103Pd: 17 days half-life, 21 keV energy, 125 Gy monotherapy, 100 Gy combo
  125I: 60 days half-life, 28 keV energy, 145 Gy monotherapy, 110 Gy combo
  192Ir: 74 days half-life, 3.8 MeV energy, several reported dose/fx

A67. A

Relative contraindications for prostate brachytherapy:
  Previous RT or transurethral resection of the prostate (TURP)
  Intermediate or high risk (consider combination therapy with supplemental EBRT)
  Seminal vesicle invasion
  Pubic arch interference
  Median lobe
  Large gland (>60 mL)
  AUA score >15 (increases risk of postbrachytherapy urinary toxicity)
  Diabetes mellitus

A68. A

Site-specific GPA:
  Breast: KPS, Luminal subtype, Age
  Lung: Age, KPS, # lesions
  Melanoma/Renal: KPS + # lesions
  GI: KPS

A69. C

Resection (marginal or wide resection) for Ewing's sarcoma is preferred because it has better local control than definitive radiation (HR of 2.41 for radiation vs. surgery).

A70. C

Adequate point A dose is usually considered to be 85 Gy (in conjunction with 45 Gy of pelvic RT).

A71. C

The expected results associated with Stage III cervix cancer include the following:
  Pelvic LN: 60%
  PA LN: 30%
  5-year LC:25%
  5-year OS: 20%

A72. B

NSABP B24: Lumpectomy + RT ±5 years of Tamoxifen:
  Tamoxifen reduced ipsilateral invasive (9%–6.6%) and noninvasive (7.6%–6.7%) breast recurrence and contralateral invasive or noninvasive cancer (8.1%–4.9%).

A73. D

Typical immunophenotype for classical HL:
  CD15+, CD30+, PAX-5+ (weak), CD3–, CD20–(majority), CD45–, CD79a–
Typical immunophenotype for NLPHL:
  CD20+, CD45+, CD79a+, BCL6+, PAX-5+, CD3–, CD15–, CD30–

A74. A

Treatment of early stage B nonbulky disease is with 30 Gy combined modality therapy.

A75. B

Surgical options for patients with MPM can include:
  Pleurectomy/decortication (P/D): Complete removal of the involved pleura and all gross tumor
  Radical (or extended) P/D: Resection of diaphragm and pericardium in addition to total pleurectomy
  Extrapleural pneumonectomy (EPP): En-bloc resection of involved pleura, lung, ipsilateral diaphragm, and pericardium

A76. A

Approximately 75% to 80% of primary cutaneous lymphomas are T-cell origin in the Western world, with mycosis fungoides (MF) the most common type, and cutaneous B-cell lymphomas accounting for approximately 20% to 25%.

A77. D

The most common paraneoplastic syndrome is SIADH (syndrome of inappropriate antidiuretic hormone) in 75% of cases.

A78. A

Pathologies with highest incidence of hemorrhage: Renal, melanoma, choriocarcinoma, thyroid.

A79. C

Standard oligodendrogliomas are Grade II; anaplastic tumors are Grade III.

A80. D

Current standard chemotherapy protocol for osteosarcoma includes: Doxorubicin, Cisplatin, MTX, ± Ifosfamide.

A81. B

Endometrioid endometrial adenocarcinoma (estrogen-related): 75% of cases.
Papillary serous (UPSC), clear cell and mucinous carcinomas (nonestrogen related): 20% of cases.
Leiyomyosarcoma/endometrial stromal sarcoma, uterine sarcoma, and adenosarcoma: approximately 5% of cases.

A82. A

Indolent B-cell lymphoma include:
    Follicular, grades 1, 2, 3a
    Small lymphocytic (CLL)
    Marginal zone, extranodal (MALT)
    Splenic marginal zone
    Marginal zone, nodal (monocytoid B-cell)
    Lymphoplasmacytic (Waldenström's macroglobulinemia)
    Primary cutaneous, follicle center
    Hairy cell leukemia

A83. C

There was no difference in recurrence or survival if chemotherapy was given either preoperatively or postoperatively (NSABP B18).

A84. C

Dose for thymomas: 45 to 50 Gy in the postoperative setting. For gross disease or positive margins, 54 to 60 Gy is generally recommended.

A85. C

There is a bimodal age distribution of Hodgkin's lymphoma (~20 years and ~65 years) but this may differ with geography, level of industrialization, and race.

A86. B

Symptoms caused by hypersecretion of ACTH include central obesity, hypertension, psychologic changes, purple skin striae, diabetes, hirsutism, and Nelson's syndrome.

A87. A

Evidence exists demonstrating an improvement in long-term OS in patients treated with long-term androgen deprivation therapy (ADT) (in addition to radiation therapy).

A88. D

Relative contraindications for bladder preservation include multifocal disease, clinical extravesicular disease, component of Tis, hydronephrosis, and subtotal TURBT.

A89. B

Bulky Hodgkin's lymphoma is defined as equal to or greater than 10 cm.

A90. A

The majority of level V nodal primaries arise from the nasopharynx.

A91. C

5-year OS of vaginal cancer:
  Stage I: 75%
  Stage II: 50%
  Stage III: 30%
  Stage IV: 20%

A92. A

The expected results associated with Stage III cervix cancer include the following:
  Pelvic LN 30%
  PA LN: 10%
  5-year LC: 80%
  5-year OS: 70%

A93. C

A published meta-analysis has demonstrated that a D2 dissection carries increased mortality risks associated with spleen and pancreas resection and no evidence of OS benefit, but possible benefit in T3+ tumors.

A94. C

Dose for primary treatment is in the range of 45 to 50 Gy in 1.8 to 2.0 Gy per fraction. For MM: Palliative RT dose range is 10 to 30 Gy in 1.5 to 2.0 Gy per fraction.

A95. B

T staging of colorectal cancer:
  T1—Tumor invades submucosa
  T2—Tumor invades muscularis propria
  T3—Tumor invades through the muscularis propria into the subserosa or into nonperitonealized pericolic or perirectal tissue
  T4—Tumor directly invades organs/structures and/or perforates the visceral peritoneum

A96. A

Subsites of hypopharynx include: pyriform sinuses (most common), posterior pharyngeal walls, and postcricoid area (least common).

A97. B

GOG99 risk factors: mod-poorly diff grade, LVI, and outer 1/3 myometrial invasion

A98. B

All these fractionation schedules are generally considered acceptable except 45 Gy in 25 fractions which was shown to be inferior to 45 Gy in 30 fractions BID in a randomized controlled trial.

A99. B

Degree of tumor necrosis is a prognostic factor in osteosarcoma; tumor necrosis is assessed as Grade I (no necrosis), II (50%–95%), III (more than 95% but less than 100%), and IV (100%).

A100. B

Factors that generally affect prognosis for Ewing's sarcoma: local versus metastatic, site of metastasis, age >14 years, bone marrow involvement, adequacy of local control of primary, and adequacy of systemic control for metastases.

A101. D

Osteosarcoma outcomes: 5-year Local control—72%, 5-year OS—67%, 5-year DFS—65%, 5-year distant metastases—26%.

A102. B

The combined regimen of cisplatin and pemetrexed improved survival compared to cisplatin alone (12.1 vs. 9.3 months) for mesothelioma.

A103. D

Risk stratification groups from RTOG 0129:
    Low-Risk: p16+, no smoking history <10 pack years
      3-year OS 94%
    Intermediate-Risk: p16+ with smoking history >10 pack years, or p16– and no smoking
      history (<10 pack years)
      3-year OS 67%
    High-Risk: p16– with smoking history >10 pack years
      3-year OS 42%

A104. D

Several phase III randomized trials have demonstrated that short-course ADT (4–6 months in intermediate-risk disease) improves long-term overall survival in patients with intermediate-risk prostate cancer by 5% to 10%.

A105. B

Oral cavity group stage:

0	Tis	N0M0	
I	T1	N0	M0
II	T2	N0	M0
III	T3	N0	M0
	T1-3	N1	M0
IVA	T4a	N0-1	M0
	T1-4a	N2	M0
IVB	Any T	N3	M0
	T4b	Any	NM0
IVC	Any T	Any	NM1

A106. B

Localized involvement of a single extralymphatic organ or site in the absence of any lymph node involvement (IE) (rare in Hodgkin's lymphoma).

A107. D

Papillary histology is better than sclerosing or nodular in terms of survival results.

A108. D

Chemoradiation therapy for glioblastoma is delivered by the Stupp Regimen: concomitant Temozolomide 75 g/m² followed by 1 month wash-out then adjuvant TMZ (150 – 200 mg/m²) × up to 12 cycles.

A109. A

Prognosis of Ewing's sarcoma:
    current 5-year OS for localized disease is 65% to 75%.
    current 5-year OS for metastatic disease to lungs only is 50%.

A110. C

Children with neurofibromatosis often have tumors that are more indolent and are at increased risk of RT complications including vascular complications and second malignancies.

A111. A

B symptoms include the following symptoms: unexplained loss of more than 10% of body weight in the 6 months before diagnosis, unexplained fever with temperatures above 38°C, drenching night sweats.

A112. B

85% of skin melanoma patients present with localized disease, 10% present with regional disease, and 5% present with metastatic disease.

A113. A

Frankel Grade(s):
    A (Complete paralysis)
    B (Sensory function only below the injury level)
    C (Incomplete motor function below injury level)
    D (fair to good motor function below injury level)
    E (normal function)

A114. D

Anaplastic Oligodendroglioma/Oligoastrocytoma:
    Median OS: 4 to 15 years
    Nondeleted: 3 years
    Codeleted: 15 years

A115. B

Audiometry must be obtained prior to therapy; often done as part of making diagnosis. Only 5% have a normal test.

A116. C

NSGCTs consist of a group of histologies:
    Embryonal carcinoma (most common)
    Yolk sac
    Choriocarcinoma
    Teratoma
    Mixed

A117. B

Metastatic disease occurs in approximately 25% of children at diagnosis of Ewing's sarcoma. Most common metastatic sites are lung, bone, and bone marrow. Lymph node and liver metastases are rare.

A118. D

Regional nodal radiation is generally indicated for four or more positive nodes.

A119. B

Chemoradiation therapy for glioblastoma is delivered by the Stupp Regimen: concomitant Temozolomide 75 g/m^2 followed by 1 month wash-out then adjuvant TMZ (150 – 200 mg/m^2) × up to 12 cycles.

A120. C

A typical dose fractionation schedule used in Grade II astrocytoma is 5,040 to 5,400 cGy in 180 cGy fractions.

A121. C

Risk of lymph node involvement is 60% for early-stage disease and 85% for advanced-stage disease in hypopharynx cancer.

A122. B

The stomach wall is made up of five layers. From the lumen out, the layers are:
Mucosa
Submucosa
Muscularis
Subserosa
Serosa

A123. B

Frequently seizure (which occurs in about 80% of cases) is a favorable prognostic feature.

A124. C

In children 10 years or older, RT is often used as initial management of low-grade astrocytoma with PFS rates of 70% to 80%. In children younger than 10 years, chemotherapy has been commonly used as initial treatment, with PFS rates in this setting of 40% to 50%.

A125. A

Based on a published meta-analysis, prophylactic cranial irradiation (PCI) improves survival by 5% in 3 years after chemoradiotherapy.

A126. B

Genetic Syndromes with increased risk of ovarian cancer:
BRCA1: 35% to 45% lifetime risk
BRCA2: 15% to 25% lifetime risk

A127. C

IPI identified five pretreatment characteristics to design a model to predict an individual patient's risk of death:
1. Age >60 years
2. Tumor Stage III or IV (advanced disease)
3. Number of extranodal sites >1
4. Performance status >2
5. Serum LDH level >1 times normal

A128. C

In adults, only 25% of ependymomas occur in the brain; 75% occur in the spine.

A129. D

GBM median survival is 14.6 months with chemoradiotherapy versus 12.1 months with radiation therapy alone.

A130. A

Typical prescription for PBI: 34 Gy BID in 10 fractions.

A131. B

Paraneoplastic syndromes occur in about 20% of patients and usually consist of elevated calcium, hypertension, and transaminitis.

A132. A

Osteosarcoma outcomes: 5-year Local control—72%, 5-year OS—67%, 5-year DFS—65%, 5-year distant metastases—26%.

A133. D

Known prognostic factors for primary recurrence:
    Margin <8 mm (1 cm fresh)
    Size >4 cm
    Grade
    Depth of invasion >5 to 9 mm
    LVI

A134. C

Four risk groups are associated with the IPI:
    Low-risk (0–1 factors, 5-year OS 73%)
    Low-intermediate (2 factors, 5-year OS 51%)
    High-intermediate (3 factors, 5-year OS 43%)
    High-risk (4–5 factors, 5-year OS 26%)

A135. B

Canadian trial: Women with lumpectomy with negative margins, pT1-2, and separation <25 cm randomized to 50 Gy in 25 fractions versus 42.6 Gy in 16 fractions (2.66 Gy). 10-year risk of local recurrence 6.7% in standard arm versus 6.2% in hypofractionation arm. No difference in cosmetic outcome.

A136. C

Dose to the primary neuroblastoma is 21.6 Gy in 1.8 Gy fractions to subclinical disease with a boost of 14.4 Gy to gross residual disease.

A137. C

Four risk groups are associated with the IPI:
    Low-risk (0–1 factors, 5-year OS 73%)
    Low-intermediate (2 factors, 5-year OS 51%)
    High-intermediate (3 factors, 5-year OS 43%)
    High-risk (4–5 factors, 5-year OS 26%)

A138. A

Lung cancer is leading cause of death in both sexes with estimated 158,040 deaths accounting for nearly one-third of all cancer deaths. Globally, the reported incidence of lung cancer in 2012 was about 1.8 million with estimated 1.59 million deaths per year.

A139. B

Chemotherapy is usually indicated only in the second trimester or postpartum.

A140. C

An unresectable Wilms' tumor is considered to be Stage III.

Wilms' tumor staging:
    Stage I—Complete resection, tumor limited to kidney, capsule intact
    Stage II—Complete resection, but tumor beyond kidney (capsule penetration, other extension beyond kidney
            including through renal vessels)
    Stage III—Any of the following factors:
      Positive lymph nodes or surgical margins
      Gross residual
      Tumor deemed unresectable
      Tumor in separate nodules
      Extension to peritoneum
      Any operative spill (flank or diffuse)
      Biopsy prior to resection
    Stage IV—Distant metastases or involved nonregional nodes
    Stage V—Bilateral disease

A141. B

Stage IIIA breast cancer:
    T0   N2 M0
    T1   N2 M0
    T2   N2 M0
    T3   N1 M0
    T3   N2 M0

A142. B

In pN1 patients following RP, median survival is improved by 2 years with ADT. In cN1 patients treated with RT, long-term OS was improved by approximately 20% with ADT.

A143. A

Assessing pathology with Breslow thickness, mitotic rate, and ulceration best predict the risk of lymph node metastases in skin melanoma.

A144. C

Ipsilateral lung: V20 ≤10%. Hypofractionation: V16 ≤15%.

A145. C

Mediastinal nodal staging: FDG-PET has better sensitivity (91%), specificity (86%), negative predictive value (95%), and positive predictive value (74%) compared to CT scan (75% sensitivity and 66% specificity).

A146. C

Staging of locally advanced prostate cancer involves the following:
   T3—through capsule
      T3a—EPE or microscopic invasion of bladder neck
      T3b—seminal vesicles
   T4—invades adjacent structures: bladder neck, external sphincter, rectum, levator muscles, and/or pelvic wall

A147. D

Lymph node drainage for larynx cancer:
   Supraglottis
      55% are node-positive at diagnosis
      Levels II to IV are most commonly involved
   Glottis
      <1% of T1 tumors, 2% to 5% of T2, and 20% to 30% of T3 to T4 are node-positive at diagnosis

A148. A

Group II consists of patients with gross total resection but residual disease.
   2A. Positive margins
   2B. Positive lymph nodes
   2C. Both positive margins and lymph nodes

A149. D

Local control is at least 95% or higher for acoustic neuroma.

A150. D

Immunohistochemical stains can be used to confirm diagnosis. Usually, AE1/AE3 which is marker for carcinoma and neuroendocrine markers such as synaptophysin, chromogranin, and CD56 are used.

A151. C

Adenocarcinoma is now the most common histologic type followed by squamous cell carcinoma and large cell carcinoma. Other less common subtypes are bronchogenic carcinoid, and adeno-squamous carcinoma.

A152. D

MGMT-methylated: OS 21.7 months with chemo-RT versus 15.3 months with RT alone
MGMT-unmethlyated: OS 11.8 months with chemo-RT versus 12.7 months with RT alone

A153. A

Molecular subtypes:
   Luminal A: ER/PR + Her2neu–
   Luminal B: ER/PR + Her2neu+
   Basal like: ER/PR – Her2 neu – (triple negative)
   Her2neu+: ER/PR – Her2 neu+

A154. C

A biologically equivalent dose (BED) >100 Gy is needed for optimum local control in early stage NSCLC.

A155. A

Parotid gland cancers account for 80% to 90% of all malignant salivary gland tumors.

A156. C

Ocular melanoma:
   80% arise in choroid
   10% to 15% in ciliary body
   <10% in iris

A157. A

This phase III trial assessed 64 Gy radiation alone versus 50 Gy (2 Gy/fx) with concurrent 5-FU/cisplatin (four cycles). The 5-year survival rate for RT alone was 0% and 27% for combined chemoradiotherapy.

A158. C

The MAGIC protocol was a European randomized trial demonstrating survival benefit associated with preoperative and postoperative ECF (epirubicin, cisplatin, and 5-FU). Preoperative chemotherapy demonstrated a 4-month improvement in median survival and 13% improvement in 5-year overall survival (both statistically significant).

A159. C

NSABP B-21: Following lumpectomy + ALND, patients with invasive breast cancer 1 cm or less randomized to (a) Tamoxifen, (b) radiation + placebo, or (c) radiation + Tamoxifen.

A160. A

Heart dose for regional breast irradiation: V25 <5%.

A161. D

Any T4 kidney cancer is staged as stage IV.

A162. C

For level VI nodes in the content of unknown primary of the head and neck, the most frequent primary sites include: anterior cervical skin, larynx, and thyroid.

A163. B

Positive ipsilateral nodes in pediatric neuroblastoma is considered to demonstrate Stage IIB disease. Positive contralateral nodes denote Stage III disease.

A164. C

In utero exposure to DES is related to clear cell adenocarcinoma, not squamous cell cancer.

A165. C

Overall 5-year survival is 50% to 60%. 5-year distant recurrence rate is 13% to 34%.

A166. A

>90% of cholangiocarcinomas are adenocarcinomas with about 10% squamous cell carcinomas.

A167. B

Prognosticators for spread of squamous cell carcinoma of the skin include:
   Anatomic site
   Duration and size of the lesion
   Depth of dermal invasion
   Perineural invasion
   Degree of differentiation

A168. B

5-year survival rate for multiple myeloma is approximately 34% according to the SEER database.

A169. A

M-protein is IgG in approximately 55% of cases and IgA in approximately 20% of multiple myeloma.

A170. D

Bilateral Wilms' tumor is separately classified as stage V disease.

A171. A

NSABP B-14: Women with ER positive invasive breast cancer s/p lumpectomy or mastectomy with negative pathologic lymph nodes randomized to 5 years of Tamoxifen or placebo.

A172. B

A 5-year OS of 48% has been reported for patients who had a complete pathologic response following neoadjuvant chemoradiation.

A173. A

Nasopharyngeal cancer has a high propensity for lymphatic spread (70%–80%). Nasopharynx cancer has highest risk of retropharyngeal and level V lymph node metastases.

A174. C

NCCN High Risk definition features:
   +LN
   +margins
   LVI
   Deep stromal invasion
   Large primary tumor
   Parametrium

A175. D

Control rates are excellent with radiation therapy after subtotal resection with greater than 90% progression-free survival.

A176. C

Staging of vulvar cancer:
   Stage I: 2 cm, confined to vulva/perineum
      IA: 1 mm stromal invasion
      IB: >1 mm stromal invasion
   Stage II: >2 cm, confined to vulva/perineum
   Stage III: spread to lower urethra, vagina, or anus and/or unilateral regional LN
   Stage IVA: spread to upper urethra, bladder mucosa, rectal mucosa, or pelvic bone and/or bilateral regional LN
   Stage IVB: DM including pelvic LN

A177. D

4-cm margins are routinely used for extremity STS, in both the preoperative and postoperative scenarios.

A178. C

Various named nodes/tumors exist in this setting including:
    Periumbilical metastasis (Sister Mary Joseph nodule)
    Enlarged left supraclavicular nodes (Virchow nodes)
    Axillary adenopathy (Irish node)
    Ovarian metastases (Kruckenberg tumor)

A179. C

Prognostic factors for poor OS:
    Site (anal canal vs. perianal skin)
    Size (size >5 cm)
    Involved nodes
    Male sex
    HPV or p16 positivity are prognostic for improved OS

A180. C

Locally advanced hypopharynx cancer is T staged as follows:
    T3: Tumor is more than 4 cm in greatest dimension or with fixation of hemilarynx or extension to esophagus
    T4a: Tumor invades thyroid/cricoid cartilage, hyoid bone, thyroid gland, or central compartment soft tissue
    T4b: Tumor invades prevertebral fascia, encases carotid artery, or involves mediastinal structures

A181. A

These are uncommon neoplasms, with approximately 4,500 new cases annually in the United States.
    55% arise in maxillary sinus
    25% in ethmoid sinus
    20% in nasal cavity

A182. D

The 5-year survival rate expected from a Stage IIIA endometrial cancer is 60%.

A183. D

IgD or IgE myeloma are uncommon, usually <1% of cases.

A184. B

Most common sites of origin are adrenal medulla, posterior mediastinum, and other paraspinal ganglia. Metastatic disease is very common, occurring in approximately 70% at diagnosis. Common metastatic sites are lymph nodes, bone and bone marrow, liver, orbits, and skin.

A185. D

T4 mesothelioma tumors are unresectable tumors including those involving the spine.

A186. C

Toxicities related to vaginal radiation:
    Vaginal dryness/atrophy
    Pubic hair loss
    Vaginal stenosis/fibrosis (50%)
    Cystitis (50%)

Proctitis (40%)
Rectovaginal or vesicovaginal fistula (<5%)
Vaginal necrosis (<5%–15%)
Urethral stricture (rare)
Bowel obstruction (rare)

A187. B

Radiation for Ewing's sarcoma can lead to secondary malignancy, (RT dose dependent, less likely if dose <48 Gy, 20-year risk of any secondary malignancy is 9.2% and risk of secondary sarcoma is 6.5%).

A188. D

Lymphedema risk is approximately 5% after SNLB, 10% with ALND, and up to 20% with ALND and regional nodal radiation.

A189. A

Pre-op EBRT is favored over post-op because:
Tumor is more easily definable
The tumor displaces critical structures
Radiation dose needed before surgery is less because the tumor is better vascularized and oxygenated
There is decreased risk of intraoperative tumor seeding

A190. A

bHCG can be elevated in some seminomas and NSGCTs with a half-life 24 hours.

A191. C

Pituitary adenomas can be categorized into microadenomas (<1 cm) or macroadenomas (≥1 cm).

A192. C

PSA bounce occurs in about 15% of patients treated with EBRT who develop a transient rise in PSA of about 15% above nadir. This usually occurs 18 to 24 months following therapy.

A193. C

Pancreaticoduodenectomy (Whipple Procedure), with/without pylorus sparing involves the removal of pancreatic head, duodenum, gallbladder, antrum of the stomach, with surgical drainage of distal pancreatic duct, and biliary system through pancreaticojejunostomy with an overall mortality rate of 6.6%.

A194. D

Syndromes that are associated with childhood CNS cancers include neurofibromatosis types I and II, tuberous sclerosis, von Hippel Lindau syndrome, and Gorlin syndrome.

A195. A

Radical mastectomy does not provide survival or local control benefit over total mastectomy based on NSABP B-04.

A196. A

Most common malignancy in the orbit is metastasis. Most common primary malignancies include ocular melanoma (eye) and orbital lymphoma (orbit).

A197. D

In relation to this staging cervix cancer question, the following staging information is relevant:

IB1 (clinically visible, confined to cervix, ≤4 cm)

IB2 (clinically visible, confined to cervix, >4 cm)

IIB (parametrial involvement)

IIIA (Lower 1/3 vagina invasion)

A198. B

The majority of pediatric CNS tumors occur intracranially, with only 5% of tumors originating in the spinal cord or cauda equina.

A199. C

75% of bladder tumors are either T1, Tis, or T1 at presentation.

A200. D

HPV type 16 leads to highest risk of squamous cell carcinoma, and HPV type 18 leads to highest risk of adenocarcinoma. HPV 6 and 11 are associated with benign warts.

Index

CPSIA information can be obtained
at www.ICGtesting.com
Printed in the USA
LVOW04s2345301117
558174LV00011B/178/P

9 781620 700631